Developmental Dyslexia

Developmental Dyslexia
Neural, Cognitive, and Genetic Mechanisms

Edited by Christopher H. Chase,
Glenn D. Rosen, and
Gordon F. Sherman

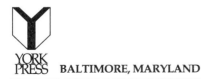

YORK PRESS   BALTIMORE, MARYLAND

This book was manufactured in the United States of America.
Typography by The Type Shoppe, Inc.
Printing and binding by McNaughton & Gunn, Inc.
Cover design by Joseph Dieter, Jr.

Library of Congress Cataloging in Publication Data

Developmental dyslexia : neural, cognitive, and genetic mechanisms /
   edited by Christopher H. Chase, Glenn D. Rosen, and Gordon F.
   Sherman.
       p. cm.
   Includes bibliographical references and index.
   ISBN 0-912752-39-4
   1. Dyslexia--Pathophysiology.   2. Developmental neurobiology.
I. Chase, Christopher H.   II. Rosen, Glenn D.   III. Sherman,
Gordon F.
RJ496.A5D486   1996   96-10323
616.85'53—dc20   CIP

CONTENTS

CONTRIBUTORS

Jocelyne Bachevalier, Ph.D.
Department of Neurobiology and Anatomy
University of Texas Health Science Center - Houston
6431 Fannin
Houston, Texas 77225

Ingrid B. Borecki, Ph.D.
Division of Biostatistics
Washington University School of Medicine
660 South Euclid Avenue, Box 8067
St Louis, Missouri 63110

Christopher H. Chase, Ph.D.
Department of Communications and Cognitive Science
Hampshire College
West Street
Amherst, Massachusetts 01002

John C. DeFries, Ph.D.
Institute for Behavioral Genetics
University of Colorado
Campus Box 447
Boulder, Colorado 80309

Victor H. Denenberg, Ph.D.
Department of Biobehavioral Sciences
University of Connecticut
Storrs, Connecticut 06269-4154

Julie Fiez, Ph.D.
Department of Neurology and Neurological Surgery
Box 8111
Washington University School of Medicine
St. Louis, Missouri 63110

Roslyn Holly Fitch, Ph.D.
Center for Molecular and Behavioral Neuroscience
Rutgers University
197 University Avenue
Newark, New Jersey 07102

Albert M. Galaburda, Ph.D.
Department of Neurology and
Charles A. Dana Research Laboratories
Beth Israel Hospital
Harvard Medical School
Boston, Massachusetts 02215

Christopher Gallen, M.D., Ph.D.
Premier Research Worldwide
124 South 15th Street
Philadelphia, Pennsylvania 19102-3010

Jeffrey Gilger, Ph.D.
Department of Speech-Language-Hearing Sciences and Disorders
University of Kansas
3031 Dole Human Development Center
Lawrence, Kansas 66045

Stephen D. Goldinger, Ph.D.
Cognitive Systems Group
Department of Psychology
Arizona State University
Tempe, Arizona 85287-1104

Steve Miller, Ph.D.
Center for Molecular and Behavioral Neuroscience
Rutgers University
197 University
Newark, New Jersey 07102

Bruce F. Pennington, Ph.D.
Department of Psychology
University of Denver
2155 South Race Street
Denver, Colorado 80208

Steven E. Peterson, Ph.D.
Department of Neurology and Neurological Surgery
Department of Radiology and
Department of Anatomy and Neurobiology
Washington University School of Medicine
St. Louis, Missouri 63110

Marcus E. Raichle, M.D.
Department of Neurology and Neurological Surgery
Department of Radiology and
Department of Anatomy and Neurobiology
Washington University School of Medicine
St. Louis, Missouri 63110

Keith Rayner, Ph.D.
Department of Psychology
University of Massachusetts
Amherst, Massachusetts 01002

Glenn D. Rosen, Ph.D.
Department of Neurology and
Charles A Dana Research Laboratories
Beth Israel Hospital
Harvard Medical School
Boston, Massachusetts 02215

Lisa M. Schrott, Ph.D.
Department of Psychiatry
University of Colorado Health Sciences Center
Box C-233
4200 East Ninth Avenue
Denver, Colorado 80262

Barry Schwartz, Ph.D.
The Scripps Research Institute
10666 North Torrey Pines Road
Mail Stop SBR-1
La Jolla, California 92037

Gordon F. Sherman, Ph.D.
Department of Neurology and
Charles A. Dana Research Laboratories
Beth Israel Hospital
Harvard Medical School
Boston, Massachusetts 02215

Shelley D. Smith, Ph.D.
Boys Town National Research Hospital
555 North 30th Street
Omaha, Nebraska 68131

John F. Stein, Ph.D.
University Laboratory of Physiology
Oxford University
South Park Road
Oxford OX1 3PT
United Kingdom

Paula Tallal, Ph.D.
Center for Molecular and Behavioral Neuroscience
Rutgers University
197 University Avenue
Newark, New Jersey 07102

Guy C. Van Orden, Ph.D.
Cognitive Systems Group
Department of Psychology
Arizona State University
Tempe, Arizona 85287-1104

PREFACE

This book is based on papers presented at the conference, "The Extraordinary Brain II: Neural and Cognitive Mechanisms Underlying Speech, Language and Reading" which took place in 1992. The conference was sponsored by the National Dyslexia Research Foundation (NDRF), Emily Fisher Landau and the Fisher-Landau Foundation, and the John Chany Trust. This conference was the second in a series of three meetings planned by William Baker, the executive director of the NDRF, to explore three areas of dyslexia research: neurobiology and neuropathology, cognitive science and neuropsychology, and education. Dr. Paula Tallal was the principal organizer for this conference.

Chapters for this book have been organized into four sections describing the study of different mechanisms that are relevant to the study of language and reading, and a fifth section describes two methods for functional neural imaging. Most of the chapters report on research on neural, genetic, and cognitive mechanisms of dyslexia. Chapters that describe important theoretical and methodological advances in developmental neurobiology, functional brain imaging, and computational modeling are also included.

This book has taken several turns before finally coming to press. The editors are particularly grateful to Elinor Hartwig of York Press for the dedication and care she provided in guiding the publication of this book. William Baker and Paula Tallal's work in arranging the conference and initially organizing the book project also are gratefully acknowledged. We especially appreciate Emily Fisher Landau's support.

Part • I

Neural Mechanisms

It is perhaps noteworthy that Samuel Torrey Orton, the physician who was responsible for the recognition of dyslexia as a specific learning disability in the United States, was also the first to consider that the disorder might have a neural substrate. His theory, based on the notion of increased cerebral hemispheric competition, spawned a wealth of papers and books, and no doubt spurred Dr. Orton toward the investigation of the brains of dyslexics. In fact, it is reported that in the 1930s he had obtained the post-mortem brain of a dyslexic with the intention of analyzing it in depth, but his butter-fingered research assistant dropped the specimen, thereby ending the study prematurely.

Even if this story is apocryphal, it can certainly be used as a metaphor for the progression of research into the neural substrates of developmental dyslexia. Thus, while the initial description of dyslexia (or "congenital word blindness") at the turn of the century presupposed an organic cause for the disease, investigators did not "pick up the brain" as it were, for nearly 70 years. Following Drake's rather sketchy description of the brain of a dyslexic in 1968, it was another decade before Galaburda and colleagues began to examine this issue in earnest. Since that time, interest in the examination of neural substrates of this disorder has steadily increased.

In the two chapters that make up this section, we are presented with a discussion of two very different types of animal models of developmental disorders. In their chapter, Galaburda et al. acknowledge the difficulty of modeling in mice and rats, language disorders with their uniquely human characteristics, yet they detail evidence showing some of the similarities between the brains of dyslexics and those of mice and rats with altered brain development. Bachevalier has elegantly demonstrated, in non-human primates, that while object discrimination tasks develop relatively quickly in infancy, object memory takes much longer. What both chapters have in common is the notion that the effects of early injury to neural systems can have profound and long-lasting behavioral implications.

Chapter • 1

Animal Models of Developmental Dyslexia

Albert M. Galaburda
Lisa M. Schrott
Gordon F. Sherman
Glenn D. Rosen
Victor H. Denenberg

The development of animal models is crucial for understanding various forms of human neuropathology, but the identification of suitable models for language and language disturbances has been hampered by the fact that language is a uniquely human attribute. We have taken the position that, even if language is uniquely human, issues thought to be important for language function, e.g., lateralization and brain asymmetry, or cortical organization and temporal processing, can be gainfully modeled in nonhuman species. Our specific focus is the explanation of language deficits in developmental dyslexia.

We begin with observations made in the brains of dyslexic individuals, from which we choose features that can be modeled in experimental animals. Specifically the human dyslexic shows absence of the ordinary pattern of leftward asymmetry of the *planum temporale* (Galaburda 1993; Larsen et al. 1990), and the perisylvian cortex (mainly frontal cortex involving the vascular watershed of the anterior and middle cerebral arteries) displays foci of ectopic neurons in the molecular layer, or more severe dysplasias (Galaburda 1993; Humphreys, Kaufmann, and Galaburda 1990). In addition two female brains and one male brain (Humphreys, Kaufmann, and Galaburda 1990) showed multiple foci of glial scarring affecting the same perisylvian and vascular territories and interspersed among the foci of ectopic cells. We have suggested that the injury leading to the scars also led to the production of minor cortical malformations, the difference being only in the time of onset during cortical development: malformations occurring earlier (at around the middle of pregnancy); scars originating later (second half of gestation and early postnatal period). With regard to the etiology, and aided by the results of related research in experimental animals (see below; [Humphreys, Kaufmann, and Galaburda 1990; Sherman et al. 1987; Sherman, Galaburda, and Geschwind 1985]), we propose that ischemic injury to the developing cortex produced by autoimmune damage of vessel walls—arteritis with predominant consequences on blood flow through vascular watersheds—leads to the cortical injury, the scars, and the malformations. A second set of observations is made on the human dyslexic thalamus. We have found that neurons in both the magnocellular layers of the lateral geniculate nucleus and in the left medial geniculate nucleus are smaller than expected (Galaburda and Livingstone 1993; Livingstone et al. 1991; Galaburda, Menard, and Rosen 1994). The former is associated with slowness in the early segments of the magnocellular pathway as assessed by evoked reponse techniques that address magnocellular function separately from parvocellular (Livingstone et al. 1991). The latter may relate to the temporal processing abnormalities described in the auditory system of language impaired children (Tallal and Piercy 1973). The relationship between the first set of findings, i.e., the anomaly in asymmetry and the cortical malformations, and the second set, i.e., the anomaly in rapid temporal processing associated with thalamic changes, is another focus of research with potential for resolution in animal models.

The animal research has also aimed at explaining the question of how minor malformations could lead to noticeable and even persistent disorders of cognitive function. For example, strains of mice that spontaneously develop autoimmune disease also may display foci of neocortical ectopic neurons and cortical scars (Sherman et al. 1987; Sherman, Galaburda, and Geschwind 1985). Associated with these ectopias there may be significant changes in some cortical neuronal subtypes (Sherman, Stone, Rosen, and Galaburda 1990), prominent alterations in cortico-cortical connectivity (Sherman, Stone, Press, Rosen, and Galaburda 1990), and modification of behavior (Denenberg, Sherman, Schrott, Rosen, and Galaburda 1991). Interestingly, affected animals show alterations in the usual pattern of brain asymmetry, thus suggesting an interaction between very early developmental events and the expression of cortical asymmetry (Rosen et al. 1989). It is also apparent that similar abnormalities can be induced in newborn rodents, which are still undergoing neuronal migration to the neocortex, by a variety of mechanisms of injury (Humphreys et al. 1989). Although this research supports the idea that injury is most likely the intervening mechanism in the production of malformations and scars in the dyslexic brain as well, the exact etiology of the injury has not been determined, and the immunopathogenic hypothesis remains unproven. Evidence has been accrued, however, that whatever the exact mechanism of the injury, it is innate rather than transferred from the mother during fetal life (Denenberg, Sherman, Schrott, Rosen, and Galaburda 1991: Sherman et al. 1994). On the other hand, despite the innate nature of the malformation, abnormal behaviors associated with them can be modified by early experience (Schrott, Denenberg, Sherman, Waters, Rosen, and Galaburda 1992).

Alterations in the pattern of asymmetry may be expected to produce changes in cognitive capacity, but the exact manner by which this occurs is not known. Thus, changes in numbers of neuronal subtypes and patterns of connectivity can readily be accepted as substrates for functional change, but animal models presently available are not sufficient for understanding the exact means by which such anatomical changes lead to changes in behavior. This aspect of the research might be better carried out on computational models where connections and processor types can be manipulated and behavioral consequences analyzed. On the other hand, changes in the temporal performance of thalamic neurons could be more easily related to temporal processing deficits, which in turn could lead to explanations of the sort needed for the phonological deficits documented in human dyslexics. This line of animal experimentation, therefore, appears promising.

FUNCTIONAL CEREBRAL LATERALIZATION, IMMUNOLOGY, AND DYSLEXIA

Continuing interest in the Geschwind hypothesis (Geschwind and Behan 1982) has led to several papers in recent years. This hypothesis proposed a positive correlation between lefthandedness (or nonrighthandedness), immune disturbances (allergic or autoimmune), and learning disabilities (mainly dyslexia or stuttering). It suggested that testosterone *in utero* leads to abnormal development of left hemisphere dominance, thus resulting in more lefthandedness and developmental language disorders, and to anomalous development of the immune system leading to autoimmune and atopic illnesses later in life.

Many studies have failed to confirm the predicted relationships between lefthandedness, learning disorders, and immune dysfunction.

Nonetheless, a French study of men between the ages of 17 and 24 years showed a higher frequency of stuttering but not of allergic disorders in lefthanders (Dellatolas et al. 1990). Extreme righthandedness, however, was associated with a diminished incidence of allergic disorders. Both right- and lefthanded stutterers exhibited an increase in the incidence of allergy, which is similar to the findings of Pennington et al. 1987 who found an increased incidence of allergic disorders among all dylexics. Furthermore, Hugdahl and colleagues (Hugdahl, Synnevag, and Satz 1990) studied 105 dyslexics and an equal number of controls and found that the dyslexics had significant increases in allergic and autoimmune diseases but there were not handedness differences between the groups. Another study (Betancur et al. 1990) found no overall association between lefthandedness and allergies, although there was a tendency toward lefthandedness in patients whose allergic symptoms started before puberty. A related area of intense research in one laboratory, which is illustrated by Neveu et al. 1991, and which may bear on the Geschwind hypothesis, looks at the relationship between immunological function and lateralization in rodents. The research found that the association between paw preference and immune reactivity varies according to the sex of the animal and the immunological parameters studied. Thus, it may require carrying out large population-based studies with uniform measures of handedness and diagnostic criteria for learning and immunological disorders before this issue will be satisfactorily settled. At the present time the relationship between learning and immune disorders appears to be stronger than that between learning disorders and lefthandedness or immune disorders and lefthandedness.

ANIMAL STUDIES

NZB/BINJ and BXSB/MpJ mice are being used as an animal model of neural-immune interactions that may be associated with the human dyslexic condition (Denenberg, Sherman, Schrott, Rosen, and Galaburda 1991; Denenberg et al. 1992; Denenberg et al. 1991; Sherman et al. 1987). Because dyslexia is a specific learning disorder and may be accompanied by enhancement of certain abilities (Geschwind and Galaburda 1985a; Geschwind and Galaburda 1985b; Geschwind and Galaburda 1985c), the use of a behavioral battery is crucial. Within such a battery, a spectrum of performance levels can be found. Furthermore, differential patterns of learning can be associated with specific components of the neural-immune interaction. The battery of behavioral tasks that we have administered includes five measures of learning (discrimination, two spatial tasks, a complex maze, and avoidance learning), as well as tests of lateralization and activity. Because of prior findings associating the presence of ectopias and a higher incidence of immune disorders in dyslexic individuals (see above), the behavior of NZB and BXSB mice has been examined from the perspective of ectopia-associated and autoimmune-associated behaviors.

Ectopia-Associated Behaviors

In working with inbred strains, one of the most difficult problems is the choice of an appropriate control group. Comparing across inbred strains is risky, since behaviors are known to be influenced by the vastly different genetics of each strain. Therefore, within-strain comparisons were used to examine the behavior of NZB and BXSB mice. In the investigation of ectopia-associated behaviors, this was easily accomplished since 40–50% of NZB and BXSB mice develop ectopias. Three measures in the behavioral battery were found to be sensitive to the presence of ectopias: a non-spatial discrimination learning task, and two spatial measures, water escape and the Morris maze.

Ectopias depressed performance on discrimination learning. This test utilized a two-arm swimming T-maze, with a grey stem, and a black and a white alley. An escape ladder hung at the end of the alley designated to be positive (Wimer and Weller 1965). Reinforcement consisted of escape from the water plus being placed in a dry box beneath a heat lamp. The left-right location of the positive stimulus was altered in a semi-random sequence, so the animals had to use an associative, rather than spatial or positional strategy, to solve the task. Measures included number of correct choices and time to reach the escape ladder. Mice received 10 trials for 5 days (Denenberg, Talgo, Schrott, and Kenner 1990). In this task, NZB mice with ectopias made fewer correct choices and took longer to find the escape ladder over the first 4 days of testing, but caught up by day 5. In ectopic NBZ mice, a significant improvement in both performance measures was seen if they were reared in an enriched environment as compared to standard cages. No such effects were seen in non-ectopic mice (Schrott, Denenberg, Sherman, Waters, Rosen, and Galaburda 1992).

A similar pattern of behavior is seen in the Morris maze. This is a complex spatial task requiring the animal to find a hidden escape platform using extra-maze cues. The starting point varies from one of four locations in a semi-random sequence. Time and distance to reach the escape platform were measured. In addition, the maze is divided into 4 quadrants and 3 annuli and the percent of time spent in each portion was also measured. Mice received 4 trials a day for 5 days (Denenberg et al. 1990). Ectopic NZB mice were slower to find the escape platform and spent more time in the outermost annulus of the maze, reflecting a different pattern of learning than NZB mice without ectopias. Rearing in an enriched environment, however, was able to compensate for the deficit in ectopic mice. Enriched ectopic NZB mice had similar performance to their enriched non-ectopic littermates (Schrott, Denenberg, Sherman, Waters, Rosen, and Galaburda 1992).

The presence of ectopias also interacts with an animal's paw preference. On the discrimination learning task, right-pawed BXSB male mice had better performance than their left-pawed ectopic littermates. The opposite relationship was seen for the spatial water escape task. In this task an animal was placed in one end of an oval tub and had to swim to find a hidden escape platform at the other end using extra-maze spatial cues. The mice received 5 trials on a single day of testing and time to reach the platform was recorded. For water escape learning, left-pawed NZB males and females and BXSB males had faster times than their right-pawed counterparts. No paw preference effects were seen in non-ectopic mice of either strain (Denenberg, Sherman, Schrott, Rosen, and Galaburda 1991).

The behavioral consequences of ectopia presence are task-specific. No main ectopia effects are seen for measures of lateralization, activity, the Lashley maze, or avoidance conditioning. Ectopic mice are capable of learning, but often at a slower rate or with poorer scores. In addition, ectopias interact with other variables, such as paw preference and environmental enrichment. Across numerous studies it has been found that the presence of an ectopia, rather than its architectonic location, hemisphere, or size, is the crucial characteristic for these associations. Most likely this is because the effect of an ectopia is widespread. The disruption of underlying fiber architecture, alterations in neuronal circuitry, and neurotransmitter abnormalities that accompany an ectopia reflect a brain that has developed abnormally (Sherman, Morrison, Rosen, Behan, and Galaburda 1990; Sherman, Press, Rosen, and Galaburda 1990; Sherman, Stone, Press, Rosen, and Galaburda 1990; Sherman, Stone, Rosen, and Galaburda 1990). Whether the learning deficits are a direct consequence of the ectopia or whether an ectopia is a marker for aberrant development in general, with concomitant learning deficits, is not known at present.

Autoimmune-Related Behavior

Poor performance in active and passive avoidance conditioning has been consistently associated with autoimmune mice (Denenberg, Sherman, Schrott, Rosen, and Galaburda 1991; Denenberg et al. 1992; Forster, Retz, and Lal 1988; Nandy et al. 1983; Schrott et al. 1994; Spencer et al. 1986). In the present set of studies, avoidance conditioning was conducted in a two-way shuttlebox. The box was separated into two compartments by a divider. Five seconds of a pulsed light served as the conditioned stimulus, while up to 20 seconds of .4mA footshock acted as the unconditioned stimulus. The number of avoidances, escapes (and the time to make them), as well as null responses were recorded. The most striking characteristic of NZB and BXSB mice is their very poor performance. Escape from the shock is their preferential response, with few avoidances made. It is interesting to note that failure to avoid or escape the shock (a null response) is not extinguished rapidly, as would typically be found in an animal learning this task. Instead, null responses and the latency to escape often increased across days.

This response pattern is associated with a high degree of autoimmunity (the more autoimmune a mouse, the poorer the avoidance performance). The native relationship between these two variables was more difficult to establish than the relationships between ectopias and behavior because of the lack of a proper control. Comparing avoidance performance across strains (an autoimmune strain vs. a strain with normal immune functioning) is problematic because an avoidance difference could result from any number of genetic differences unrelated to immune functioning. Comparing avoidance performance within a strain was not possible, because all mice within a strain develop autoimmune disorders and there is insufficient variability in avoidance performance (all mice have poor performance). This difficulty was solved in a rather complicated way. A set of embryo transfer studies permitted comparison of genetically identical mice who differed with regard to their immune status, as a function of the uterine environment in which they were raised. Transfer of a non-autoimmune DBA embryo to an autoimmune BXSB maternal host induced autoimmune disease in the adult animal, as well as impaired avoidance performance. Conversely, when the severity of the disease was reduced by transferring a NZB embryo to a non-autoimmune hybrid mother, avoidance performance was improved (Denenberg, Sherman, Schrott, Rosen, and Galaburda 1991).

Further support for this association was provided by a study with BXSB-DBA reciprocal hybrids. The hybrid offspring were autosomally identical but differed in degrees of immune reactivity. The DBA x BXSB cross yielded offspring with greater immune reactivity and poorer avoidance performance than the BXSB x DBA cross (Denenberg et al. 1992). Finally, in a group of genetically related mice, NXRF recombinant inbred lines, the line with the greatest degree of autoimmunity had the poorest avoidance performance (Schrott et al. 1994). Thus, in four groups of mice with vastly different rearing histories, the degree of autoimmunity was negatively related to performance on an active avoidance conditioning task.

The degree of autoimmunity was not associated with any of the other tasks in the behavioral battery. Environmental enrichment had no effect on avoidance learning, nor were any ectopia interactions present (Denenberg, Sherman, Schrott, Rosen, and Galaburda 1991; Denenberg et al. 1992; Schrott, Denenberg, Sherman, Waters, Rosen, and Galaburda 1992). In addition, pharmacological manipulations including cholinomimetics, nootropics and anti-depressants failed to improve performance (Schrott 1992). Although the negative neuroanatomical and neurochemical findings cannot conclusively prove that immune dysregulation mediates active avoidance deficits in autoimmune mice, they are consistent with this hypothesis. Possible immune mechanisms include (1) immune complex deposition on brain membranes and subsequent alterations in the permeability of the blood-brain barrier, (2) effects of circulating autoantibodies or other autoimmune factors, (3) cytokine effects, (4) altered stress responses and/or hormonal interactions, and (5) developmental aspects. These possible mechanisms are by no means mutually exclusive.

Finally, we have recently shown that DBA (non-immune disordered) mice who had induced minor malformations of the cortex (Humphreys et al. 1991; Rosen et al. 1992)—including ectopias and microgyria—were similarly affected on the battery of behavioral tests as NZB and BXSB mice. Specifically, lesioned mice performed poorly when compared to sham-operated animals in discrimination learning and in a spatial Morris Maze Match-to-Sample task. In shuttlebox avoidance conditioning, where immunological disorder has been shown to compromise behavioral performance in autoimmune mice, there was no difference between lesioned and sham animals. These results further support the dissociation between the effects of developmental neocortical anomalies and autoimmune disease on behavior (Rosen et al. 1995).

Other Behaviors

One behavior that does not fit into either of these categories is the Lashley maze, a complex maze that can be solved using spatial and/or associative learning strategies (Denenberg, Talgo, Carroll, Fretter, and Deni 1991). BXSB mice have excellent performance on this task, while NZB have great difficulty learning it, even when given additional trials and cues (Schrott, Denenberg, Sherman, Rosen, and Galaburda 1992). NZB mice are known to have abnormalities of the hippocampus, including the formation of ectopias and a small infrapyramidal mossy fiber tract system (Anstätt 1988; Fink, Zilles, and Schleicher 1991; Nowakowski 1988). These abnormalities are not seen in BXSB mice (Sherman et al. unpublished data) and may account for the poor performance of NXBs in the Lashley maze. In addition, NZB mice have a low incidence of callosal agenesis (approximately 7%). Certain recombinant inbred lines with NZB as one of the progenitors develop a higher incidence of callosal agenesis, and this abnormality affects spatial learning (Schrott et al., submitted).

Temporal Processing in Rats

Language impaired individuals exhibit severe deficits in the discrimination of rapidly presented auditory stimuli, including phonological and non-verbal stimuli (i.e., sequential tones; [Tallal 1984; Tallal and Piercy 1973]). In an effort to relate these results, male rats with neonatally induced microgyria (Humphreys et al. 1991) were tested in an operant paradigm for auditory discrimination of stimuli consisting of 2 sequential tones. Subjects were shaped to perform a go-no go target identification, using water reinforcement. Stimuli were reduced in duration from 540 to 249 ms across 24 days of testing. Results showed that all subjects were able to discriminate at longer stimulus durations. However, bilaterally lesioned subjects showed specific impairment at stimulus durations of 332 ms or less, and were significantly depressed in comparison to shams. Right and left lesioned subjects were significantly depressed in comparison to shams at the shortest duration (249 ms). Interestingly, the neonatal lesion did not substantially involve the auditory pathways, thus suggesting that any nearby lesion may propagate along connectionally related areas to result in changes in those areas incompatible with normal temporal processing capacity. The experiments could not address the question of whether the cortical lesion propagates upstream and results in temporal processing anomalies early in the process, or whether all the results could be explained by late slowing. These questions are, however, amenable to further experimental testing (Fitch et al. 1994).

SUMMARY AND CONCLUSIONS

Dyslexia is associated with changes in the brain consisting of anomalous cerebral asymmetries in language areas, minor cortical malformations, including molecular layer ectopias and focal microgyria, and small neurons in the lateral and medial geniculate nuclei. The latter may be associated with slowed temporal processing beginning early in the processing streams of both the visual and auditory systems. Substantial usefulness has been derived from modeling the anatomical findings in the brains of genetically inbred or early manipulated mice and rats. More recently, these rodent anatomical models have been tested behaviorally and a variety of behaviors can be linked to the anomalies of brain asymmetry and to minor cortical malformations seen in these animals. These abnormal behaviors include lateralization changes, problems with associate learning, and slowness of temporal processing. The identification of these component behavioral phenotypes, in association with specific anatomical phenotypes, is apt to be useful in identifying responsible genes, which can then be pursued in affected human populations.

REFERENCES

Anstätt, T. 1988. Quantitative and cytoarchitectonic studies of the entorhinal region and the hippocampus of New Zealand Black mice. *Journal of Neural Transmission* 73:249–57.

Betancur, C., Vélez, A., Cabanieu, G., Le Moal, M., and Neveu, P. J. 1990. Association between left-handedness and allergy: A reappraisal. *Neuropsychologia* 28:223–27.

Dellatolas, G., Annesi, I., Jallon, P., Chavance, M., and Lellough, J. 1990. An epidemiological reconsideration of the Geschwind-Galaburda theory of cerebral lateralization. *Archives of Neurology* 47:778–82.

Denenberg, V., Talgo, N., Schrott, L., and Kenner, G. 1990. A computer-aided procedure for measuring discrimination learning. *Physiology and Behavior* 47:1031–34.

Denenberg, V. H., Morbraaten, L. E., Sherman, G. F., Morrison, L., Shchrott, L. M., Waters, N. S., Rosen, G. D., Behan, P. O., and Galaburda, A. M. 1991. Effects of the autoimmune uterine/maternal environment upon cortical ectopias, behavior and autoimmunity. *Brain Research* 563(1-2):114–22.

Denenberg, V. H., Sherman, G. F., Morrison, L., Schrott, L. M., Waters, N. S., Rosen, G. D., Behan, P. O., and Galaburda, A. M. 1992. Behavior, ectopias and immunity in BD/DB reciprocal crosses. *Brain Research* 571:323–29.

Denenberg, V. H., Sherman, G. F., Schrott, L. M., Rosen, G. D., and Galaburda, A. M. 1991. Spatial learning, discrimination learning, paw preference and neocortical ectopias in two autoimmune strains of mice. *Brain Research* 562(1):98–104.

Denenberg, V. H., Talgo, N. W., Carroll, D. A., Fretter, S., and Deni, R. A. 1991. A computer-aided procedure for measuring Lashley III maze performance. *Physiology and Behavior* 50:857–61.

Fink, G. R., Zilles, K., and Schleicher, A. 1991. Postnatal development of forebrain regions in the autoimmune NZB-mouse: A model for degeneration in neuronal systems. *Anatomy and Embryology* 183(6):579–88.

Fitch, R. H., Tallal, P., Brown, C., Galaburda, A. M., and Rosen, G. D. 1994. Induced microgyria and auditory temporal processing in rats: A model for language impairment? *Cerebral Cortex* 4(3):260–70.

Forster, M. J., Retz, K. C., and Lal, H. 1988. Learning and memory deficits associated with autoimmunity: Significance in aging and Alzheimer's disease. *Drug Development Research* 15:253–73.

Galaburda, A. M. 1993. Neurology of developmental dyslexia: An update. *Current Opinions in Neurobiology* 3:237–42.

Galaburda, A. M., and Livingstone, M. S. 1993. Evidence for a magnocellular defect in developmental dyslexia. *Annals of the New York Academy of Sciences* 682:70–82

Galaburda, A. M., Menard, M. T., and Rosen, G. D. 1994. Evidence for aberrant auditory anatomy in developmental dyslexia. *Proceedings of the National Academy of Sciences (USA)* 91(17):8010–13.

Geschwind, N, and Behan, P. O. 1982. Left-handedness: Association with immune disease, migraine, and developmental disorder. *Proceedings of the National Academy of Sciences (USA)* 79:5097–5100.

Geschwind, N., and Galaburda, A. M. 1985a. Cerebral lateralization. Biological mechanisms, associations, and pathology: I. A hypothesis and a program for research. *Archives of Neurology*. 42:428–521.

Geschwind, N., and Galaburda, A. M. 1985b. Cerebral lateralization. Biological mechanisms, associations, and pathology: II. A hypothesis and a program for research. *Archives of Neurology*. 42:521–52.

Geschwind, N., and Galaburda, A. M. 1985c. Cerebral lateralization. Biological mechanisms, associations, and pathology: III. A hypothesis and a program for research. *Archives of Neurology* 42:634–54.

Hugdahl, K., Synnevag, B., and Satz, P. 1990. Immune and autoimmune diseases in dyslexic children. *Neuropsychologia* 28(7):673–79.

Humphreys, P., Kaufmann, W. E., and Galaburda, A. M. 1990. Developmental dyslexia in women: Neuropathological findings in three cases. *Annals of Neurology* 28:727–38.

Humphreys, P., Rosen, G. D., Press, D. M., Sherman, G. F., and Galaburda, A. M. 1991. Freezing lesions of the newborn rat brain: A model for cerebrocortical microgyria. *Journal of Neuropathology and Experimental Neurology* 50:145–60.

Humphreys, P., Rosen, G. D., Sherman, G. F., and Galaburda, A. M. 1989. Freezing lesions of the newborn rat brain: A model for cerebrocortical microdysgenesis. *Society of Neuroscience Abstracts* 15:1120.

Larsen, J., Hoien, T., Lundberg, I., and Odegaard, H. 1990. MRI evaluation of the size and symmetry of the planum temporale in adolescents with developmental dyslexia. *Brain and Language* 39:289–301.

Livingstone, M. S., Rosen, G. D., Drislane, F. W., and Galaburda, A. M. 1991. Physiological and anatomical evidence for a magnocellular defect in developmental dyslexia. *Proceedings of the National Academy of Sciences (USA)* 88:7943–47.

Nandy, K., Lal, H., Bennett, M., and Bennett, D. 1983. Correlation between a learning disorder and elevated brain-reactive antibodies in aged C57BL/6 and young NZB mice. *Life Sciences* 33:1499–1503.

Neveu, P. J., Betancur, C., Barneoud, P., Vitiello, S., and Le Moal, M. 1991. Functional brain asymmetry and lymphocyte proliferation in female mice: Effects of right and left cortical ablation. *Brain Research* 550(1):125–28.

Nowakowski, R. S. 1988. Development of the hippocampal formation in mutant mice. *Drug Development Research* 15:315–36.

Pennington, B. F., Smith, S. D., Kimberling, W. J., Green, P. A., and Haith, M. M. 1987. Lefthandedness and immune disorders in familial dyslexics. *Archives of Neurology* 44:634–39.

Rosen, G. D., Waters, N. S., Galaburda, A. M., and Denenberg, V. H. 1995. Behavioral consequences of neonatal injury of the neocortex. *Brain Research* 681:177–89.

Rosen, G. D., Sherman, G. F., Mehler, C., Emsbo, K., and Galaburda, A. M. 1989. The effect of developmental neuropathology on neocortical asymmetry in New Zealand Black mice. *International Journal of Neuroscience* 45:247–54.

Rosen, G. D., Sherman, G. F., Richman, J. M., Stone, L. V., and Galaburda, A. M. 1992. Induction of molecular layer ectopias by puncture wounds in newborn rats and mice. *Developmental Brain Research* 67(2):285–91.

Schrott, L. M. 1992. Behavior in autoimmune mice: Neural immune interactions. Dissertation submitted at the University of Connecticut.

Schrott, L. M., Denenberg, V. H., Sherman, G. F., Rosen, G. D., and Galaburda, A. M. 1992. Lashley maze deficits in NZB mice. *Physiology and Behavior* 52:1085–89.

Schrott, L. M., Denenberg, V. H., Sherman, G. F., Waters, N. S., Rosen, G. D., and Galaburda, A. M. 1992. Environmental enrichment, neocortical ectopias, and behavior in the autoimmune NZB mouse. *Developmental Brain Research* 67(1):85–93.

Schrott, L. M., Morrison, L., Wimer, R., Wimer, C., Behan, O., and Denenberg, V. H. 1994. Autoimmunity and avoidance learning in NXRF recombinant inbred strains. *Brain, Behavior and Immunity* 8:100-110.

Sherman, G. F., Galaburda, A. M., Behan, P. O., and Rosen, G. D. 1987. Neuro-anatomical anomalies in autoimmune mice. *Acta Neuropathologica (Berlin)* 74:239–42.

Sherman, G.F., Galaburda, A. M., and Geschwind, N. 1985. Cortical anomalies in brains of New Zealand mice: A neuropathologic model of dyslexia? *Proceedings of the National Academy of Sciences (USA)* 82:8072–74.

Sherman, G. F., Morrison, L., Rosen, G. D., Behan, P. O., and Galaburda, A. M. 1990. Brain abnormalities in immune defective mice. *Brain Research* 532:25–33.

Sherman, G. F., Press, D. M., Rosen, G. D., and Galaburda, A. M. 1990. Radial glial immunoreactive fibers in the region of spontaneous microdysgenesis in newborn New Zealand Black mice. *Society for Neuroscience Abstracts* 16:1152.

Sherman, G. F., Stone, J. S., Press, D. M., Rosen, G. D., and Galaburda, A. M. 1990. Abnormal architecture and connections disclosed by neurofilament staining in the cerebral cortex of autoimmune mice. *Brain Research* 529:202–7.

Sherman, G. F., Stone, J. S., Rosen, G. D., and Galaburda, A. M. 1990. Neocortical VIP neurons are increased in the hemisphere containing focal cerebrocortical microdysgenesis in New Zealand Black Mice. *Brain Research* 532:232–36.

Sherman, G. F., Stone, L. V., Denenberg, V. H., and Beier, D. R. 1994. A genetic analysis of neocortical ectopias in New Zealand Black mice. *NeuroReport* 5:721–4.

Spencer, D. G., Humphries, K., Mathis, D., and Lal, H. 1986. Behavioral impairments related to cognitive dysfunction in the autoimmune New Zealand Black mouse. *Behavioral Neuroscience* 100:353–58.

Tallal, P. 1984. Temporal or phonetic processing deficit in dyslexia? That is the question. *Applied Psycholinguistics* 5:167–69.

Tallal, P., and Piercy, M. 1973. Defects of non-verbal auditory perception in children with developmental aphasia. *Nature* 241:468–69.

Wimer, R., and Weller, S. 1965. Evaluation of a visual discrimination task for the analysis of the genetics of mouse behavior. *Perceptual and Motor Skills* 20:203–8.

Chapter • 2

The Maturation of the Occipitotemporal Pathway for Object Discrimination and Object Recognition in Rhesus Monkeys

Jocelyne Bachevalier

In primates, cortical tissue essential for visual perception extends far beyond the primary visual area, striate cortex, to include not only the prestriate regions of the occipital lobe but also large portions of the temporal and parietal lobes. There exist at least 20 cortical areas with visual functions in monkeys and these multiple visual areas appear to be organized hierarchically into two separate cortical pathways, each having the striate cortex as the source of its initial input (figure 1). As originally proposed by Ungerleider and Mishkin (1982), one of the pathways is directed dorsally into the parietal lobe and is crucial for spatial perception and visuomotor performance. The other is directed ventrally into the temporal lobe and is crucial for object recognition. The issue of the ontogenetic maturation of the occipitotemporal pathway in nonhuman primates is addressed in the present chapter.

Much of what we know about the occipitotemporal pathway for object perception derives from studies that have explored: (a) the flow of information through the cortical areas in the pathway by neuroanatomical tracing techniques (Jones and Powell 1970; Kuypers et al. 1965; Pandya and Kuypers 1969; Ungerleider 1985; Felleman and Van Essen 1991; Zeki 1973); (b) the contribution of particular stations to visual perception by surgically damaging the ventral pathway in monkeys and then testing the animals on visual tasks (e.g., Dean, 1976; Gaffan, Harrison, and Gaffan 1986a, 1986b; Gross 1973, 1992; Mishkin 1966,

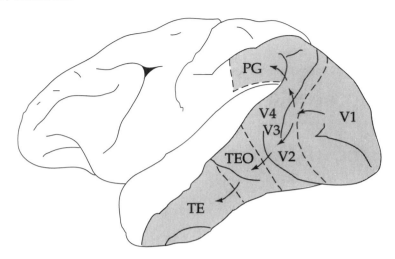

Figure 1.   Lateral view of the left hemisphere of a rhesus monkey brain. The shaded area defines the cortical visual tissue in the occipital, temporal, and parietal lobes. Arrows schematize two cortical pathways, each originating in striate cortex (V1), passing through extrastriate areas (V2, V3, and V4) and then coursing either dorsally into the inferior parietal cortex (area PG) or ventrally into the inferior temporal cortex (areas TEO and TE). Modified from Mishkin, Ungerleider, and Macko (1983).

1972; Mishkin and Phillips 1990); (c) by recording electrical activity from neurons at each cortical station in animals exposed to various visual stimuli (Desimone et al. 1985; Desimone and Ungerleider 1989; Gross 1973; Gross et al. 1993). Converging information from these numerous studies have led to a neural model for object vision. As proposed by Mishkin (1982), visual perception of an object depends on the sequential processing of its physical attributes along a chain of visual cortical areas beginning in the striate cortex (V1), through the extrastriate cortical areas (V2, V3, and V4), and finally inferior temporal cortical areas (TEO and TE). Neurons in the different cortical areas along the ventral visual pathway integrate an object's physical properties, such as size, shape, color, and texture, until the final cortical station (area TE), a cytoarchitectonic division that occupies approximately the anterior two-thirds of the inferior temporal cortex (Bonin and Bailey 1947), synthesizes a complete representation of the object. This postulated integration of the coded visual properties of an object within area TE suggests that this cortical area is especially well suited to serve not only as the higher-order area for object perception but also as the storehouse for their central representations and, hence, for their later recognition.

   That area TE is important for the retention of some form of visual experience has been inferred from lesion studies that have shown that, in macaques, bilateral ablations of the inferior temporal cortex yield marked impairment in either the retention of visual discrimination learned prior to surgery or the acquisition of new visual discrimination postsurgery (Mishkin 1954; see also reviews by Dean 1976 and Gross 1973, 1992). This learning and retention deficit occurs even though visual perceptual abilities, such as visual acuity, color vision, and discrimination of stimuli differing in orientation (Dean 1976; Holmes and Gross 1984; Gross 1992), remain intact. These findings led to the view that inferior temporal cortex is probably involved in higher-order mechanisms, though the exact nature of these mechanisms remains unknown.

Dean (1976, 1982) has argued that the fundamental impairment of monkeys with inferior temporal cortical lesions is in visual classification, a notion that has been elaborated more recently by Gaffan and colleagues (1986a, b). According to this view, the underlying impairment following bilateral lesions of inferior temporal cortex is not a loss of visual associative learning but rather a lack of discrimination among objects within the same perceptual category, i.e., a decrease in the number of the object's attributes. An alternative hypothesis is that inferior temporal cortex is connected not purely with visual analyses, but with mnemonic or associative processes (Gross 1973; Cowey and Gross 1970) that require the convergence of visual information with the central representation of motivational or emotional system (Geschwind 1965; Mishkin 1982). Strong evidence in favor of this proposal is given by the findings that bilateral inferior temporal lesions in monkeys severely impairs their ability to recognize objects seen just a few seconds earlier (Mishkin 1982). In addition, there exist neurophysiological data suggesting that inferior temporal cortex could be the site of memory storage (Fuster and Jervey 1981; Brown, Wilson and Riches 1987; Desimone et al. 1991).

The neural model elaborated by Mishkin (1982) entails that neurons in area TE form a neuronal network in which the central representations of visual stimuli are formed and stored with the participation of additional brain stations. Indeed, inferior temporal cortical areas provide integrated visual inputs to two independent circuits: a *corticostriatal pathway*, involving the basal ganglia, and a *corticolimbic pathway*, involving the medial temporal, medial diencephalic, medial prefrontal areas as well as basal forebrain (Mishkin 1982; Mishkin, Malamut, and Bachevalier 1984; Mishkin and Petri 1984; Mishkin and Appenzeller 1987; Mishkin and Petri 1994). In the corticostriatal pathway (figure 2), visual inputs from area TE (and visual areas posterior to area TE, such as area TEO) are processed through a series of stations from the striatum to the globus pallidus and substantia nigra, then to the ventral thalamus, and, finally, to the premotor cortex. Through this pathway, cortically processed visual inputs could become associated with extrapyramidally generated motor outputs to yield the stimulus-response bonds that constitute the formation of visual habits. Behavioral evidence in support of this corticostriatal habit system comes from studies demonstrating impairment in visual discrimination following damage to either the inferior temporal cortex (Mishkin 1954; Phillips et al. 1988), the projections from the visual areas to the neostriatum (Horel 1978; Zola-Morgan, Squire, and Mishkin 1982) or the striatal regions (Buerger, Gross, and Rocha-Miranda 1974; Divac, Rosvold, and Szwarcbart 1967; Wang, Aigner, and Mishkin 1990). In the corticolimbic pathway (figure 2), storage of the object's representation (and assignment of some meaning or association to it) is realized each time a perception formed in the final station of the visual cortex (area TE) interacts with the medial temporal lobe structures. Inferior temporal cortical area TE projects heavily to this medial temporal lobe region, sending efferents directly to the perirhinal cortex and amygdala and indirectly to the hippocampus via the perirhinal and entorhinal cortex (Aggleton, Burton, and Passingham 1980; Amaral and Price 1984; Iwai and Yukie 1987; Iwai et al. 1987; Jones and Powell 1970; Seltzer and Pandya 1976; Turner, Mishkin, and Knapp 1980; Van Hoessen and Pandya 1975; Webster, Ungerleider, and Bachevalier 1991a). Furthermore, bilateral damage to either area TE,

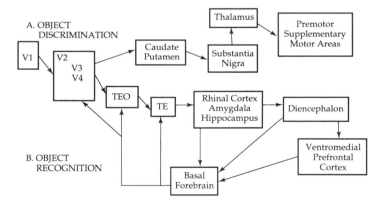

Figure 2.   The postulated neural circuits for visual habit formation (a form of procedural memory) and visual object recognition (a form of declarative memory). The arrows schematize the flow of visual information originating in striate cortex (V1), passing through extrastriate areas (V2, V3, and V4), and then coursing ventrally into the inferior temporal cortex (areas TEO and TE). Visual information is next processed via two independent pathways, one (A) coursing through the basal ganglia (caudate, putamen), substantia nigra, and thalamus to end onto the premotor supplementary motor areas, and the other (B) coursing through the medial temporal structures (rhinal cortex, hippocampal formation and amygdala), the medial diencephalon, the medial prefrontal cortex, and finally from the basal forebrain back onto the cortical areas in which perception of an object has taken place. From Bachevalier, Malkova, and Beauregard (1996).

the medial temporal lobe structures, or the temporal stem white matter containing the efferents from area TE to the medial temporal lobe structures, results in a severe loss of object recognition (Mishkin 1978, 1982; Zola-Morgan, Squire, and Mishkin 1982; Mishkin and Phillips 1990). It is thus postulated that the role of the medial temporal lobe structures and their projection targets to the diencephalon, prefrontal cortex, and basal forebrain is to facilitate consolidation of new memories within the inferior temporal cortex.

To summarize, the brain of adult monkeys appears to possess two independent mechanisms for the storage of visual information, each having inferior temporal cortex as an important source of its initial visual input: a corticostriatal habit system, which operates as an incremental build-up of stimulus-response associations through reinforcement and repeated trials, and a corticolimbic system, which stores sensory representations and their associations. The first part of this review will summarize behavioral data on the maturation of visual discrimination and visual recognition abilities in primates. The second part will consider neurobehavioral, neurobiological, and electrophysiological findings in infant monkeys suggesting that delayed maturation of the cortical association areas of the brain, and more specifically area TE, appears to be responsible for the delayed maturation of some object memory abilities.

THE DEVELOPMENT OF OBJECT DISCRIMINATION ABILITY

The acquisition of visual discriminations is known to occur very early in life in infant monkeys (Harlow 1959; Zimmerman and Torrey 1965). Monkeys younger than one month of age can readily acquire visual discriminations when the discriminations are presented one object-pair at a time with massed practice and short intertrial intervals (Zimmerman and Torrey 1965), and by two months of age, they can learn short lists of 8 object pairs presented with massed practice at short intertrial intervals (Mahut and Zola-Morgan 1977). We recently demonstrated (Bachevalier and Mishkin 1984) that, by 3 months of age, they are as efficient as adults in mastering a discrimination task in which long lists of 20 object-pairs were presented with distributed practice at extremely long intertrial intervals (24 hours). These early visual discrimination abilities despite long intertrial intervals were shown by testing 3- and 6-month-old monkeys in a multiple-trial concurrent discrimination task (24-hr ITI task). Performance on this task is known to be preserved in adult monkeys with medial temporal lobe lesions (Malamut, Saunders, and Mishkin 1984) but to be severely impaired in adult monkeys with removals of inferior temporal cortical area TE (Phillips et al. 1988). In this task, a set consisting of 20 pairs of objects was presented just once a day. A positive and a negative object (i.e., one baited and one not) were presented simultaneously over the lateral wells of the test tray. After the animal made a choice by displacing one of the objects, there was a 20-sec. delay, following which the second pair of objects was presented for choice, and so on until all 20 pairs had been presented once each. The same series of objects was then repeated once every 24 hours. The positive and negative objects within each pair, as well as the serial order of the pairs, remained constant across sessions, but the objects' left-right positions were randomized daily. Testing was continued in this way until the monkeys attained a learning criterion of 90 correct responses in 100 trials. Three-month-old female monkeys learned as rapidly as male and female adult monkeys (Bachevalier, Hagger, and Bercu 1989). By contrast, the 3-month-old male monkeys required significantly more sessions and made more errors to reach criterion on the task than did the females (figure 3). This sex difference was absent in the 6-month-old group, in which both the male and female animals performed as efficiently as the male and female adults. Additional evidence of sexual dimorphism in visual discrimination learning by infant macaques comes from a study showing that 4- to 5-month-old males learned both single and concurrent visual discriminations with short intertrial intervals at a slower rate than females (H. Mahut, personal communication).

In neuroendocrinological studies, we demonstrated further that the androgen levels in male monkeys, which are elevated before birth and then progressively decline to reach a nadir around 6 months of

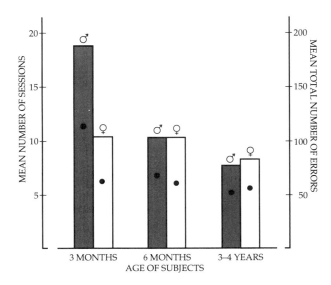

Figure 3.   Mean number of sessions (bars) and errors (circles) preceding criterion on the 24-hr ITI task. Numbers of animals were 8 males and 5 females at the age of 3 months, 6 males and 3 females at the age of 6 months, and 7 males and 3 females at the age of 3-4 years. From Bachevalier (1990a).

age (Bercu et al. 1983, 1987; Resko 1970; Phoenix 1974), are probably responsible for the sex differences in object discrimination learning. In the first of two experiments (Bachevalier, Hagger, and Bercu 1989), plasma gonadal hormone levels were determined in the 3- and 6-month-old animals from the study reported above, after they had reached criterion on the task. In the 3-month-old male monkeys, a significant correlation ($r_s = -0.95$, $p<0.01$) was found between circulating levels of testosterone and learning scores, such that the higher the level, the poorer the score. By contrast, no significant correlations were found between plasma testosterone levels and learning scores in either the 3-month-old female monkeys or in the 6-month olds of either sex. Similarly, there were no significant correlations between plasma estradiol levels and learning scores in male and female monkeys at any age. Thus, the postnatal decline of circulating androgen levels, which reaches a nadir around 6 months, could account for the lack of sex differences in the 6-month olds. In a second experiment (Hagger and Bachevalier 1991), we found that this sex difference in object discrimination learning can be reversed in the two sexes by perinatal manipulation of androgen levels. Thus, 3-month-old males orchiectomized neonatally required significantly fewer sessions than intact males and performed at the same rate as intact females. By contrast, 3-month-old females treated neonatally with dihydrotestosterone significantly needed more sessions than normal females and performed at the same rate as intact males. Our experimental evidence thus far seems to indicate that the presence of perinatal androgens can affect performance on the concurrent object discrimination task by some, as yet, unspecified action on the maturing neural circuit underlying object discrimination learning. One hint as to where in this circuit (figure 2) androgens might exert their influence has come from studies of the effects of neonatal ablations of the anterior portion of the inferior temporal cortex (area TE). As shown in figure 4, whereas both male and female adult monkeys with area TE lesions are severely impaired in learning the object discrimination task, only the 3-month-old female infants with neonatal area TE lesions were impaired as compared to the unoperated females. The 3-month-old male infants, by contrast, did not differ from the unoperated male infants. Thus, such neonatal lesions affect performance of 3-month-old female monkeys more than that of 3-month-old males, presumably because at that age area TE is more fully developed in females than in the males (Bachevalier and Hagger 1991; Bachevalier et al. 1990). Together with the finding of our neuroendocrinological study, these data suggest that the high levels of androgens found in infant male monkeys before and shortly after birth retard the development of object discrimination ability, presumably by slowing the maturation of either cortical area TE, or its projection targets in the striatum, or both.

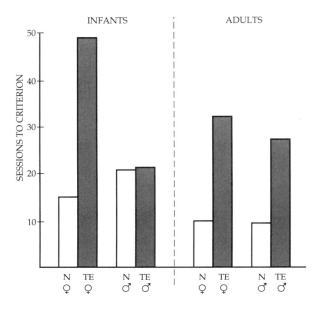

Figure 4. Average number of sessions to attain criterion on the 24-hr ITI task by 3-month-old (operated neonatally) and adult monkeys (operated in adulthood) of both sexes. N, normal controls; TE, animals with bilateral area TE lesions. From Bachevalier (1990b).

Similarly, the ability to acquire object discrimination has been found to emerge very early in life in humans (Zeaman and House 1963; Overman et al. 1992). Recent studies also demonstrate the presence of a transient sex difference in the ability to learn object discrimination in human infants (Overman et al. 1994). Interestingly, young boys (between 13-35 months of age), like 3-month-old infant monkeys, required significantly more trials to learn an object discrimination task than girls. By contrast, no sex differences occurred in older children (between 36-54 months of age). This parallel in learning performance in the two species favors the view that the biological substrate underlying the sex differences in human infants and in infant monkeys might be similar.

THE DEVELOPMENT OF OBJECT RECOGNITION

The development of object recognition memory was first assessed by testing infant monkeys at different ages in a one-trial object recognition test (delayed nonmatching-to-sample, DNMS) that was used to demonstrate anterograde amnesia in adult monkeys with either area TE or medial temporal lobe lesions (Mishkin 1978). In this task, on each sample (or familiarization) trial, one object is presented over the test tray's central well, which the animal uncovered to obtain a concealed food reward. Ten seconds later, the sample object and a new object are presented simultaneously over the test tray's lateral wells, and now the animal finds the reward only if it chooses the new one. Thirty seconds later, another set of trials is presented in the same way, but with a new pair of objects, and so on for 20 trials a day, each with a completely new pair of objects chosen from a stock of several hundred (Mishkin and Delacour 1975). Groups of rhesus monkeys varying in age from 3 months to 3 years were trained in this way until they reached a learning criterion of 90 percent correct responses in 100 trials. As indicated by the learning curves (figure 5A), speed of learning varied systematically with age. The 2- and 3-year olds showed a sharp improvement in score from the first 2-day block to the second and continued to improve rapidly thereafter, whereas both the one-year and the 6-month groups improved significantly only on the third block. The 4-month group showed a greater retardation; their scores improving only on the sixth block. The most striking result, however, was found in the 3-month group, which failed to improve through the first nine blocks of training. It was only on the 10th block that the mean scores of these animals differed from their initial scores, after which they showed slow but progressive improvement to criterion. In short, infant rhesus monkeys failed to solve the DNMS task until they were approximately 4 months of age. With further maturation, there was a gradual improvement in learning ability, yet it did not reach the adult level of proficiency even at one year. Only at about 2 years of age do monkeys master the recognition task as efficiently as adult animals.

A similar delay in the maturation of abilities to solve the DNMS task was recently demonstrated in human infants (Diamond 1990; Overman 1990). When human subjects were tested with the same one-trial visual recognition task that we used to test infant monkeys (Overman et al. 1992), it was found that infants of 12 months of age did very poorly on this visual recognition task, although they were easily able to solve a visual discrimination problem. Also, in human infants as in infant monkeys, ability to perform on the DNMS task increased progressively with age. Thus, there is an age at which the DNMS task can first be solved and a considerably greater age at which it can be solved with full adult proficiency.

This slow ontogenetic development of object recognition memory in infant monkeys was also shown in the memory performance test. That is, after each individual attained criterion on the basic delayed non-matching principle with 10 sec delay, it was given a performance test (Gaffan 1974) in which, first, the delay interval between familiarization and test was lengthened in stages from 10 sec to 30 sec, then to 60 sec, and finally to 120 sec. Then, the list of objects to be remembered was increased in stages from one object to three objects, then to five objects, and finally to ten objects. In this last stage, for example, all ten sample objects were presented one at a time for familiarization, after which each of the ten was paired with a different novel object for the test trials. Since there was a 20-sec interval between presentations throughout the performance test, the minimum retention interval for the list of ten objects was 200 sec, or more than 3 min. The overall averaged performance across the three delays and the three lists conditions for the five age groups tested in this portion of the task is shown in figure 5B. The data indicate

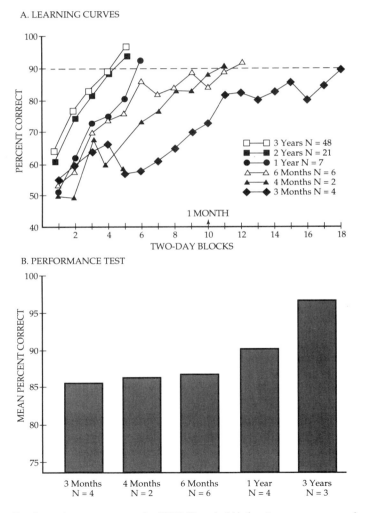

Figure 5. Learning curves on the DNMS task (A) for 6 age groups and mean performance scores (B) in the 6 conditions of the performance test (3 delays and 3 lists) for the 5 age groups tested in that part of the task. From Bachevalier (1990a).

that scores on the memory performance test declined systematically in inverse relation to age, suggesting a slow ontogenetic development of recognition memory to adult levels of function. These findings suggested that this protracted maturation of object recognition ability in primates presumably resulted from a relatively slow ontogenetic development of the neural circuit on which it depends (figure 2B). They also led to the speculation that one or more of the structures in the medial temporal lobe (Bachevalier and Mishkin 1984), and perhaps more specifically the hippocampal formation (Rose 1980; Nadel and Zola-Morgan 1984; Schacter and Moscovitch 1984) may not be fully functional at birth. Our more recent neurobehavioral data have now cast serious doubts on this view (Bachevalier 1990a; Bachevalier and Mishkin 1994; Malkova, Mishkin, and Bachevalier 1995).

DEVELOPMENTAL NEUROBEHAVIORAL STUDIES

One set of results emerged from an investigation of the effects of early lesions at different neural stations in the neural pathway underlying visual recognition memory. We began our behavioral investigation by comparing the effects of neonatal damage to either the medial temporal lobe structures (including the amygdaloid complex, hippocampal formation, and adjacent cortical areas), known to be critical for the formation of new memories, or the inferior temporal cortical area TE, known to be critical for the storage of visual memories. When tested at 10 months of age on the visual DNMS task, infant monkeys with neonatal temporal lobe lesions were severely impaired in visual recognition, whereas those with neonatal ablation of area TE showed significant sparing (Bachevalier and Mishkin 1993). As shown in figure 6, both early and late damage to the medial temporal lobe yielded a severe impairment in visual recognition, reflected in drops in performance of 22% for infants and 32% for adults (as compared with their unoperated controls). By contrast, although late damage to area TE resulted in a drop in performance of 29%, early lesions of this cortical area resulted in a drop of only 8%. All behavioral data gathered so far indicate that early damage to the medial temporal lobe structures yields a behavioral syndrome strikingly similar to that found earlier after late damage to the medial temporal lobe. That is, like large medial temporal lobe lesions in adulthood, those in infancy result in a global and long-lasting memory deficit, affecting not only memory for visual information (Bachevalier and Mishkin 1993) but also memory for tactile stimuli and spatial locations (Malkova et al. 1995). Similar profound memory loss was recently reported in several clinical studies of children who sustained medial temporal lobe damage (Ostergaard 1987; Rossitch and Oakes 1989; Tongstard, Harwicke, and Levine

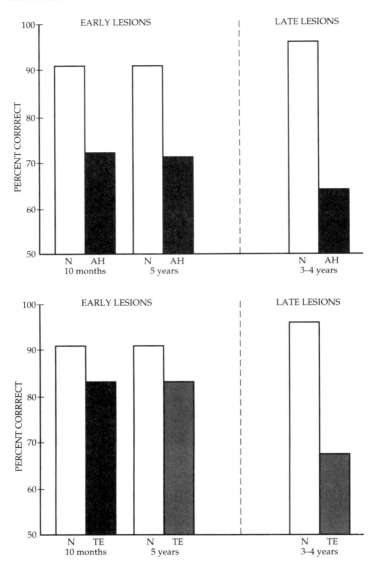

Figure 6. Average scores on the recognition performance test of the DNMS by 10-month-old and 5-year-old monkeys (operated neonatally) and 3- to 4-year-old adult monkeys (operated in adulthood). N, normal controls; AH, animals with medial temporal lobe removals; TE, animals with area TE removals.

1987; Vargha-Khadem, Isaacs, and Watkins 1992, Wood, Brown, and Felton. 1989).

Another indication that the medial temporal lobe structures develop early in infancy came from an investigation of recognition memory in infant monkeys using a paired-comparison preferential viewing task

(Bachevalier 1990a; Bachevalier, Brickson, and Haggar 1993). In this task, originally designed to test recognition memory in human infants (Fantz 1956; Fagan 1970), recognition memory is inferred from the infant's tendency to look more at a novel than at a previously exposed target. Between 15 to 30 days of age (figure 7), infant monkeys showed a strong preference for viewing novel objects at least for a short time (Bachevalier, Brickson, and Haggar 1993; Gunderson and Sackett 1984). Moreover, this early developing recognition ability was absent after both early and late damage to the medial temporal lobe (Bachevalier, Brickson, and Haggar 1993; Saunders 1989; McKee and Squire 1993). By contrast, early damage to area TE, unlike late damage, yielded a significant sparing of preference for novelty.

These neurobehavioral data indicate further that the degree of recognition loss after neonatal area TE lesions differs sharply from that after neonatal medial temporal removals. These findings have several implications. Firstly, they demonstrate that the medial temporal lobe structures operate early in life to sustain object recognition memory and that other regions cannot assume this function even when the damage occurs neonatally. Secondly, the significant and permanent sparing of

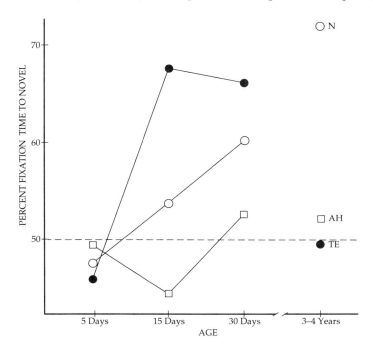

Figure 7.   Scores are percent fixation to novel stimuli on the visual paired-comparison task by 5-day-old, 15-day-old, and 30-day-old monkeys (operated neonatally) and adult monkeys. N, normal controls; AH, animals with medial temporal lobe removals; TE, animals with area TE removals.

visual recognition memory after early area TE lesions suggests that, at the time of the early lesion, area TE was functionally immature and, therefore, not critically committed to visual recognition. Hence, early in infancy, in the absence of area TE, other visual areas can apparently assume much of area TE's visual memory functions. Finally, the protracted development of object recognition memory as measured by the DNMS task cannot be attributable to an immaturity of the medial temporal lobe structures (see also Nelson 1993); rather it is the functional immaturity of association areas, such as area TE, which is the limiting factor. Recent neurobiological and electrophysiological studies have provided direct evidence of functional immaturity of the neocortex in the infant macaque.

DEVELOPMENTAL NEUROANATOMICAL, NEUROBIOLOGICAL, AND ELECTROPHYSIOLOGICAL STUDIES

Recent neuroanatomical studies in infant monkeys have shown that while many of the connections of inferior temporal cortex are similar in infant and adult monkeys (Webster, Ungerleider, and Bachevalier 1991a; Webster, Bachevalier, and Ungerleider 1994a, 1994b; Rodman and Consuelos 1994), there is also considerable elimination of normally transient projections and refinement of initially widespread projection fields during the early postnatal period. For example, we have found that area TEO, a cortical area just posterior to area TE in the inferior temporal cortex, projects to the lateral basal nucleus of the amygdala in infant monkeys but not in adults. Similarly, we found that area TEO projects to parahippocampal area TF in infant but not in adult monkeys. This different pattern of neuronal connectivity in infant and adult monkeys indicates that there exist, early in life, exuberant connections between visual areas, other than area TE, and the medial temporal lobe structures which must retract with maturation, since they do not exist in adult monkeys. Furthermore, not only do transient projections exist in early infancy, but also, for many of those that are retained, the laminar distribution of their terminals, which is initially widespread, becomes more restricted during maturation to achieve the adult-like pattern. For example, whereas area TE in adults projects to layer I in perirhinal areas 35 and 36, in infants the projection is to layers I and IV. Likewise, there are projections from area TE to various subcortical structures, e.g., superior colliculus, nucleus medialis dorsalis, and the genu of the caudate nucleus, that are more widespread in infants than in adults. Together, this anatomical evidence points to a relative immaturity of association areas of the cortex in neonates, and to its potential for reorganization as a result of early neural insult. Our most recent results

(Webster, Ungerleider, and Bachevalier 1991b; Webster, Bachevalier, and Ungerleider 1995) actually demonstrate that a lesion of area TE early in development leads to maintenance of normally transient projections and to reorganization in other cortical areas outside the inferior temporal lobe, thereby accounting at least in part for the sparing of object memory.

In an earlier study (Bachevalier et al. 1986), the distribution of opiate receptors in the brain of a newborn monkey was mapped by in vivo autoradiographic localization of [^{3}H] naloxone binding to tissue sections and compared to that found in adult monkeys. The distribution of opiate receptors appeared adult-like in subcortical structures (both limbic and nonlimbic) and allocortical areas. By contrast, major differences between the infant and adult brains were seen in the neocortex. The first distinction is that, whereas in the adult brains the density of receptor bindings varied from field to field, in the newborn it was distributed uniformly throughout the neocortex. The second important difference is that, whereas the adult brain was characterized by area-specific laminar patterns across the six layers of cortex, the newborn brain was not. In the newborn, all neocortical areas, except the primary visual cortex, had a unimodal laminar distribution. These findings suggest that postnatal redistribution of opiate binding sites takes place mostly in the cortical mantle. This late development of opiate receptor distribution together with the data on the protracted period of dendritic growth and synaptic density (Boothe et al. 1979; Kemper, Caveness, and Yakovlev 1973; Lund, Boothe, and Lund 1977; Rakic 1978; Rakic et al. 1986) suggest that neocortical maturation continues well after birth in monkeys.

Furthermore, in collaboration with the Laboratory of Cerebral Metabolism at NIMH, we have applied the 2-deoxyglucose method postoperatively to a series of infant monkeys that had received unilateral optic tract section combined with forebrain commissurotomy at one day, one week, and one, 2, 3, 4, and 6 months of age (Bachevalier, Hagger, and Mishkin 1991). With this surgical procedure and the 2-deoxyglucose injection applied when the animals were passively looking at geometric patterns, metabolic activity produced by direct retinal stimulation was thereby limited to one hemisphere, and it was thus possible to compare local cerebral glucose utilization in a "seeing" and a "blind" hemisphere in the same animal. In all occipitotemporal cortical areas of the intact ("seeing") hemisphere, absolute local cerebral glucose utilization values were lowest in the youngest subjects, peaked at 4 months, and then declined in the 6-month-old subject to levels found in adults. Differences in the rate of glucose utilization between the "seeing" and "blind" hemispheres (figure 8) indicated that, although adult levels of metabolic activity are attained in all striate and prestriate areas as early as 3 months of age, they are not attained in inferior tem-

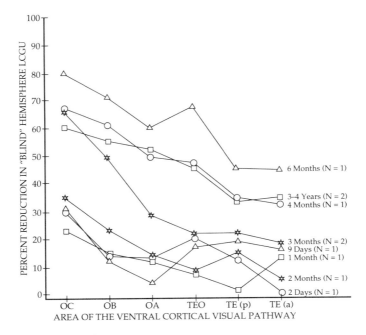

Figure 8.   Percent reduction of local cerebral glucose utilization (LCGU) in the "blind" as compared to the "seeing" hemisphere in monkeys from 2 days to 4 years of age. For each animal, the percent reduction was calculated by dividing the absolute LCGU in the "blind" hemisphere by the absolute LCGU in the "seeing" hemisphere, and multiplying this ration by 100. Adapted from Bachevalier, Hagger, and Mishkin (1991).

poral cortical areas (TEO and TE) until the animals are about 4 months of age (figure 8). This reduction in metabolic activity also corroborates the immaturity of electrophysiological responses of area TE.

Electrophysiological recordings of inferotemporal neurons in alert infant monkeys (for review see Rodman 1994) revealed that TE neurons showed adult-like response properties as early as the second month of life. At this early age, TE neurons showed stimulus selectivity, particularly for boundary curvature, but also for color and faces, although their responses were in general weaker and of longer latency than the responses recorded in adult monkeys. Also, as in adult monkeys, neuronal responses were strongest at the fovea when compared with responses at other locations. By contrast, TE neurons were not responsive at this early age when the animals were anesthetized, despite the presence of normal neuronal activity in striate cortex (Rodman, Skelly, and Gross 1988). This absence of responsiveness of inferior temporal neurons under anesthesia persisted up to 4 months of age, indicating that developmental changes in cellular metabolism, extrinsic modulating influences, or other factors last up to this age.

CONCLUSION

The behavioral data summarized in this paper indicate that the ability to perform on either object discrimination tasks, such as concurrent visual discrimination, or some of the object recognition tasks, such as paired-comparison preferential viewing, emerges very early in infancy. By contrast, the ability to solve a delayed nonmatching-to-sample task develops slowly during the first year in monkeys. This protracted development appears to be related to an immaturity of the last cortical stations into the occipitotemporal pathway for object memory.

Thus, the data of the developmental neurobehavioral and neurobiological studies indicate substantial postnatal changes in the ventral occipitotemporal pathway for object memory in monkeys. The neuroanatomical findings indicate the presence of both transient projections as well as more widespread connections between temporal cortical areas TE and TEO and other cortical and subcortical structures. In addition, the data of the metabolic and electrophysiological studies suggest that, within the first 4 months of life in monkeys, reduced metabolic activity in TE neurons might not be sufficient for the generation of action potentials necessary to sustain visual recognition. Since the emergence of adult-like levels of metabolic activity in area TE coincides with the emergence of abilities to perform on the DNMS task, we may assume that the protracted emergence of recognition ability in primates is likely to be due to an immaturity of inferior temporal cortical areas. Given the functions of area TE reviewed above, the slow development of this visual cortical area might yield an inability in either the formation of the complete representation of the object itself, or the storage of this neural representation through the feedback action of the medial temporal lobe structures onto area TE, or both.

ACKNOWLEGEMENTS

The work discussed in this chapter was supported in part by NIMH Grant No. MH49728.

REFERENCES

Aggleton, J. P., Burton M. J., and Passingham, R. E. 1980. Cortical and subcortical afferents to the amygdala of the rhesus monkey (*Macaca mulatta*). *Brain Research* 190:347–68.

Amaral, D. G. and Price, J. L. 1984. Amygdalo-cortical projections in the monkey (*Macaca fascicularis*). *Journal of Comparative Neurology* 230:465–96.

Bachevalier, J. 1990a. Ontogenetic development of habit and memory formation in primates. In *Development and Neural Bases of Higher Cognitive Functions*, ed. A. Diamond. New York: Academic Press.

Bachevalier, J. 1990b. Memory loss and socio-emotional disturbances following neonatal damage of the limbic system in monkeys: An animal model for childhood autism. In *Advances in Psychiatry: Schizophrenia*, eds. C. A. Tamminga and S. C. Schulz. New York: Raven Press.

Bachevalier, J., Malkova, L., and Beauregard, M. 1996. Multiple memory systems: A neuropsychological and developmental perspective. In *Attention, Memory, and Executive Functions*, eds. G. R. Lyon and N. A. Krasnegor. Baltimore: Brookes Publishing Co.

Bachevalier, J., Brickson, M., and Hagger, C. S. 1993. Limbic-dependent recognition memory in monkeys develops early in infancy. *NeuroReport* 4:77–80.

Bachevalier, J., Brickson, M., Hagger, C. S., and Mishkin, M. 1990. Age and sex differences in the effects of selective temporal lobe lesion on the formation of visual discrimination habits in rhesus monkeys (Macaca mulatta). *Behavioral Neuroscience* 104:885–99.

Bachevalier, J. and Hagger, C. 1991. Sex differences in the development of learning abilities in primates. *Psychoneuroendocrinology* 16:177–88.

Bachevalier, J., Hagger, C. S., and Bercu, B. B. 1989. Gender differences in visual habit formation in 3-month-old rhesus monkeys. *Developmental Psychobiology* 22:585–99.

Bachevalier, J., Hagger, C., and Mishkin, M. 1991. Functional maturation of the occipitotemporal pathway in infant rhesus monkeys. In *Brain Work and Mental Activity: Alfred Benzon Symposium 31*, eds. N. A. Lassen, D. H. Ingvar, M. E. Raichle, and L. Friberg. Copenhagen: Munksgaard.

Bachevalier, J., and Mishkin, M. 1984. An early and a late developing system for learning and retention in infant monkeys. *Behavioral Neuroscience* 98:770–78.

Bachevalier, J., and Mishkin, M. 1994. Effects of selective neonatal temporal lobe lesions on visual recognition memory in rhesus monkeys. *Journal of Neuroscience* 14:2128–39.

Bachevalier, J., Ungerleider, L. G., O'Neill, B., and Friedman, D. P. Regional distribution of [^{3}H]naloxone binding in the brain of a newborn rhesus monkey. *Developmental Brain Research* 25:302–8.

Bercu, B. B., Lee, B. C., Pineda, J. L., Spiliotis, B. E., Denman, D. W. III, Hoffman, H. J., Brown, T. J., and Sachs, H. C. 1983. Male sexual development in the monkey: I- Cross-sectional analysis of pulsatile hypothalamic-pituitary-testicular function. *Journal of Clinical Endocrinology and Metabolism* 56:1214–26.

Bercu, B. B., Spiliotis, B. E., Reed, G. F., and Lee, B. C. 1987. Male sexual development in the monkey: IV- Further analysis of hypothalamic pituitary-testicular function and correlation with electron and light microscopy of the testis. *Journal of Pediatric Endocrinology* 2:7–22.

Bonin, G. Von, and Bailey, P. 1947. *The Neocortex of Macaca Mulatta*, Urbana: University Illinois Press.

Boothe, R. G., Greenough, W. T., Lund, J. S. and Wrege, K. 1979. A quantitative investigation of spine and dendrite development of neurons in visual cortex (area 17) of Macaca nemestrina monkeys. *Journal of Comparative Neurology* 186:473–90.

Brown, M. W., Wilson, F. A. W., and Riches, I. P. 1987. Neuronal evidence that inferotemporal cortex is more important than hippocampus in certain process underlying recognition memory. *Brain Research* 409:158–62.

Buerger, A. A., Gross, C. G., and Rocha-Miranda, C. E. 1974. Effects of ventral putamen lesions on discrimination learning by monkeys. *Journal of Comparative and Physiological Psychology* 86:440–46.

Cowey, A. and Gross, C. G. 1970. Effects of foveal prestriate and inferotemporal lesions on visual discrimination by rhesus monkeys. *Experimental Brain Research* 11:128–44.

Dean, P. 1976. Effects of inferotemporal lesions on the behavior of monkeys. *Psychology Bulletin* 83:41–71.

Dean, P. 1982. Visual behavior in monkeys with inferotemporal lesions. In *Analysis of Visual Behavior*, eds. D. J. Ingle, M. A. Goodale, and R. J. W. Mansfield. Cambridge: MIT Press.

Desimone, R., Schein, S. J., Moran, J., and Ungerleider, L. G. 1985. Contour, color and shape analysis beyond the striate cortex. *Vision Research* 25:441–52.

Desimone, R., and Ungerleider, L. G. 1989. Neural mechanisms of visual processing in monkeys. In *Handbook of Neurophysiology*, Vol. 2., eds. F. Boller and J. Grafman. Amsterdam: Elsevier Science Publishers.

Diamond, A. 1990. Rate of maturation of the hippocampus and the developmental progression of children's performance on the delayed non-matching to sample and visual paired comparison tasks. In *The Development and Neural Bases of Higher Cognitive Functions*, ed. A. Diamond. New York: Academic Press.

Divac, I., Rosvold, H. E., and Szwarcbart, M. K. 1967. Behavioral effects of selective ablation of the caudate nucleus. *Journal of Comparative and Physiological Psychology* 63:184–90.

Fagan, J. F. III 1970. Memory in the infant. *Journal of Experimental Child Psychology* 9:217–26.

Fantz, R. L. 1956. A method for studying early visual development. *Perceptual and Motor Skills* 6:13–15.

Felleman, D. J. and Van Essen D. C. 1991. Distributed hierarchical processing in the primate cerebral cortex. *Cerebral Cortex*, 1:1–47.

Fuster, J. M., and Jervey, J. P. 1981. Inferotemporal neurons distinguish and retain behaviorally relevant features of visual stimuli. *Science* 212:952–54.

Gaffan, D. 1974. Recognition impaired and association intact in the memory of monkeys after transection of the fornix. *Journal of Comparative and Physiological Psychology* 86:1100–09.

Gaffan, D., Harrison, S., and Gaffan, E. A. 1986a. Visual identification following inferotemporal ablation in the monkey. *The Quarterly Journal of Experimental Psychology* 38B:5–30.

Gaffan, E. A., Harrison, S., and Gaffan, D. 1986b. Single and concurrent discrimination learning by monkeys after lesions of inferotemporal cortex. *The Quarterly Journal of Experimental Medicine* 38B:31–51.

Geschwind, N. 1965. Disconnection syndromes in animals and man. *Brain* 88:237–94.

Gross, C. G. 1973. Visual functions of inferotemporal cortex. In *Handbook of Sensory Physiology VII/3B*, ed. R. Jung. Berlin:Springer-Verlag.

Gross, C. G. 1992. Representation of visual stimuli in inferior temporal cortex. *Phylosophical Transactions of the Royal Society of London* 335:3–10.

Gross, C. G., Rodman, H. R., Gochin, P. M. and Colombo M. W. 1993. Inferior temporal cortex as a pattern recognition device. In *Proceedings of the 3rd Annual NEC Research Symposium*, ed. E. Baum. Philadelphia: SIAM.

Gunderson, V. M. and Sackett, G. P. 1984. Development of pattern recognition in infant pigtailed macaques (*Macaca nemestrina*). *Developmental Psychology* 20:418–26.

Hagger, C., and Bachevalier, J. 1991. Visual habit formation in 3-month-old monkeys (*Macaca mulatta*): Reversal of sex difference following neonatal manipulations of androgens. *Behavioural Brain Research* 45:57–63.

Harlow, H. F. 1959. The development of learning in rhesus monkeys. *American Scientist* 47:458–79.

Holmes, E. J., and Gross, C. G. 1984. Effects of inferior temporal lesions on discriminations of stimuli differing in orientation. *Journal of Neuroscience* 4:3063–8.

Horel, J. A. 1978. The neuroanatomy of amnesia: A critique of the hippocampal memory hypothesis. *Brain* 101:403–45.

Iwai, E., and Yukie, M. 1987. Amygdalofugal and amygdalopetal connections with modality-specific visual cortical areas in macaques (*Macaca fuscata, Macaca mulatta*, and *Macaca fascicularis*). *Journal of Comparative Neurology* 261:362–87.

Iwai, E., Yukie, M., Suyama, H., and Shirakawa, S. 1987. Amygdala connections with middle and inferior temporal gyri of the monkey. *Neuroscience Letters* 83:25–29.

Jones, E. G., and Powell, T. P. S. 1970. An anatomical study of converging sensory pathways within the cerebral cortex. *Brain* 993:793–820.

Kemper, T. L., Caveness, W. F., and Yakovlev, P. I. 1973. The neuronographic and metric study of the dendritic arbours of neurons in the motor cortex of *Macaca mulatta* at birth and at 24-months of age, *Brain* 96:765–82.

Kuypers, H. G. J. M., Szwarcbart, M. K., Mishkin, M., and Rosvold, H. E. 1965. Occipitotemporal corticocortical connections in the rhesus monkey. *Experimental Neurology* 11:245–62.

Lund. J. S., Boothe, R. G., and Lund R. D. 1977. Development of neurons in the visual cortex (area 17) of the monkey (*Macaca nemestrina*): A Golgi study from fetal day 127 to postnatal maturity. *Journal of Comparative Neurology* 176:149–88.

Mahut, H., and Zola-Morgan, S. 1977. Ontogenetic time-table for the development of three functions in infant macaques and the effects of early hippocampal damage upon them. *Society for Neuroscience Abstracts* 3:428.

Malamut, B. L., Saunders, R. C., and Mishkin, M. 1984. Monkeys with combined amygdalo-hippocampal lesions succeed in object discrimination learning despite 24-hour intertrial intervals. *Behavioral Neuroscience* 98:759–69.

Malkova, L., Mishkin, M., and Bachevalier, J. 1995. Long-term effects of selective neonatal temporal lobe lesions on learning and memory in monkeys. *Behavioral Neuroscience* 109:212–26.

McKee, R. D., and Squire, L. R. 1993. On the development of declarative memory. *Journal of Experimental Psychology: Learning, Memory and Cognition* 19:397–404.

Miller, E. K., Li, L., and Desimone, R. 1991. A neural mechanism for working and recognition memory in inferior temporal cortex. *Science* 254:1377–9.

Mishkin, M. 1954. Visual discrimination performance following partial ablations of the temporal lobe: II- Ventral surface vs. hippocampus. *Journal of Comparative and Physiological Psychology* 47:187–93.

Mishkin, M. 1966. Visual mechanisms beyond the striate cortex. In *Frontiers of Physiological Psychology*, ed. R. Russell. New York: Academic Press.

Mishkin, M. 1972. Cortical visual areas and their interactions. In *Brain and Human Behavior*, eds. A. G. Karczmar and J. C. Eccles. Berlin: Springer-Verlag.

Mishkin, M. 1978. Memory in monkeys severely impaired by combined but not by separate removal of amygdala and hippocampus. *Nature (London)* 273:297–98.

Mishkin, M. 1982. A memory system in the monkey. *Philosophical Transactions of the Royal Society of London* B298:85–95.

Mishkin, M., and Appenzeller, T. 1987. The anatomy of memory. *Scientific American* 256:80–89.

Mishkin, M., and Delacour J. 1975. An analysis of short-term visual memory in the monkey. *Journal of Experimental Psychology: Animal Behavior Processes* 1:326–34.

Mishkin, M., Malamut, B. L., and Bachevalier, J. 1984. Memories and Habits: Two neural systems. In *Neurobiology of Learning and Memory*, eds. G. Lynch, L. McGaugh, and N. M. Weinberger. New York: Guilford Press.

Mishkin, M., and Petri, H. L. 1984. Memories and Habits: Some implications for the analysis of learning and retention. In *Neuropsychology of Memory*, eds. N. Butters and L. Squire. New York: Guilford Press.

Mishkin, M., and Phillips, R. R. 1990. A corticolimbic memory path revealed through its disconnection. In *Brain Circuits and Functions of the Mind: Essays in Honor of Roger W. Sperry*, ed. E. Trevarthen. Cambridge: Cambridge University Press.

Mishkin, M., Ungerleider, L. G., and Macko, K. A. 1983. Object vision and spatial vision: Two cortical pathways. *Trends in Neuroscience* October:414–17.

Nadel, L. and Zola-Morgan, S. 1984. Infantile amnesia: A neurobiological perspective. In *Infant Memory*, ed. M. Moscovitch. New York: Plenum.

Nelson, C. A. 1993. Neural correlates of recognition memory in the first postnatal year of life. In *Human Development and the Developing Brain*, eds. G. Dawson and K. Fischer. New York: Guilford Press.

Ostergaard, A. L. 1987. Episodic, semantic and procedural memory in a case of amnesia at an early age. *Neuropsychologia* 25:341–57.

Overman, W. H. 1990. Performance on traditional match-to-sample, non-match-to-sample, and object discrimination task by 12 to 32 month-old children: A developmental progression. In *The Development and Neural Bases of Higher Cognitive Functions*, ed. A. Diamond. New York: Academic Press.

Overman, W. H., Bachevalier, J., Turner, M., and Peuster, A. 1992. Object recognition versus object discrimination: Comparison between human infants and infant monkeys. *Behavioral Neuroscience* 106:15–29.

Overman, W. H., Schuhmann, E. Ryan, P. Epting, K., and Bates, K. 1994. Cognitive gender differences in children parallel biologically based cognitive gender differences found in monkeys. *Society for Neuroscience Abstracts* 24:363.

Pandya, D. N., and Kuypers, H. G. J. M. 1969. Cortico-cortical connection in the rhesus monkey. *Brain Research* 13:13–36.

Petri, H. L., and Mishkin, M. 1994. Behaviorism, cognitivism, and the neuropsychology of memory. *American Scientist* 82:30–37.

Phillips, R. R., Malamut, B. L., Bachevalier, J., and Mishkin, M. 1988. Dissociation of the effects of inferior temporal and limbic lesions on object discrimination learning with 24-hr. intertrial intervals. *Behavioural Brain Research* 27:99–107.

Phoenix, C. H. 1974. Effects of dihydrotestosterone on sexual behavior of castrated male rhesus monkey. *Physiology & Behavior* 12:1045–55.

Rakic, P. 1978. Neuronal migration and contact guidance in primate telencephalon. *Postgraduate Medical Journal* 54:25–40.

Rakic, P., Bourgeois, J-P., Eckenhoff, M. F., Zecevic, N. and Goldman-Rakic, P. S. 1986. Concurrent overproduction of synapses in diverse regions of the primate cerebral cortex. *Science* 232: 232–35.

Resko, J. A. 1970. Androgen secretion by the fetal and neonatal rhesus monkey. *Endocrinology* 87:680–87.

Rodman, H. R. 1994. Development of inferior temporal cortex in monkey. *Cerebral Cortex* 5:484–98.

Rodman, H. R., and Consuelos, M. C. 1994. Cortical projections to anterior inferior temporal cortex in infant macaque monkeys. *Visual Neuroscience* 11:119–33.

Rodman, H. R., Skelly, J. P., and Gross, C. G. 1988. Absence of visual responsiveness in inferior temporal cortex in macaques less than four months of age. *Society for Neuroscience Abstracts* 14:11.

Rose, D. 1980. Some functional correlates of the maturation of neural systems. In *Biological Studies of Mental Processes*, ed. D. Caplan. Cambridge: MIT Press.

Rossitch, E. and Oakes, W. J. 1989. Kluver-Bucy syndrome in a child with bilateral arachnoid cysts: Report of a case. *Neurosurgery* 24:110–12.

Saunders, R. C. 1989. Monkeys demonstrate high level of recognition memory in delayed non-matching to sample with retention intervals of 6 weeks. *Society for Neuroscience Abstracts* 15:342.

Schacter, D. L. and Moscovitch, M. 1984. Infants, amnesics and dissociable memory systems. In *Infant Memory*, ed. M. Moscovitch. New York: Plenum.

Seltzer, B. and Pandya, D. N. 1976. Some cortical projections to the parahippocampal area in the rhesus monkey. *Experimental Neurology* 50:146–60.

Tonsgard, J. H., Harwicke, N., and Levine, S. C. 1987. Kluver-Bucy syndrome in children. Pediatric Neurology 3:162–65.

Turner, B. H., Mishkin, M., and Knapp, M. 1980. Organization of the amygdalopetal projections from modality-specific cortical association areas in the monkey. *Journal of Comparative Neurology* 191:515–43.

Ungerleider, L. G. 1985. The corticocortical pathways for object recognition and spatial perception. In *Pattern Recognition Mechanisms*, eds. C. Chagas, R. Gattass, and C. Gross. Vatican City: Pontifical Academy of Sciences.

Ungerleider, L. G., and Mishkin, M. 1982. Two cortical visual systems. In *Analysis of Visual Behavior*, eds. D. J. Ingle, M. A. Goodale, and R. J. W. Mansfield. Cambridge: MIT Press.

Van Essen, D. C. and Maunsell, J. R. 1983. Hierarchical organization and functional streams in the visual cortex. *Trends in Neuroscience* 6:414–17.

Van Hoesen, G. W., and Pandya, D. N. 1975. Some connections of the entorhinal (area 28) and perirhinal (area 35) cortices of the rhesus monkey: I-Temporal lobe afferents. *Brain Research* 95:1–24.

Varga-Khadem, F., Isaacs, E. B., and Watkins, K. E. 1992. Medial temporal-lobe versus diencephalic amnesia in childhood. *Journal of Clinical and Experimental Neuropsychology* 14:371–2.

Wang, J., Aigner, T., and Mishkin, M. 1990. Effects of neostriatal lesions on visual habit formation in rhesus monkeys. *Society for Neuroscience Abstracts* 16:617.

Webster, M. J., Bachevalier, J., and Ungerleider, L. G. 1994. Connections of inferior temporal areas TEO and TE with parietal and frontal cortex in macaque monkeys. *Cerebral Cortex* 5:470–83.

Webster, M. J., Bachevalier, J., and Ungerleider, L. G. 1994. Development and plasticity of visual memory circuits. In *Maturational Windows and Cortical Plasticity in Human Development: Is There a Reason for an Optimistic View?*, eds. B. Julesz, G. Cowan, and I. Kovacs. Proceedings volume in the Santa Fe Studies in the Sciences of Complexity. Redwood City, CA: Addison-Wesley Publishing Co.

Webster, M. J., Ungerleider, L. G., and Bachevalier, J. 1991a. Connections of inferior temporal areas TE and TEO with medial temporal-lobe structures in infant and adult monkeys. *The Journal of Neuroscience* 11:1095–1116.

Webster, M. J., Ungerleider, L. G., and Bachevalier, J. 1991b. Lesions of inferior temporal area TE in infant monkeys alter cortico-amygdalar projections, *NeuroReport* 2:769–72.

Wood, F. B., Brown, I. S., and Felton R. H. 1989. Long-term follow-up of a childhood amnesic syndrome. *Brain and Cognition* 10:76–86.

Zeaman, D., and House, B. J. 1963. The role of attention in retardate discrimination learning. In *Handbook of Mental Deficiency*, ed. N. R. Ellis. New York: McGraw-Hill.

Zeki, S. M. 1973. Comparison of the cortical degeneration in the visual region of the temporal lobe of the monkey following section of the anterior commissure and the splenium. *Journal of Comparative Neurology* 148:167–76.

Zimmermann, R. R., and Torrey, C. C. 1965. Ontogeny of learning. *Behavior of Nonhuman Primates: Modern Research Trends*, Vol. 2. New York: Academic Press.

Zola-Morgan, S., Squire, L. R., and Mishkin, M. 1982. The neuroanatomy of amnesia: Amygdalohippocampus versus temporal stem. *Science* 218:1337–9.

Part • II

Genetic Mechanisms

Extraordinary progress in the field of genetics has taken place in the past decade. Genetic mapping techniques have played a crucial role in determining the molecular description of a number of human disorders including cystic fibrosis, neurofibromatosis, and Huntington's disease. Although developmental dyslexia runs in families and is heritable, a thorough genetic understanding of this learning disability has been hampered by the heterogeneity of the disorder, the lack of available neurobiological markers, and the environmental effects on the expression of the reading problems.

Identification of genes that predispose individuals to dyslexia would further our understanding of this complex learning problem. An earlier report indicated that an area on chromosome 15 might be linked to developmental dyslexia (Smith et al. 1983), but the focus has now shifted to chromosome 6 (Cardon et al. 1994). In the next two related chapters, Pennington, Gilger, and colleagues review basic genetic concepts applicable to the study of developmental dyslexia and explore the latest data implicating chromosome 6. The distinction between a disorder produced by genes that affect normal variation of the phenotype versus a disorder that is produced by a separate set of genes is discussed. Further, the authors dissect and creatively analyze issues raised by Shaywitz et al. (1992). They explain some of the confusion produced by the aforementioned article by dissociating issues concerning (1) whether developmental dyslexia is a discrete disorder or is the tail end of the normal distribution, and (2) whether it has a distinct etiology or is affected by factors that affect reading skills in the population in general. Most importantly, these chapters provide the context with which to interpret and evaluate future genetic results on developmental learning disabilities.

Cardon, L., Smith, S., Fulker, D., Kimberling, W., Pennington, B., and DeFries, J. 1994. Quantitative trait locus for reading disability on chromosome 6. *Science* 266:276–79.

Shaywitz, S. E., Escobar, M. D., Shaywitz, B. A., Fletcher, J. M., and Makuch, R. 1992. Evidence that dyslexia may represent the lower tail of a normal distribution of reading ability. *New England Journal of Medicine* 326:145–50.

Smith, S. D., Kimberling, W. J., Pennington, B. F., and Lubs, H. A. 1983. Specific reading disability: Identification of an inherited form through linkage analysis. *Science* 219:1345–47.

Chapter • 3

How is Dyslexia Transmitted?

Bruce F. Pennington
Jeffrey W. Gilger

In this paper, we review what is currently known about how developmental dyslexia is transmitted in families. In other words, what do we know about the genetic and environmental mechanisms that underlie the well-established concentration of dyslexia in families? We also review what is known about the transmission of normal reading skill in families, since the comparison of the mechanisms of transmission in normal and abnormal reading skill begins to address what has been a fundamental and contentious issue among both dyslexia researchers and students of abnormal behavior more generally. This issue is whether dyslexia is a discrete disorder with a distinct etiology or whether it is just the tail of the normal distribution of reading ability and is caused by the same factors that cause normal variation in reading skill (Miles and Haslam 1986; Rodgers 1983; Shaywitz et al. 1992; Stevenson 1988; Yule and Rutter 1975).

Notice that there are really two issues here. One is whether dyslexia is distributionally distinct (i.e., is there a "hump" or unexpected excess of cases on the lower tail of the distribution of reading scores?). The other is whether dyslexia is etiologically distinct. Previous work has conflated the two issues, with studies appropriate to the first question used to answer the second. However, since these are separate issues, it is possible to find no "hump" but still to find evidence of a distinct etiology (Pennington and Gilger 1992).

In what follows, we will (1) briefly review the evidence for familiality and heritability of dyslexia; (2) address sex effects on transmission and show why classic, X-linked transmission can be ruled out; (3) review the evidence bearing on major locus transmission; (4) review the familiality, heritability, and transmission of normal reading skill; and (5) consider what model of transmission best fits all the data. We will also consider what implications that model has for whether dyslexia is a discrete disorder with a distinct etiology.

We conclude our review with a discussion of the implications of the transmission results for genetic linkage studies of dyslexia.

Familiality and Heritability

The observation that dyslexia aggregates in families is nearly as old as the description of the disorder itself; this observation has been repeatedly replicated, both in case reports and in formal family studies. Soon after developmental dyslexia was first described at the end of the last century by Kerr (1897) and Morgan (1896), several reports of familial aggregation appeared (Fisher 1905; Hinshelwood 1907, 1911; Thomas 1905), one of which described a kindred with three affected generations (Stephenson 1907). Similar reports, including several with larger numbers of families, continued to appear over subsequent decades. As part of his classic study of the transmission of dyslexia, Hallgren (1950) reviewed these later reports. Several aspects of these later reports are particularly noteworthy: (1) a substantial majority of affected children had affected relatives; (2) the average recurrence rate among first degree relatives, in those studies that report it, is high, about 30%; (3) there is frequently transmission across two or more generations; and (4) several reports note that dyslexia co-occurs with other language disorders.

Three later studies of population samples of children also reported significant familial recurrence of reading problems (Owen et al. 1971; Yule and Rutter 1975; Walker and Cole 1965). These results indicate that familial recurrence in the earlier reports is not just an artifact of clinic ascertainment, that is, a rare phenomenon found only in highly selected cases. Two of these studies (Owen et al. 1971; Walker and Cole 1965) were among the first to use formal tests instead of history to determine the presence of reading and spelling problems in relatives; thus their findings indicate that familiality is not just an artifact of potentially biased or subjective history measures. The Walker and Cole study examined only siblings, not parents, and found a non-random distribution of disabled readers across sibships; that is, affected children were concentrated in a subset of families. The Owen et al. study examined both parents and siblings, yet examined only mean differences between relatives of probands versus relatives of controls on reading and spelling measures. They did not examine rates of affected relatives. Their results demonstrate familiality in that relatives of probands had significantly lower scores than relatives of control children.

Four formal family studies have addressed rates of recurrence and possible mechanisms of transmission. These studies also have (1) adequately large samples, (2) generally appropriate sampling schemes, and (3) systematic study of all ascertained families. Hallgren's study (1950) is the first of four, although some criticisms can be raised with respect to criteria (2) and (3). There have been three subsequent, methodologically adequate family studies. The findings of all four studies are summarized in table 1.

Several results in table 1 are noteworthy. First, sibling recurrence is high and very consistent across studies, ranging from 38.5% to 43%. Parent recurrence is likewise high, ranging from 27% to 49%, and is generally consistent across studies.

Since the definition of dyslexia phenotype differed across these four samples, the similarity in values is all the more striking. These findings are consistent with those of earlier case reports, and indicate strong evidence of familiality of dyslexia. In fact, the median relative increase in risk to a child having an affected parent is about *8 times* the population risk of 5% (Gilger, Pennington, and DeFries 1991, tables 2 and 3). This relative increase in risk is higher than that found in many familial behavior disorders. Second, the recurrence rates for first

Table 1. Studies of familial recurrence in the first degree relatives of dyslexic probands

Study	Families	Ascertainment	Diagnosis	% Affected Sibs (N)	% Affected Parents (N)	Mating Types* 0	1	2
Hallgren (1950)	112	Special school, Clinic	History, Records, Interviews	40.8 (174)	42.4 (224)	.17	.80	.03
Finucci, et al. (1976)	20	Special schools	Tests	42.5 (40)	47.2 (36)	.19	.62	.19
CFRS (Vogler et al. 1985)	133	Public schools	Tests, History	43.0 (168)	49.0 (265)	.27	.48	.24
Iowa (Gilger, et al. 1991)	39	LD Clinic	Tests, History	38.5 (52)	27.0 (77)	.47	.50	.03

* None, one, or both parents affected.

degree relatives approach the value expected (50%) under a simple autosomal dominant model of transmission, although as we will see, other mechanisms of transmission are also consistent with these data. Third, this high recurrence rate, the fact that the parent and sib recurrence rates are essentially equal, and the preponderance of matings with one affected parent (as opposed to none or both), together argue strongly against a simple autosomal recessive model. Under this latter model, sibling recurrence should be around 25% and considerably higher than parent recurrence, and there should be considerably more matings with neither parent affected. Obviously familial transmission may be entirely environmental, but if separate evidence indicates genetic influence, then family data constrains what the mechanism of genetic transmission can be. Having established that dyslexia is robustly familial, we can next ask whether that familiality is due, at least in part, to heritable influences. Although both twin and adoption studies can address this issue, we only have data for dyslexia from twin studies.

Earlier twin studies include those reviewed by Zerbin-Rudin (1967) and that of Bakwin (1973), both of which found significantly greater monozygotic (MZ) than dizygotic (DZ) concordance for the trait of dyslexia, thus indicating heritability (i.e., genetic influence as part of the etiology of extreme low scores in reading, denoted as h^2g). However, these earlier studies had methodological problems. The studies reviewed by Zerbin-Rudin (1967) recruited twins from clinics, thus introducing a possible ascertainment bias. Bakwin's study utilized parent interviews and questionnaires for the diagnosis of dyslexia, rather than test scores. Both studies failed to analyze separately same and opposite sex DZ twins; analyzing them together may depress the DZ concordance rate if the trait in question has a sex difference in prevalence.

Two methodologically adequate twin studies of dyslexia have since appeared, both of which have produced reasonably similar results. One is the Twin Family Reading Study (TFRS) being conducted at the Institute for Behavior Genetics (IBG) in Boulder, Colorado. The other is a twin study conducted in London at the Institute for Psychiatry. The basic results in the TFRS sample (DeFries, Fulker, and LaBuda 1987; DeFries et al. 1991a; Olson et al. 1991) are that deficits in reading and spelling are substantially heritable ($h^2g \pm SE = 0.44 \pm .11$ and $0.62 \pm .14$, respectively), as are deficits in nonword reading ($0.75 \pm .15$), whereas deficits in orthographic coding were not significantly heritable ($0.31 \pm .20$), but were significantly influenced by the common family environment ($c^2g = 0.48 \pm .17$). (The terms h^2g and c^2g refer to the etiology of extreme group deficits and are thus distinct from the more familiar symbols, h^2 and c^2, which refer respectively to the heritability and common environmentality of normal variations. We will compare h^2 and h^2g values for reading and related phenotypes in a later section.)

In the London study, there was likewise significant heritability for deficits in spelling (h^2g = 0.61±.39) and greater heritability for deficits in nonword reading than for deficits in orthographic coding (De Fries et al. 1991a). However, deficits in reading were *not* significantly heritable. The reason for this one disparity in the results of the two studies is not clear; it is important to note that the TFRS includes a much larger sample of dyslexic twins (MZ = 86 pairs, DZ = 73 pairs as compared with 23 and 42, respectively, in the London sample).

In summary, we have strong evidence that dyslexia is both familial and heritable. Thus, it is appropriate to ask next what genetic mechanisms underlie its transmission.

Sex Effects on Transmission

Traditional wisdom has long held that there is a strong male predominance (about 4 to 1) in the rates of dyslexia. Consequently, there has been a longstanding interest in possible sex effects on transmission. However, it is now clear that most of the apparent male predominance was an artifact of clinical ascertainment, and that the sex ratio in population samples is often not substantially different from unity, although across samples the male/female ratio is always greater than one, averaging about 1.5/1.0 (Shaywitz et al. 1990; Wadsworth et al. 1992). Thus, although there may be a sex difference in the rates of dyslexia, it is much smaller than previously supposed.

It is still worth asking if there are sex effects on transmission, since some of these could yield nearly equal sex ratios. Moreover, modern genetics has recently uncovered novel sex effects on transmission in some disorders, and it is therefore important to ask if any of these pertain to dyslexia. Specifically, we will consider four sex effects on transmission: (1) classic X-linked inheritance, such as is seen in color blindness or hemophilia; (2) sex-influenced transmission, such as is seen in male pattern baldness; (3) non-nuclear DNA or mitochondrial inheritance, which appears to occur in some dementing illnesses; and (4) imprinting, which occurs in fragile X syndrome, among others.

In a classic X-linked recessive disorder, there is a large excess of affected males and no transmission from fathers to sons, who receive their only X chromosome from their mother. (In an X-linked dominant disorder, there is likewise no father to son transmission; in contrast, there is commonly an excess of affected *females*.) In sex-influenced transmission, the gene(s) for the disorder are not on the X chromosome (hence, they are *autosomal*,) but their phenotypic expression is still influenced by the sex of the person who carries them. In mitochondrial inheritance, transmission is exclusively from mothers to offspring, since only the eggs, not the sperm, transmit mitochondrial DNA. Finally, in imprinting, phenotypic expression can vary considerably depending on the sex of the transmitting parent, because germ cell DNA is methylated in a sex-specific way that affects genetic expression in the offspring.

To test these four possible sex effects on transmission, we can examine rates (and severity) of transmission for each of the four possible combinations of parent and child sex. Table 2 presents such data on rates of transmission from three studies reviewed by Gilger, Pennington, and DeFries (1991).

We can immediately see there is robust evidence of transmission from fathers to sons, allowing us to reject both recessive and dominant X-linked transmission. We can also reject mitochondrial transmission, since the transmission rates for each parental sex are essentially equal (.344 for fathers and .343 for mothers). This result also argues against an imprinting effect, at least on the rates of dyslexia. Since the average rates in male and female offspring are about equal in this table, there is also little evidence here for sex-influenced transmission. However, the finding mentioned above of a slight excess of affected males does suggest a sex influence on transmission; we will see below that a sex difference in penetrance was found across several samples in a segregation analysis of dyslexia. In summary, we can clearly reject classic, X-linked transmission, mitochondrial transmission, and an imprinting effect on either rates or severity of dyslexia. Sex-influenced transmission remains a possibility. There is also some indication in twin data that the degree of heritability (h^2g) may vary with the sex of the dyslexic offspring with females possibly exhibiting higher heritability (Bakwin 1973; De Fries, Gillis, and Wadsworth 1993).

Table 2. Transmission probabilities in dyslexic families as a function of sex of affected parent and child's sex*

	Fa Affected	Mo Affected	
Iowa Study			
Male Child	0.315	0.174	
Female Child	0.182	0.424	
Linkage Study			
Male Child	0.411	0.540	
Female Child	0.522	0.367	
Colorado Study			
Male Child	0.283	0.208	
Female Child	0.350	0.345	
Unweighted Averages			
Male	.336	.307	.322
Female	.351	.378	.364
	.344	.343	

* Sex ratio assumed to be 1:1 and population prevalence to be 0.05.

Before closing this section, it is important to mention briefly another possible sex effect that has been examined in dyslexia. Tallal, Ross, and Curtis (1989) reported the surprising finding of a disproportionate number of male offspring born to mothers who had a developmental language disorder (DLD). Since there is some degree of overlap between DLD and dyslexia, it made sense to examine whether this phenomenon occurred in dyslexic families as well. Wadsworth et al. (1992) reported on five independent samples of dyslexic families and did not find an excess number of male offspring born to dyslexic mothers. Combining across samples, the sex ratios in sibships (including probands) were 1.10, 1.15, 1.28, and 1.59 across the four parental affection types (neither affected, mother only, father only, and both, respectively). Excluding probands, the four ratios were 0.89, 1.19, 1.11, and 1.46. Therefore, maternal dyslexia does not appear to exert an effect on the sex ratio of offspring, unlike the results reported for DLD.

Major Locus Versus Polygenic Transmission

As discussed above, the available family data argue strongly against X-linked or simple autosomal recessive transmission, but are consistent with an additive or dominant major locus effect because of the high and similar recurrence rates in parents and siblings. There are several more searching tests of the mode of transmission, the most important of which is complex segregation analysis. Before reviewing segregation studies of dyslexia, it is instructive to review the results from less powerful, but more intuitively accessible methods. If transmission is polygenic, one would expect the rates of affection in relatives to drop off systematically with decreasing degrees of genetic relation to the proband. In contrast, if transmission is due to one or a few major loci, then rates of affection should be fairly constant across decreasing degrees of genetic relation, but only on the affected side of the family (or on both sides, if both parents are affected). Thus comparing affection rates across generations or collateral branches in a pedigree is one intuitively straightforward test of major locus transmission.

A second test concerns the distribution of continuous scores in the relatives of a proband. If transmission is polygenic (or multifactorial), then this distribution should be unimodal, because relatives should have continuously varying mixtures of the many polygenes (or multifactors) that additively affect the continuous phenotype. In contrast, if the phenotype is largely due to one or few segregating loci, then some relatives will have the critical allele or alleles and others will not, producing discontinuity (i.e., multimodality) in the distribution of relatives' scores. Because there are more sensitive tests of major locus effects, the results of this test are asymmetrical in their implications: a positive result supports a major locus effect, but a null result does not exclude it.

What are the results of these two tests in family studies of dyslexia? With regard to the first, we lack sufficient data. Of the four family studies listed in table 1, only the Iowa has systematic data on non-primary relatives of probands, and that has not yet been analyzed with regard to this question. However, as Hallgren (1950) discovered, many dyslexic families have three or more generations of affecteds; 29 of his 112 (26%) families had three generation of affecteds. Of course under a polygenic model, three generations of affecteds will occur in some proportion of cases. On the other hand, since it can be difficult to diagnose grand-parents, the true proportion of families with three generations of affecteds may actually be higher.

With regard to the second test, we have clearer results. We per-formed a commingling analysis using SKUMIX (MacLean et al. 1976) on a weighted composite of Peabody Individual Achievement Test (PIAT) scores (Reading Recognition, Reading Comprehension, and Spelling) obtained by the siblings and parents of dyslexic probands in the 133 families in the CFRS sample. To control for possible age and sex effects on these scores, they were age adjusted and standardized within sex relative to the mean and SD of control family scores. The SKUMIX analyses revealed that the best fitting model was one with *two* com-mingled distributions with residual skewness (skew = $-.645\pm.12$); the estimated z-score means and proportion of cases for each of the two dis-tributions were -0.51 (68%) and 0.84 (32%). These results are consistent with the expected effects of a segregating major locus and inconsistent with multifactorial transmission.

We turn now to the results of formal segregation analyses of dyslexia. There have been three of these: Hallgren's (1950), that of Lewitter, DeFries, and Elston (1980), and our recent study (Pennington et al. 1991), which included a re-analysis of the CFRS data studied by Lewitter et al. Hallgren used the method of segregation analysis available at that time, specifically the Weinberg proband method, to test an auto-somal dominant model of transmission in the 90 (of 112) families that had one affected parent. Essentially this method compares the observed Mendelian ratio (based on the recurrence rate in siblings) to that expected under a given model of transmission. Since this value (45.7% ± 4.3%) was within two standard errors of the expected value for dominant transmission, he concluded that this model of transmission fit the data from these 90 families. However, a high recurrence rate in siblings and parents does not by itself compel such a conclusion, because other mechanisms could produce a high recurrence rate. Other weaknesses of his study were that he did not use formal tests to diagnose parents and siblings and he tended to discount non-genetic contributors to read-ing problems in diagnosing individuals with other affected relatives.

The study of Lewitter, DeFries, and Elston (1980) included 133 nuclear families, all members of which were tested. Rather than a discrete phenotype definition, a continuous phenotype measure based on a discriminant analysis was employed. A shortcoming of this study was that adults with a positive history of dyslexia but normal test scores (compensated adults) were not counted as affected.

In the population as a whole, no support was found for a single major locus (autosomal dominant, autosomal recessive, or co-dominant transmission), but the null hypothesis of no vertical transmission was likewise rejected. These investigators also tested different models of transmission in subpopulations, including families with probands of a given sex, families with severely affected probands, and children considered alone because of possible unreliability of the measures in adults. Autosomal recessive inheritance could not be rejected in families with female probands and co-dominant inheritance was supported when children were considered alone. The authors concluded that their results most likely indicated genetic heterogeneity. This conclusion is similar to that reached by Finucci et al. (1976) in a well-conducted study of 20 extended families, all members of which were tested. Unfortunately, this sample was too small to permit a formal, complex segregation analysis.

Our recent study used a more powerful method of complex segregation analysis, the program POINTER (Lalouel et al. 1984), which allows a test of the "mixed" model. (In the mixed model, there is both a major locus effect *and* a multifactorial background.) We also allowed for parental compensation in the phenotype definition of dyslexia. We studied four samples of families, the CFRS and Iowa samples discussed earlier, a Linkage sample of 23 extended families (N = 342) selected to be consistent with autosomal dominant transmission, and a small sample of 9 extended families (N = 131), whose probands had been identified as learning disabled through their schools' special education programs in Washington state. The point of including the Linkage sample was to see to what extent the results from the three samples not selected for a mode of transmission would match those for a sample selected to exhibit dominant transmission. In other words, because the data in table 1 suggest that apparent dominant transmission may be very common in the families of dyslexic probands, we wanted to test this possibility more formally by comparing the segregation results across these samples.

These results are displayed in tables 3 and 4. As can be seen, two of the three samples had similar results to those of the Linkage sample. In both the CFRS and Washington samples, as in the Linkage sample, sex-influenced autosomal dominant or additive transmission best fit the data and both polygenic and recessive transmission could be rejected. The estimated gene frequency of the hypothesized major locus was between 3 and 5% across samples. Penetrance was estimated to be complete in males, but incomplete in females (ranging from 55-89%

Table 3. Summary of conclusions drawn from segregation analyses of dyslexic families*

| | Samples | | | |
| | Colorado Family | | | |
Null Hypothesis	Reading Study	Washington	Linkage	Iowa
No transmission	Rejected	Rejected	Rejected	Rejected
No major gene	Rejected	Rejected	Rejected	Consistent
No multifactorial/ polygenic effect	Consistent	Consistent	Consistent	Rejected
No dominant gene effect	Rejected	Rejected	Rejected	Not applicable
No recessive gene effect	Consistent	Consistent	Consistent	Not applicable
No additive gene effect	Rejected	Rejected	Rejected	Not applicable

* These results are based on a population prevalence of 7.5%, a male-to-female ratio of 1.8:1, and appropriate ascertainment corrections.

Table 4. Dominant and additive model parameter estimates

| | Parameters* | | Gene |
Study	Dominance	Threshold	Frequency
Colorado Reading Study			
Dominant	[1.00]	3.20	.049
Additive	[0.50] (0.99)	6.10	.049
Washington			
Dominant	[1.00]	3.52	.030
Additive	(0.50) (0.67)	6.80	.035
Linkage			
Dominant	[1.00]	3.43	.039
Additive	[0.50] (0.58)	6.20	.043

* Threshold is the distance in SD units between the means of the two homozygote (AA and aa) distributions, $t = U_{aa} - U_{AA}$. Dominance is the position of the mean of the heterozygote (Aa) distribution relative to both homozygote means, $d = U_{Aa} - U_{AA}/U_{aa} - U_{AA}$. In the pure recessive case, $U_{Aa} = U_{AA}$, and dominance thus equals zero. In the pure dominant case, $U_{Aa} = U_{aa}$, and dominance thus equals one. Gene frequency is the estimated population frequency of the abnormal allele, a. Results are based on a population prevalence of 7.5%, a male-to-female ratio of 1.8:1, and appropriate ascertainment corrections. Values in brackets are set according to additive/dominant Mendelian expectations. Values of dominance in parentheses are derived from general Mendelian models, where dominance is allowed to vary.

across samples and models, with a median of about 65%). When penetrance was forced to be equal by sex, the fit of the model worsened significantly, further supporting the hypothesis of sex influenced transmission. A sex difference in penetrance of this magnitude would produce the slight excess of males observed among affected relatives of probands and in population samples, yielding the sex ratio of about 1.5/1.0 mentioned above. Both Hallgren (1950) and Sladen (1970) hypothesized sex-influenced, transmission of dyslexia; our results provide empirical support for this hypothesis.

In contrast to the results for the other three samples, those for the Iowa sample were not consistent with major locus transmission, and instead best fit a polygenic or multifactorial model. This result may be due to the use of group rather than individual tests in that study, as well as to a broader phenotype definition, which may have been affected by cognitive and academic problems besides dyslexia.

In summary, our recent report is the most comprehensive study of the transmission of dyslexia to date. It provides strong evidence for sex-influenced, major locus transmission in a large proportion of dyslexic families, a hypothesis that is consistent with the data reviewed in the previous sections.

The Transmission of Normal Reading Skill

Another more searching test of the single major locus hypothesis of the transmission of dyslexia tests an implicit corollary of this hypothesis: that the etiology of dyslexia is not only discrete but also distinct from the etiology of normal variations in reading skill. Therefore, it is useful to examine what is known about the genetics of normal reading skill; is it likewise familial and heritable? If so, what is the mode of transmission and does it differ from that found for dyslexia?

Reading skill, like most cognitive traits, exhibits substantial kinship correlations. For instance, primary relatives (who share half their genes in common) have a correlation for reading skill of about .40 (in the CFRS sample). Thus, reading skill, like dyslexia is familial.

That some of this familiality is due to genes is demonstrated by the results of twin studies of normal reading skill. Harris (1986) reviewed such studies and found a high degree of similarity in results across six studies. The median MZ intraclass correlation was 0.89 and the median DZ intraclass correlation was 0.61. Using Falconer's method of doubling the MZ-DZ difference, we obtain an estimate of broad heritability (h^2) of .56, suggesting that about half the variance in normal reading skill is due to genetic influences. More recently, the heritability of reading and reading-related measures was examined in both the dyslexic and control twin samples in the previously discussed TFRS (Olson et al. 1991). These investigators found h^2 values of .35 and .59 for PIAT Reading

Recognition and values of .52 and .41 for a nonword reading task, in the control and dyslexic samples, respectively. Because these values were fairly similar across the two samples, these authors suggest that the genetic influences on individual differences in reading may be similar both within the normal range and in the low tail of the distribution.

This twin study has also been used to address the question of whether there is a significant difference between h^2g, the heritability of a group deficit in reading, and h^2, the heritability of normal variation in reading (DeFries et al. 1991b). Finding such a difference would be consistent with the hypothesis that the etiology differs in the two cases. In this analysis, the two values ($h^2g = 0.47$ and $h^2 = 0.73$) were not significantly different, though clearly not identical. If similar and significantly different values were obtained in a larger sample, it would at least indicate that *environmental* factors were more important in the etiology of extreme scores. However, it would not necessarily indicate that different genetic influences were operating in the two cases, although such a result would be consistent with this hypothesis.

In summary, available data indicate significant familiality and heritability for normal variations in reading skill, just as we found for dyslexia. The data do not clearly tell us whether the same or different genetic influences are operating in the two cases. One way to approach that question is through a complex segregation analysis of the transmission of reading skill in non-dyslexic families.

We have completed such an analysis of the control families in the CFRS sample (Gilger et al. 1994). The phenotype was the weighted PIAT composite score mentioned above, which was adjusted for sex and age and standardized. Because SKUMIX found a single distribution with significant skewness, the data were also adjusted for skewness before POINTER was run, making this a conservative test for a major locus effect.

Much to our surprise, we found that the best fitting model was autosomal dominant transmission for the continuous reading composite scores in *control* families. Table 5 presents the results of the segregation analysis and figure 1 graphically depicts the major locus effect on the distribution of reading composite scores. Notice that the dominant allele acts to push scores up toward the threshold for dyslexia. (In this figure, higher scores indicate *worse* reading skill).

Several additional tests were run to test the validity of these results. Specifically, we ran further tests of Mendelian transmission: the general transmission model (GTM) and the no transmission model (NTM). The GTM allows the three transmission probabilities, or taus, to be estimated rather than fixed at their expected Mendelian values (of 1.0, 0.50, and 0.0 for the aa, Aa, and AA genotypes, respectively). If the GTM fits the data significantly better than the major locus model, then Mendelian transmission is not supported, because the best estimates of

Table 5. Summary of conclusions drawn from segregation analysis of reading skill in normal families.

Null Hypothesis	X^2 (df)	p	Interpretation
No transmission	24.78(4)	<.001	Rejected
No major gene	7.13(2-3)	.028-.068	Rejected*
No multifactoral/			
polygenic effect	0.32(1)	NS	Consistent
No dominant gene effect:			
a) d = 0	5.56(1)	<.05	Rejected
b) d = 0.5	4.20(1)	<.05	Rejected
No Mendelian transmission			
GTM vs. Mixed	7.43(3)	>.05	Ambiguous
GTM vs. NTM	2.77(2)	>.05	
No Mendelian transmission			
(H = 0.0)			Rejected
GTM vs. Major Locus	5.96(3)	>.05	
GTM vs. NTM	17.58(1)	<.001	

*This result approached significance with df = 3, and was significant with df = 2. The true df is probably less than 3.

the transmission probabilities deviate from Mendelian expectations. The NTM constrains the three taus to be equal, a distinctly non-Mendelian situation; thus the GTM (and the major locus model) should fit the data better than the NTM if transmission is indeed Mendelian. The results of both of these further tests were consistent with Mendelian expectations, but only when H, the heritability of the multifactorial background, was constrained to be zero (consistent with the fact that

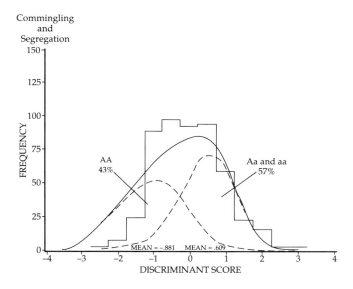

Figure 1. Discriminant Reading Scores

we were unable to reject the null hypothesis of no multifactorial/polygenic effect—see table 5). However, when H was free to vary, the results were ambiguous. The GTM model was not significantly better than the mixed model (which is consistent with Mendelian transmission), but the GTM was not significantly better than the NTM (which, of course, is inconsistent with Mendelian transmission).

We also tested whether the assumption of similar correlations between siblings and between parents and offspring was valid. The ratio of these correlations is represented by the parameter Z; allowing Z to vary tests the validity of the assumption of similar correlations. Allowing Z to vary did not significantly improve the fit of any relevant model.

In summary, these results argue against simple multifactorial/polygenic transmission for normal individual differences in reading skill and argue for a major locus effect that meets most, but not all, Mendelian expectations. The estimated gene frequency of this hypothesized major locus for poor reading is .35; thus about 57% of the population would have at least one copy of the allele for poor reading. The model estimates that about 54% of the phenotypic variance in normal reading is accounted for by this major locus; thus, about half of the variance is unexplained. The companion, normal allele is recessive and positive with respect to reading skill. Also, this hypothesized allele does not make someone dyslexic; it depresses reading scores by a small amount. Most of these control subjects hypothesized to have this allele had scores that were not close to threshold for dyslexia. Also, there could be other undetected loci whose effect is to *increase* reading skill; there are undoubtedly environmental factors that have this effect.

Moreover, it would be a mistake to take either the *single* part of the single major locus result, or its effect size, too literally. POINTER cannot resolve genetic heterogeneity; it only has access to phenotypic distributions. If there are a few major loci, each exerting a similar, sizeable effect but in different families, then POINTER will, of course, call this the effect of a single major locus. Indeed, if there are even a few genes of sizeable effect being transmitted in the *same* families, with their joint effect being in the range of what we have detected here, then POINTER could possibly still clump their effects together and call this a single major locus effect. Experts in segregation analysis are just beginning to explore how segregation analysis programs like POINTER interpret such a situation; since a few genes of sizeable effect is not one of the explicit hypotheses that these programs test, programs like POINTER will have to find that some other model provides the best fit. Finally, the effect size (54% of the phenotypic variance) seems too large for what is usually found for a single QTL.

Therefore, the important conclusion from this study is that there appear to be genes of major effect that affect the transmission of *normal* reading skill. In the next section, we will consider the possible relations of these genes to those involved in the transmission of dyslexia.

Summary of Transmission Results

Given all these results, what can we say with confidence about the transmission of dyslexia? How much scientific progress has there been since 1950, when Hallgren's classic study was published?

Table 6 lists the conclusions from previous sections. Unlike the situation in Hallgren's time, we now have very strong, converging evidence that dyslexia is both familial and heritable. We can also reject the hypotheses of classic, X-linked or simple recessive transmission, at least in the vast majority of cases. We also have evidence that dyslexia is genetically heterogeneous (Smith et al. 1990). Perhaps most importantly, we have evidence that supports Hallgren's observation that what looks like autosomal dominant transmission occurs in many dyslexic families. There do appear to be the effects of major loci, acting in a dominant or additive fashion, on the transmission of reading problems.

However, we can place several important constraints on Hallgren's hypothesis of a monohybrid, autosomal dominant gene for dyslexia. First, it is unlikely to be *one* gene, because of the evidence of genetic heterogeneity. Second, it may not be a gene for dyslexia per se, since the familiality, heritability, and transmission results for *normal* variations in reading skill are not clearly different from those for dyslexia. If valid, the finding of a major locus effect on the transmission of normal reading skill, which acts to depress reading scores, suggests that the same loci may be involved in the transmission of both normal reading skill and dyslexia. If this is true, then dyslexics would have more of

Table 6. Status of Hypotheses Regarding the Transmission of Dyslexia

Hypothesis	Status
No transmission	Rejected
Completely environmental	Rejected
X-linked	Rejected
Depends on sex of parent	Rejected
Depends on sex of child	Supported
Multifactoral background	Equivocal
Major locus effect	Supported
Recessive	Rejected
Additive	Supported
Dominant	Supported
Same as transmission of normal reading	Supported
Genetically heterogeneous	Supported

the unfavorable alleles at these loci and/or additional environmental risk factors, so that their reading scores are pushed beyond the cutoff for dyslexia. In this case, the locus (or loci) is not a necessary "disease" locus, but is better conceptualized as a susceptibility locus.

Therefore, instead of a classic, autosomal dominant disease gene, which is rare in the population and which is by itself necessary and sufficient to produce the disorder of dyslexia, we may be dealing with several, more frequent quantitative trait loci (QTLs), which are involved in the transmission of both dyslexia and normal variations in reading skill. No one QTL is likely to be necessary to produce dyslexia. Whether one QTL has an effect size *sufficient* to produce dyslexia is an open, empirical question that only linkage methods can answer.

Figure 2 graphically depicts the relation between QTLs and the two, traditional extreme possibilities for genetic transmission, a single major locus and polygenic transmission. It is important to point out that these extremes are not dichotomous, but form the endpoints of a continuum. This continuum has been recognized by workers in behavior genetics for a long time. Fisher's (1918) classic paper addressed an early controversy between proponents of these extreme positions, by demonstrating mathematically that the inheritance of continuous traits was consistent with Mendelian principles. More recently, but still two decades ago, empirical work in behavior genetics found major gene effects on quantitative, behavioral traits (e.g., open field behavior in mice, DeFries and Hegmann 1970), with these major gene effects accounting for a portion of genetic variance, the rest being due to other, genetic loci. A recent study of QTLs for alcohol-related behaviors in mice identified 7-8 QTLs for each of three such behaviors, which jointly accounted for about 50% of the phenotypic variance in each behavior, (McClearn et al. 1991). Therefore, it may well be the case that QTLs best describe the genetic influences of many continuous, behavioral traits.

The concept of QTLs and the results reviewed in this chapter bring us back to our opening question concerning whether dyslexia is a discrete disorder with a distinct etiology. Figure 3 presents some of the possible answers in a 2x2 table. Most researchers have focused on the two possibilities in the right column; either there is a disease locus for dyslexia, or both dyslexia and normal variation in reading are

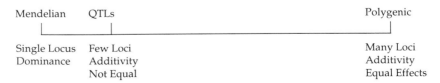

Figure 2.   Quantitative Trait Loci

Major Locus for Normal?

		Yes	No
Major Locus for abnormal?	Yes	QTLs	"Disease" Locus
	No	RD environmental polygenic	RD not discrete

Figure 3.   Multifactorial vs. Major Locus Transmission of Normal and Abnormal Reading

multifactorial, with no major locus effects on either. Hence, the answer that best fits the results presented here is an unexpected one, namely that there are major locus effects on *both* normal variation and dyslexia. If these major loci are the same, then we would say that the etiology of dyslexia is not distinct from that of normal variation, but contrary to what might be expected, both are due to a small number of discrete factors (Gilger et al. 1994). Dyslexics would only be distinct from normal readers in their distribution of alleles and environmental risk factors, not in possessing a single "disease" allele or a single pathogenetic, environmental risk factor, either of which would be sufficient to cause dyslexia.

In terms of whether dyslexia is distributionally distinct, we have argued that this is a less important issue, since the shape of the phenotypic distribution does not necessarily dictate the underlying etiological mechanisms. We presented distributional analyses using SKUMIX of reading composite scores in both dyslexic and non-dyslexic families. There was bimodality in the first case, but not in the second, yet segregation analyses of both data sets found evidence for a major locus effect. Therefore, it is perhaps not surprising that the empirical results are mixed regarding a possible "hump" on the lower tail of the distribution of reading scores. Most importantly, the presence or absence of a hump does not entail strong conclusions about the nature of underlying etiological mechanisms.

Implications for Linkage Studies of Dyslexia

Given the strong possibility that the major loci contributing to dyslexia are quantitative trait loci, and given the evidence for genetic heterogeneity, traditional linkage analysis (of large extended dyslexic families) is not the most appropriate method to identify these loci. Instead, a type of sibling pair linkage analysis is more appropriate. By selecting sibling pairs in which at least one sibling has an extreme score, one can perform linkage analyses that screen for genetic loci influencing extreme scores on a continuous measure (Fulker et al. 1991). We have used this and another sibling pair linkage method (Smith, Kimberling, and Pennington 1991) to begin to identify possible loci affecting dyslexia in the sibling pairs from the families in the Linkage sample. We are now testing whether those results, which were significant for markers on chromosomes 15 and 6, replicate in an independent and differently ascertained sib pair sample, namely dizygotic twin pairs with at least one affected member from the Twin Family Reading Study sample.

We have just completed a replication test for the chromosome 6 results using new, polymerase chain reaction markers in both the Kindred and Twin Family Reading Study samples of sib pairs, analyzing the data with a new interval mapping technique (Cardon and Fulker 1994). Each sample gave significant evidence of a quantitative trait locus located in a two centimorgan (2cM) region of the interval between the D65105 and TNFB markers, which are situated in 6p21.3. The significance of the combined results strongly supported the existence of a quantitative trait locus for dyslexia within the HLA complex (Cardon et al. 1994). This exciting finding will eventually allow us to address how much variance in reading scores this locus accounts for, and how frequently unaffected sibs have unfavorable alleles for this locus. If a similar, sib pair linkage study were conducted using probands selected for extremely *high* reading scores, we could see whether the same quantitative trait loci are affecting reading scores across the whole distribution. If they are, then our speculation that the same genes are influencing normal and extreme individual differences in reading would be supported. If not, then we would have direct evidence that dyslexia is etiologically distinct. Once we have a better understanding of these genetic mechanisms, we can also conduct much more revealing studies of environmental factors, both risk factors and protective ones, which are also undoubtedly operative in the transmission of both abnormal and normal reading skill. Most importantly, once this gene is clearly identified, we can begin to trace the dynamic, developmental pathway that runs from gene to brain to behavior.

ACKNOWLEDGEMENTS

Dr. Pennington was supported by a NIMH RSA (MH00419), MERIT award (MH38820), and grants from the March of Dimes (12-135) and The Orton Dyslexia Society. Dr. Gilger was supported in part by an NIMH training grant (MH 15442).The twin research reported in this paper was supported in part by NICHD Grants HD 11681 and HD 27802.

REFERENCES

Bakwin, H. 1973. Reading disability in twins. Developmental Medicine and Child Neurology 15:184–87.

Cardon, L. R., DeFries, J. C., Fulker, D. W., Kimberling, W. J., Pennington, B. F., and Smith, S. D. 1994. Quantitative trait locus for reading disability on chromosome 6. *Science* 266:276–79.

Cardon, L. R., and Fulker, D. W. 1994. A sibling pair approach to internal mapping of quantitative trait loci. *American Journal of Human Genetics* 55:825–31.

DeFries, J. C., Fulker, D. W., and LaBuda, M. C. 1987. Reading disability in twins: Evidence for a genetic etiology. *Nature* 329:537–39.

DeFries, J. C., Gillis, J., and Wadsworth, S. J. in press. Genes and genders: A twin study of reading disability. In *The Extrordinary Brain: Neurobiologic Issues in Developmental Dyslexia*, ed. A. M. Galaburda. Cambridge, MA: Harvard University Press.

DeFries, J. C., and Hegmann, J. P. 1970. Genetic analysis of open-field behavior. In *Contributions to Behavior-genetic Analysis—The Mouse as a Prototype*, eds. G. Lindzey and D. D. Thiessen. New York: Meridith Corporation.

DeFries, J. C., Olson, R. K., Pennington, B. F., and Smith, S. D. 1991. Colorado reading project: Past, present, and future. *Learning Disabilities: A Multidisciplinary Journal* 2(2):37–46.

DeFries, J. C., Stevenson, J., Gillis, J., and Wadsworth, S. J. 1991. Genetic etiology of spelling deficits in the Colorado and London twin studies of reading disability. *Reading and Writing* 3:271–83.

Finucci, J. M., Gutherie, J. T., Childs, A. L. Abbey, H. and Childs, B. 1976. The genetics of specific reading disability. *Annual Review of Human Genetics* 40:1–23.

Fisher, J. H. 1905. Case of congenital word-blindness (inability to learn to read). *Ophthalmological Review* 24:315.

Fisher, R. A. 1918. The correlation between relatives on the supposition of Mendelian inheritance. *Transactions of the Royal Society of Edinbourgh* 52:399–433.

Fulker, D. W., Cardon, L. R., DeFries, L. R., Kimberling, W. J., Pennington, B. F., and Smith, S. D. 1991. Multiple regression analysis of sib-pair data on reading to detect quantitative trait loci. *Reading and Writing* 3:235–313.

Gilger, J. W., Borecki, I., DeFries, J. C., and Pennington, B. F. 1994. Commingling and segregation analysis of reading performance in families of normal reading probands. *Behavior Genetics* 24:345–55.

Gilger, J. W., Pennington, B. F., and DeFries, J. C. 1991. Risk for reading disabilities as a function of parental history of learning problems: Data from three samples of families demonstrating genetic transmission. *Reading and Writing* 3: 205–17.

Hallgren, B. 1950. Specific dyslexia (congenital word-blindness): A clinical and genetic study. *Acta Psychiatrica et Neurologica Supplement* 65:1–287.

Harris, E. L. 1986. The contribution of twin research to the study of the etiology of reading disability. In *Genetics and Learning Disabilities*, ed. S. D. Smith. San Diego, CA: College-Hill Press.

Hinshelwood, J. 1907. Four cases of congenital word-blindness occurring in the same family. *British Medical Journal* 2:1229–32.

Hinshelwood, J. 1911. Two cases of hereditary word-blindness. *British Medical Journal* 1:608–9.

Kerr, J. 1897. School hygiene, in its mental, moral, and physical aspects. Howard Medical Prize Essay. *Journal of the Royal Statistical Society* 60:613–80.

Lalouel, J. M., Rao, D. C., Morton, N. E., and Elston, R. C. 1983. A unified model for complex segregation analysis. *American Journal of Human Genetics* 35:816–26.

Lewitter, F. I., DeFries, J. C., and Elston, R. C. 1980. Genetic models of reading disability. *Behavior Genetics* 10:9–30.

MacLean, C. J., Morton, N. E., Elston, R. C., and Yee, S. 1976. Skewness in commingled distributions. *Biometrics* 32:694–99.

McClearn, G. E., Plomin, R., Gora-Maslak, G., and Crabbe, J. C. 1991. The gene chase in behavioral science. *Psychological Science* 2:222–29.

Miles, T. R., and Haslam, M. N. 1986. Dyslexia: Anomaly or normal variation? *Annals of Dyslexia* 36:103–17.

Morgan, W. 1896. A case of congenital word-blindness. *British Medical Journal* 2:1378.

Olson, R. K., Gillis, J. J., Rack, J. P., DeFries, J. C., and Fulker, D. W. 1991. Confirmatory factor analysis of word recognition and process measures in the Colorado reading project. *Reading and Writing* 3:235–48.

Owen, F., Adams, P., Forrest, T., Stolz, L., and Fisher, S. 1971. Learning disorders in children: Sibling studies. *Monographs of the Society for Research in Child Development* 36:No. 4.

Pennington, B. F., Gilger, J., Pauls, D., Smith, S. A., Smith, S. D., and DeFries, J. C. 1991. Evidence for major gene transmission of developmental dyslexia. *Journal of the American Medical Association* 266(11):1527–34.

Pennington, B. F., and Gilger, J. W. 1992. In response to Shaywitz et al. article (326:145–50) [Letter to the editor]. *New England Journal of Medicine*.

Rodgers, B. 1983. The identification and prevalence of specific reading retardation. *British Journal of Educational Psychology* 53:369–73.

Shaywitz, S. E., Escobar, M. D., Shaywitz, B. A., Fletcher, J. M., and Makuch, R. 1992. Evidence that dyslexia may represent the lower tail of a normal distribution of reading ability. *New England Journal of Medicine* 326:145–50.

Shaywitz, S. E., Shaywitz, B. A., Fletcher, J. M., and Escobar, M. D. 1990. Prevalence of reading disability in boys and girls. *Journal of the American Medical Association* 264:998–1002.

Sladen, B. K. 1970. Inheritance of dyslexia. *Bulletin of The Orton Society* 20:30–40.

Smith, S. D., Kimberling, W. J., and Pennington, B. F. 1991. Screening for multiple genes influencing dyslexia. *Reading and Writing* 3:285–98.

Smith, S. D., Pennington, B. F., Kimberling, W. J., and Ing, P. 1990. Familial dyslexia: Use of genetic linkage data to define subtypes. *Journal of the American Academy of Child and Adolescent Psychiatry* 29:204–13.

Stephenson, S. 1907. Six cases of congenital word-blindness affecting three generations of one family. *Ophthalmoscope* 5:482–84.

Stevenson, J., Graham, P., Fredman, G., and McLoughlin, V. 1986. A twin study of genetic influences on reading and spelling ability and disability. *Journal of Child Psychology and Psychiatry* 28:231–47.

Stevenson, J. 1988. Which aspects of reading ability show a "hump" in their distribution? *Applied Cognitive Psychology* 2:77–85.

Tallal, P., Ross, R., and Curtiss, S. 1989. Familial aggregation in specific language impairment. *Journal of Speech and Hearing Disorders* 54:167–73.

Thomas, C. J. 1905. Congenital "word-blindness" and its treatment. *Ophthalmoscope* 3:380–85.

Wadsworth, S. J., DeFries, J. C., Stevenson, J., Gilger, J. W., and Pennington, B. F. 1992. Gender ratios among reading-disabled children and their siblings as a function of parental impairment. *Journal of Child Psychology and Psychiatry* 33:1229–1239.

Walker, L., and Cole, E. 1965. Familial patterns of expression of specific reading disability in a population sample. *Bulletin of The Orton Society* 15:12–24.

Yule, W., and Rutter, M. 1975. The concept of specific reading retardation. *Journal of Child Psychology and Psychiatry* 16:181–97.

Zerbin-Rudin, E. 1967. Congenital word-blindness. *Bulletin of The Orton Society* 17:47–54.

Chapter • **4**

The Etiology of Extreme Scores for Complex Phenotypes: An Illustration Using Reading Performance

Jeffrey W. Gilger
Ingrid B. Borecki
Shelley D. Smith
John C. DeFries
Bruce F. Pennington

Many psychometrically assessed traits yield a continuous distribution from low to high. This continuum is often unimodal and fairly normal, with the fewest percentage of individuals scoring at the extreme ends. Examples of such traits include intelligence, quantitatively measured personality constructs such as depression and extroversion, and specific cognitive or academic abilities such as reading and expressive vocabulary (Matarazzo and Pankeratz 1980; Eaves, Eysenck and Martin 1989; Minton and Schneider 1985). Depending on the scale, the higher or lower a person's score is on these tests, the more likely he or she is to have clinically significant problems. Indeed, an important part of the operational definition of many clinical disorders is falling beyond an extreme threshold on the trait distribution.

Traditional psychiatry once considered the genetic contribution to a severe disorder to be greater than that of milder forms. However, there are data to suggest that psychiatrically disordered subjects may simply represent the extreme values on a normal continuum, where all points on the scale are influenced by the same multifactorial etiologic agents (Eysenck 1952; Eaves, Eysenck, and Martin 1989; Kendler and

Send reprint requests to JWG at the University of Kansas, Department of Speech-Language-Hearing: Sciences and Disorders, 3031 Dole Human Development Center, Lawrence, KS, 66045 (email = gilger@falcon.cc.ukans.edu).

Eaves 1986). In fact, for complex human cognitive and personality traits, the assumption of most behavioral geneticists has been that such traits are under multifactorial-polygenic (MFP) control (Plomin and Rende 1991; Plomin, DeFries, and McClearn 1990; McClearn et al. 1991; Eaves, Eysenck, and Martin 1989; Fulker and Eysenck 1979). Such a quantitative genetic model assumes that many genes, with small effects, act together along with a variety of environmental factors to produce the range of phenotypes observed. Evidence for such a theoretical position comes from a variety of nonhuman and human research, where the data are consistent with the assumptions of an MFP model (Eaves, Eysenck, and Martin 1989; Plomin, DeFries, and McClearn 1990; McClearn et al. 1991).

The controversy is whether or not the etiology of, say, the extreme lower tail of a trait continuum is distinct from the so called "normal" variation in the rest of the distribution. For example, there is evidence that the etiology of general intelligence in the population differs from the etiology of intelligence in people with IQs less than 50 (Penrose 1963; Achenbach 1982). Whether the extremes in other behavioral dimensions are etiologically unique is still at issue.

Developmental dyslexia or reading disability (RD) is among the many disorders where the question of unique etiology arises. Epidemiologic studies have questioned whether RD is just the lower tail of the multifactorially determined normal distribution of reading skill, or instead represents an etiologically distinct disorder. The goal of this paper is to summarize the current thinking on the distinct etiology question for developmental reading disorder and to show how techniques of behavioral genetics can be used to conceptualize the problem and resolve whether or not extremes of a trait, such as reading, result from unique and nonnormal etiologies. While RD will be the focus of this paper, the methods and commentary are equally applicable to almost any other complex psychological or psychiatric phenotype (e.g., language disorders, see Leonard 1991; Tomblin 1991).

THE ETIOLOGICAL UNIQUENESS OF RD: TRADITIONAL APPROACHES

To address the issue of unique etiology in the past, many researchers have looked for a distinct collection of RD persons by examining distributions of reading scores for an excess of cases beyond normal curve expectancies on the lower end (Yule et al. 1974; Shaywitz et al. 1992). Other researchers have taken a more psychometric approach to the problem (e.g., Minton and Schneider 1985). While psychometrics (i.e., the way reading is measured and statistical decisions are made) are an important variable in the etiology problem, space does not permit a thorough discussion of these issues. Thus, this paper will focus on the distributional approach to the etiology question, the logic of which remains essentially the same irrespective of the tests or definitional criteria for RD that is used.

As we will describe later, the logical basis of the distributional approach is easily related to genetics and predictions under genetic models. Note, however, that when the distinct etiology question is addressed by looking for separate distributions of cases, that there are really two issues being confounded. One is whether RD is *distributionally* distinct (i.e., whether there is an excess of cases at the lower tail of a reading distribution), and the other issue is whether RD is *etiologically* distinct. Previous work has tended to confuse these two issues by performing studies appropriate to the first, in order to address the second. However, because of the possible separateness of these two concerns, it is possible to find no excess of cases at the extreme, yet find evidence suggestive of a distinct etiology of these extremes.

Survey of Prior Work

Studies examining reading score distributions for evidence of excess have yielded inconsistent results. A selection of these studies are summarized in table 1. In an early classic study, Yule and colleagues (Yule et al. 1974) examined the distributions of individual and group reading tests in two different samples of school aged children (N = 1100-2100 subjects). Using a 2 SD below the mean criterion for RD, they found a range of percentages in the RD tail depending on the test and sample examined. The percentages found often significantly exceeded 2.28% predicted by the normal curve, and were as high as 9.26%. Their conclusion was that children with RD reflect unique pathologic determinants of reading, and that they belong to a distribution separate from the normal distribution of low to high readers (e.g., similar to those with IQs below 50).

Table I Summary of Selected Epidemiological Studies of Reading Test Distributions

Study	Excess of Poor Readers in Distribution For Some or All of Tests Examined?
Yule et al. 1974	Yes
Rodgers 1983	No
vander Wissel and Zegers 1985	No
Silva, McGee, and Williams 1985	No
Share et al. 1987	No
Stevenson 1988	Yes
Shaywitz et al. 1992	No

Note: See references for complete citation.

In a later study, Shaywitz and colleagues (Shaywitz et al. 1992) did not find an excess of cases at the low end. While they agree that a small, etiologically distinct subtype of RD may exist, they argue that general reading ability and disability share the same multifactorial etiology. However, as we have argued above and elsewhere (Gilger et al. 1994; Pennington and Gilger 1992), failure to find an excess of RD cases or a mixture of distributions is not necessarily indicative of a common multifactorial etiology. Simple epidemiologic techniques used by the authors in table 1 may lack the power to resolve groups with distinct distributional etiologies.

THE ETIOLOGICAL UNIQUENESS OF RD: THE THEORY OF SOME GENETIC MODELS

Instead of the traditional epidemiological methods, the unique etiology question may be better conceptualized in terms of genetic models. Such models are more powerful and can also help disentangle the related issues of distinct etiology and distinct distribution that have been confused in previous work. Recall that previous research assumes that if RD *is not* etiologically unique, a distribution of reading test scores should follow a fairly normal, unimodal distribution.

In other words, if we assume that the entire distribution of reading test scores represents the effects of the same set of etiological factors, then for a complex trait like reading where a MFP model has long been assumed, we expect to observe relatively continuous variation in a single unimodal distribution. The MFP model is in fact a logical conclusion of researchers who fail to find an excess of poor readers, yet who believe in some heritable component in reading.

The classic MFP model of quantitative genetics stipulates that there are many genes acting to influence reading, each with small, primarily additive effects in combination with environmental variation (Falconer 1981). That is, people in the population will have continuously varying mixtures of the many genetic and nongenetic factors that affect the continuous reading phenotype. While the actual number of genes in a classic MFP system is assumed to be "many," it is also generally agreed that for a trait reflecting as few as three or four bi-allelic loci (i.e., three or four genes with two different forms such as A and a), each with fairly small effects, and some environmental variance, the trait distribution can still appear quite normal (Falconer 1981; Plomin, DeFries, and McClearn 1990).

If, on the other hand, a single major gene was responsible for a significant proportion of the variation present in reading, then a Mendelian genetic model may better fit the distributional data (Falconer 1981). Mendelian genetics is primarily concerned with traits yielding discontinuous distributions, where there are distinct classes of people in the trait distribution that are defined by a genotype at the major locus (e.g., ABO blood group, single gene disorders such as PKU, etc.). While we speak of discontinuous traits, major genes can in theory also influence quantitatively measured phenotypes (e.g., level of cholesterol in members of families with genetic hypercholesteremia).

Figures 1a and 1b show the hypothetical cases where a dominant single gene is acting to cause RD. The larger distribution to the right represents the normal range of readers. To the left is a smaller distinct distribution of individuals where a single deleterious allele (A) has reduced scores below some threshold, T, T1, or T2 (e.g., where clinically significant RD is identified). There are two important features illustrated in figures 1a and 1b. First, the distinction between the RD and normal reading groups is clearer in figure 1a than in figure 1b. This is because the figures have been drawn such that 1a shows a greater *penetrance* of the hypothesized major gene for RD. That is, of the people that carry the RD gene, more of them show the gene's effects, or at least show effects that are detectable. The distributions in figure 1b, on the other hand, overlap because the major gene contributing to reading variance has a smaller effect and is less penetrant in the clinical sense. Second, the number of readers clinically identified as disabled varies substantially with where the threshold is set. Use of T1 for example, is more specific but less sensitive to RD than is T2. These types of gene penetrance effects and threshold differences can make identification of distinct collections of individuals difficult.

Another complexity is *variable expressivity* of the genes for reading and reading disability, which no doubt occurs (Pennington 1990). Gene expressivity should be contrasted with penetrance, where in the former case it is not so much whether or not a gene has an effect, but additionally it is the variability in the qualitative or quantitative characteristics of that same gene in different people. Thus, in the context of the current dis-

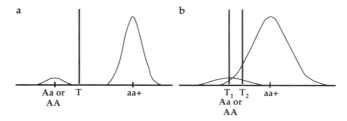

Figure 1.   Distributions of reading scores expected under a single gene model for RD when there is complete (a) and incomplete (b) penetrance, and variable expressivity. (Adapted from Fain, Spuhler, and Kimberling 1986, pg. 31). Gene "A" is dominant and acts to push people down on the reading continuum and towards the liability for reading disability.

cussion, a gene has variable expressivity if it "causes" a range of reading abilities or disabilities in people. In figures 1a and 1b, the distributions of phenotypes around the Aa and aa phenotypes are due in part to the variable expressivity of the hypothesized RD gene. The figures make it clear that this variability in expression complicates diagnostic accuracy.

Still more complex, is the situation depicted in figure 2, where the two distributions of RD and normal readers overlap even more extensively. This illustrates how a fairly normal and continuous phenotypic distribution may actually be an admixture of etiologically distinct groups—etiologically distinct in terms of whether the people in the groups inherited "good" or "bad" forms of the major gene or genes for reading. A further complication is shown by the broken line surrounding the two curves. This line represents the observed phenotypic distribution, which can appear normal. The variation around the two genotypic means, shown by the broken line, can be modeled as MFP effects, and thus, figure 2 represents the "mixed model" for RD (e.g., major gene effects *plus* MFP effects). Because MFP effects include genetic as well as environmental variance, nongenetic effects such as measurement error can also have a substantial effect on the ability to detect distributional admixture.

In addition to formal Mendelian and MFP mechanisms, genes may operate as Quantitative Trait Loci (QTL; sometimes also called oligogenic systems). If, for example, there are a limited number of key bi-allelic loci that are responsible for a major portion of variance in a quantitative trait like reading, QTL may apply (Gelderman 1975; Plomin 1990; McClearn et al. 1991). The key difference between a classic MFP system and QTL, is that in the latter case, genes of varying effect size are responsible for the heritable aspects of the variance in a quantitative phenotype. In other words, there may be an unknown number of genes underlying reading ability/disability (e.g., similar to the polygenic model), but there may be substantial variability in the proportion of additive trait variance each gene accounts for: Some of the key loci can

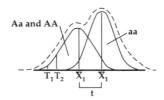

Figure 2.   Single locus (dominant), mixed model of inheritance for complex traits. Liability to reading disability is increased with the "A" allele that tends to push individuals down on the reading continuum. Multifactorial background is show by the broken line. T1 and T2 are two disease thresholds. Means of the two genotypic distributions are indicate by X1-X2; t is the distance in standard units between the two genotypic means.

have large effects and some can have small effects. One way to think about the relationship between classic MFP, Mendelian (single gene), and QTL models is simplified in figure 3. For ease of presentation and clarity we have purposely limited ourselves to the assumption of bi-allelic loci. It is noteworthy however, that in reality the distinctions between these three models may be even more complex and arbitrary when we consider tri- and multi-allelic loci (Falconer 1981).

The possibility of QTL for complex traits such as IQ and reading has received a lot of attention lately (Plomin 1990; McClearn et al. 1991; Plomin and Rende 1991; Plomin, Owen, and McGuffin 1994). As was mentioned earlier, the long held idea in behavioral genetics was that such traits were MFP in origin. The idea that several major genes could be responsible for a significant proportion of, say, reading variance, did not seem very likely, though it had long been recognized that some genes may contribute more to the observed phenotypic variance than others. In this way, QTL, in a sense, bridge the gap between the MFP models and the single major gene models (see figure 3). One exciting prospect of models invoking QTL is that as the number of gene markers available increases with advances in molecular genetics, we should be able to screen the genome for loci that are the more significant contributors to trait variance. For example, the action of QTL has already been demonstrated for apparently continuous traits in plants and non-human animals (Botstein et al. 1980; Lander and Botstein 1989; McClearn et al. 1991; DeFries and Hegman 1970; Johnson, DeFries, and Markel 1992), and some early research suggests that it may be successfully applied to complex human traits as well (e.g., Fulker et al. 1991; Cardon et al. 1994; Plomin et al. 1994; Smith Kimberling, and Pennington 1991).

Etiologic Versus Distributional Uniqueness

Figures 1 and 2 illustrate the problem that may arise when the assumption is made that failing to find a distributional excess of poor readers

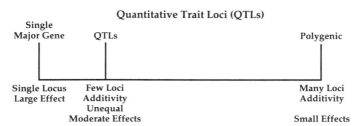

Figure 3. Line diagram of the relationship among Mendelian, Multifactorial-polygenic, and Quantitative Trait Loci models. Adapted from Pennington and Gilger (this volume).

indicates that they are similar in etiology to normal readers. The prior work cited in table 1 assumed that if there is a unique etiologic factor in RD, a clear and distinct distribution of RD individuals could be identified. But more accurately stated, failure to find an excess of cases only *excludes* genetic (or nongenetic) models where gene parameters and environmental effects are such that a statistical excess of cases *could be* identified. It does not rule out genetic models in which a unique etiology may yet exist for the *liability* to RD, but where distributional admixture is not readily recognized. Among the parameters modifying the probability of a clear separation of reader distributions are gene penetrance, gene effect size, variable expressivity, and gene frequency (Morton 1982; Falconer 1981; Gilger et al. 1994; Pennington and Gilger 1992).

Thus, in theory, failing to find a distinct class of readers only rejects certain etiologic models assumed by a statistical comparison of frequencies beyond normal curve expectations. It does not rule out other, more complicated, etiologic models that may produce a frequency of poor readers not obviously divergent from normal expectations. Techniques more powerful and flexible than those used in the studies in table 1 should take into account the many different parameters possibly operating in a distribution of reading test scores in an attempt to find the "best fitting" etiologic model. Certain tools from genetics provide a means to conduct such analyses. Two genetic techniques that are particularly relevant to distributional analyses are called commingling and genetic segregation analyses, and we will discuss these below. Other techniques we will discuss later that also address the distinct etiology question but do not do so directly through distributional analyses are the DeFries-Fulker (DeFries and Fulker 1985, 1988; DeFries and Gillis 1993) regression approaches to heritability analysis and the linkage and QTL molecular studies of RD by Smith and colleagues (Cardon et al. 1994; Fulker et al. 1991; Smith, Kimberling, and Pennington 1991).

Before closing this section, however, another important, and sometimes confusing concept in the area of genetics and etiological uniqueness deserves brief attention. In writings, the concept of "unique genetic etiology" often blurs the important difference between what might be called unique "allelic determinants for RD," or susceptibility alleles, and a unique "pathological disease locus" for RD. The first concept, as we will develop it further in this paper, is where RD is due to deleterious reading alleles at several key QTL, whose alternate alleles have a positive or neutral effect on variance in reading. The more deleterious alleles individuals inherit, the closer they get to the phenotypic disease threshold for RD. That is, a person's theoretical biological liability is modified (e.g., Greenberg 1993). In contrast, the concept of a pathological disease locus assumes either: (1) the uncommon situation where the disease locus is a pathological gene separate from the genes that influence reading skill in the normal population (i.e., a gene not otherwise involved in the developmental processes needed for normal reading); or, (2) the situation where the disease gene is a single pathological mutant gene with a very powerful effect, that was once part of the group of genes that contributed to the normal variance in reading. By "powerful effect" we mean an effect much larger than any of the other genes for reading (i.e., "megaphenic"; Morton 1982). In either case, the disease locus idea implies a single gene that by itself is generally sufficient and necessary to produce the condition of RD, and classic Mendelian genetics best fit this type of situation (e.g., Greenberg 1993). However, as our understanding of how genes work for complex traits increases, the traditional boundaries between concepts like "disease gene," "quantitative trait locus," "major gene," and so on, are blurring. For example, if one of several QTL for a disease such as hypertension or even RD should exert a moderately powerful push toward liability, it might be appropriate to think of this locus as carrying a major gene, or even a disease gene for these disorders. So, again, these terms must be considered in context and in a trait-by-trait manner.

THE ETIOLOGICAL UNIQUENESS OF RD: THE APPLICATION OF SOME GENETIC MODELS

Reading disability is one of the most thoroughly studied complex neuropsychological disorders of childhood, and it has been the focus of a great deal of genetic research (Pennington 1990, 1991). While there is still much to learn, we now have fairly clear ideas about which genetic models best fit the pattern of RD transmission in families, and perhaps said more accurately, which models do not (Pennington and Gilger this volume; DeFries et al. 1991; Pennington 1990).

If we suspect that the discrete etiologic factor affecting the extremes of a trait might be genetic, then formal genetic tests for this factor are appropriate. This is particularly true when variation in the trait has already been shown to be familial, as it has for RD. In terms of the distinct etiology question of RD, several classes of previous studies are relevant: Commingling and segregation analyses of RD and normally reading families, twin analyses of the heritability of group versus individual differences in reading, and linkage analyses of RD.

Commingling and Genetic Segregation

While these types of analyses are not typically applied to the genetics of complex human traits like IQ, reading, and personality, they have contributed greatly to our understanding of other complex human traits including anthropometric characters, medical conditions, and more, and a variety of genetic and etiologic hypotheses about a disorder like RD can be examined with these analyses given the necessary family data. Because segregation and commingling deal directly with the distributional properties of data, they are therefore the next logical step in our discussion of previous methods that look for a "hump" in the distribution of reading performance as evidence of unique etiology. While the complexities of human cognitive phenotypes like RD may make segregation and commingling difficult to perform and interpret, an understanding of how these methods can contribute to the study of the unique etiology question is still important.

For example, tests for major gene influence on a trait can be directly carried out via complex segregation analysis rather than inferring major gene involvement (or lack thereof) simply on the basis of the presence or absence of a clear excess of cases on the low end of the reading distribution (Morton 1982; MacLean et al. 1976; Lalouel et al. 1984; Morton and MacLean 1974; Smith 1986). If significant major gene influence is found by segregation analysis, then the implication is that there is some form of multi-distributional admixture in the population being studied, though it may not be clearly visible, and that the phenotypic segregation in families follows Mendelian expectations (Morton 1982). That is, that there is some discrete genetic factor traveling in families that contributes significantly to the phenotypic correlations and covariance observed among family members.

Another test for the presence of multiple distributions is commingling analysis, where tests for normal distributional components are made assuming a major gene hypothesis (MacLean et al. 1976). These analyses can be applied to family data, or to data from unrelated persons such as that used in the studies cited in table I. However, commingling analysis relies only on distributional properties of the data, and because segregation analysis also takes into account the transmission patterns from parents to offspring (i.e., trait correlations among relatives), it is a more powerful and specific test for major gene effects.

Using commingling and segregation, we can test whether the assumed etiologic factor in RD is genetic and unique from "normal" variability in reading. First, if RD is part of the normal continuum and there are no major discrete etiologic factors in its origin, then a commingling analyses of a quantitative reading phenotype should find that there is no admixture of distributions and that a single distribution model best fits the set of reading scores. Second, the best fitting genetic model as determined by segregation analyses of quantitative family data should be MFP. On the other hand, if there is a distinct genetic factor with major effect involved in RD, then commingling of distributions should be found and segregation analysis should indicate significant major gene or mixed model transmission of the reading phenotype.

In an earlier paper we reported a segregation analysis performed on several sets of families ascertained through an RD child (Pennington et al. 1991). We found that the best fitting model for the transmission of a *qualitative* (i.e., presence-absence) RD phenotype in these pedigrees was autosomal major gene. While finding a major gene effect is consistent with RD being of distinct genetic etiology, it is not necessarily conclusive. It is possible, for instance, that the major genetic effect detected for RD in these families is one member of, or a cluster of, alleles of QTL that act throughout the reading distribution, and not a single disease gene in the classic sense. If this were the case, then a segregation analysis of reading scores in families ascertained through normal readers may also show evidence of major gene effects that operate to shift a person up or down on the liability scale for reading problems. If, on the other hand, RD is distinct from general reading ability because of some discrete genetic factor (i.e., a major disease gene), and normal variability in reading is MFP in origin, the segregation analysis of reading in normal families should yield results consistent with an MFP model. This expected difference in results is primarily due to the manner in which the two types of families were selected: In one case families were selected for RD and hence the RD gene (if it exists), while in the other case, families were selected to represent normal variation in reading, with an incidence of RD roughly equal to that of the general population.

Because we had access to a group of 125 families ascertained through normal readers, we were able to test the commingling and segregation predictions for RD and nonRD family comparisons. In fact, these 125 normal families had been matched to a set of RD families analyzed in Pennington et al. (1991). Our basic question was: Are there major gene effects for the transmission of the reading phenotype in normal families as there was for the transmission of an RD phenotype in RD families? Results of these analyses have been recently reported by Gilger et al. (1994).

In brief, commingling analysis showed skewness in our data, though evidence for an admixture of separate distributions only approached statistical significance. In contrast, results of segregation analysis suggested that a dominant allele with major effect may increase a person's liability for reading difficulties (Gilger et al. 1994).

In figure 4 we present a histogram of the raw reading data, as well as an overlay of the two hypothetical genotypic distributions caused by the major gene influences detected by the segregation analysis. The reader should note that the two distributions overlap substantially, making detection of admixture difficult via commingling analysis, and especially via the common method of testing for a simple excess of cases beyond some arbitrary threshold.

What do these results indicate about the distinct etiology issue surrounding RD? Because analyses of both the RD and nonRD families

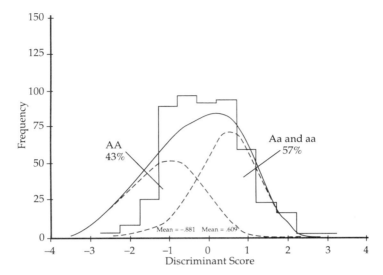

Figure 4. Outline of observed frequency distribution (histogram) and two pre-dicted component distributions for the standardized discriminant reading scores. Genotypic means and percentages are based on the dominant gene model applied to power transformed data with variance due to age, age^2, age^3, and sex removed. Note that the deleterious allele is now "a" and it acts to push an individual towards the reading disability threshold. This is represented by an *increase* on this scale and was necessary due to the statistical properties of the analyses run by Gilger et al. (1994). Adapted from J. W. Gilger et al. (1994). Commingling and segregation analysis of reading performance in families of normal reading probands. *Behavior Genetics* 24 (4), pg. 351. Reprinted with permission.

yielded similar results (i.e., major gene effects), we are less confident that RD is etiologically distinct, at least in terms of a disease gene hypothe-sis for abnormal reading and an MFP etiology for the normal range. If the gene detected in the normal families was the "RD disease gene" its prevalence would dictate a much higher number of poor readers in the normal families than the 2.5% actually found (based on a 2 SD below the mean criterion; Gilger et al. 1994).[1] However, these data do not rule out the possibility of QTL acting upon reading, where RD individuals may inherit a few *susceptibility alleles* (Greenberg 1993) that add substan-tially to reading test variance and that can make persons possessing them unique from their normal reading counterparts. Such alleles may have shown up in our analysis as a major genetic effect or "signal" that stood out from the background of other effects on reading, and that was transmitted in a fashion consistent with Mendelian models.

---

[1]It is noteworthy that for comparison purposes we also tested for unique etiology using the epidemiologic methods of Yule and others (Yule et al. 1972). This involves a z test for an excess of cases beyond the 2.28% expected when a

Twin Studies

Twin studies have often been used to estimate the extent to which variation in a trait is due to heritable influences. Specifically, the classic twin model compares the within-pair resemblance of monozygotic (MZ) twins to that of dizygotic (DZ) twins. Given a variety of statistical and theoretical assumptions (Plomin, DeFries, and McClearn 1990), any increase in resemblance of MZs over DZs is attributed to their greater genetic similarity: MZs have all of their genes in common, while DZs have on average, only half in common.

Reports of twin studies often use an index of the extent to which individual differences in a phenotype can be attributed to individual differences in genetic make-up called broad-sense heritability, or $h_B{}^2$ (Falconer 1981; Plomin, DeFries, and McClearn 1990). One way to calculate this quantity is to take twice the difference between MZ and DZ intraclass correlations. Olson et al. (1991) report $h_B{}^2$ estimates for a reading recognition test for RD and nonRD twins of the Colorado Reading Project. The $h_B{}^2$ estimate for reading in nonRD twins was .35, a value not significantly different from the $h_B{}^2$ of .59 that was obtained for the RD sample of twins. Because the difference between the $h_B{}^2$ estimate was not *statistically* significant, the authors suggested that the genetic influences on individual differences in reading may be the same for poor and normal readers. Bear in mind, however, that the heritability estimates are *actually* different, and that the study may have lacked the power to achieve conventional levels of statistical signifi-

1.96 standard deviation below the mean cut-off is used to identify a subject as RD. Briefly, we did this test using the 511 subjects making up the members of the control families examined with segregation and commingling procedures just discussed. Three different phenotypes were used: One phenotype was an IQ regression formula derived from a separate sample of 140 control normal children (see Pennington et al. 1992) and then applied to the 511 subjects to obtain standardized reading deviation scores from IQ expectancy. A second phenotype was another IQ regression formula derived from the 511 control family members themselves and then re-applied to the sample to obtain IQ deviation scores. Finally, the reading scores of the subjects were simply standardized based on the mean and standard deviation of the 511 family members, and a –1.96 cutoff was then used to identify a subject as RD. The only phenotype displaying a statistically significant excess was the IQ discrepant formula derived from the independent sample of 140 control children. It is perhaps relevant that much of the earlier work (see table 1) have used an IQ discrepant formula derived from and then re-applied to same sample. Their failure to find a significant excess of cases may have been a consequence of the conservativeness of this method, where regression weights and residuals are based on a least squares criterion such that the residuals will have a mean of 0, and be as normally distributed as possible (Cohen and Cohen 1983). Thus, except for extreme situations, deriving and applying regression formula from and then to the same sample yields a very conservative test for an excess.

cance. Thus, we need to be cautious when we essentially "accept the null" and then make statements that there is no evidence for the unique etiology of reading in abnormally reading groups.

While twin studies can be used to test a variety of genetic models, they are best and most frequently used to study traits believed to be of MFP origin. That is, they are not very useful in modeling and testing single gene hypotheses. However, DeFries and Fulker (1985, 1988) have advocated a unique use of the twin methodology that allows us to assess the distinct etiology question more directly than simply comparing $h_B{}^2$ values across separate RD and nonRD samples of twins. The process can be used for many complex phenotypes, and it begins by selecting a sample of MZ and DZ twins in which at least one member of each pair (i.e., the probands) exceeds a predetermined extreme on the continuum of interest. For example, the Colorado Twin Study of DeFries and colleagues (DeFries et al. 1991; DeFries and Gillis 1993), selects MZ and DZ twin pairs with at least one member being RD, as well as a matched sample of control twins. The design of the study permits a test between the heritability of normal variation in reading ability ($h_B{}^2$ as described above) and the heritability of a group deficit in reading (h^2g) (DeFries and Fulker 1985, 1988). Because h^2g is an estimate of the extent to which deviant reading (i.e., RD) is heritable, it may differ significantly from the extent to which normal individual differences in reading are heritable (i.e., $h_B{}^2$) if extreme low scores in reading (i.e., RD) are indeed etiologically unique.

When selected on the basis of performance on a quantitative reading test, the extent to which the low reading performance of the twin probands is heritable will effect the degree to which MZ and DZ co-twins regress towards the unselected population mean. Specifically, if reading and reading deficits are to some extent heritable, MZ co-twins should regress *less* than their DZ counterparts. These regression effects can be modelled and an estimate of $h_g{}^2$ can be obtained that represents the degree to which the difference between probands and the population mean is heritable, or the extent to which the etiology of extreme scores is genetic (DeFries and Fulker 1985, 1988). An extension of the DeFries-Fulker model also provides a test for difference between $h_g{}^2$ and $h_B{}^2$, which if significant, suggests that the etiology of extremes may differ from that of the normal continuum.

For a composite psychometric tests score of reading ability, the Colorado Twin Study reports an h^2g value of approximately .50 (SE = .11) and an $h_B{}^2$ value of approximately .73 (SE = .35) (DeFries and Gillis 1993; DeFries et al. 1991). The difference, though large, did not achieve statistical significance, and in part, this may have been a reflection of a relatively small sample and resultant low power ($h_g{}^2$ - $h_B{}^2$ test = -.23, SE = .37, $p > .50$). In fact, the statistical test for $h_B{}^2$-$h_g{}^2$ requires a large N for sufficient power.

Further work is required using the DeFries-Fulker model, in that we are again faced with the complexities inherent when the null hypothesis is "accepted" (i.e., that the etiologies of normal and abnormal reading are the same), and there have been no formal modeling studies to ascertain how often major gene or unique genetic effects would be missed when in reality they are present in the population. However, even if a significant difference was found it would not *necessarily* indicate that different genes are responsible for performance in different parts of the reading continuum, but rather, it would indicate that genetic and environmental influences in general, operate differently for normal and low readers. In sum then, the DeFries-Fulker twin application *thus far suggests* that the genetics of RD and normal variation in reading are not perfectly distinct (i.e., there is not a distinct disease gene for RD), although future work with larger numbers of subjects is needed to see if any h_B^2-h_g^2 difference that remains is reliable.

Another study utilizing the Colorado twins also addresses the unique etiology question. This study is particularly interesting because it deals with the diagnostic debate that was an intrinsic part of the distinct etiology question posed early on by the authors listed in table 1: Are there etiological differences between "garden variety poor readers" (defined by an age discrepancy based formula) and readers with "true dyslexia" (defined by an IQ discrepancy based formula)?

Pennington et al. (1992) examined the genetic evidence for the external validity of the age versus IQ discrepant method for RD diagnosis. An IQ discrepant formula quite similar to that used in the studies cited in table I (see also footnote 1) was compared to an age discrepant RD criterion on several attributes relevant to the distinct etiology question, including: (1) If there is an etiological distinction between specifically reading disabled (IQ discrepant) and simply backward readers (age discrepant), the two definitions may yield different heritability estimates, and (2) If the two definitions are tapping different etiological factors, then they should not share a large proportion of their genetic variance.

The first question was addressed by obtaining and comparing h_g^2 estimates for the IQ and age based phenotypes in the Colorado twin sample. The second question was examined by testing the extent to which the genes effecting one definition were related to the genes effecting the other definition. The results indicated that both definitions are highly heritable, with h_g^2 quotients of approximately .47 each. Furthermore, the two phenotypes were highly phenotypically correlated ($r = .93$), and this correlation was primarily due to shared genes (92% of the covariance between the two diagnoses was explained by a common genetic origin). Thus, it appears that age and IQ diagnostic phenotypes may have a common genetic etiology, and thus the argument for an etiological distinction between backward readers and specific dyslexics may not be as tenable as was once proposed (Yule et al. 1974).

Similar conclusions have been reached in the psychometric literature using different methods (Fletcher 1992).

Linkage Studies

Genes are organized linearly into chromosomes. Genes on the same chromosome will tend to be inherited together as that chromosome is passed from generation to generation, and this is called linkage. However, the meiotic process of crossing over and recombination makes linkage a probabilistic event: linkage is less likely to occur for genes far apart on a chromosome, and more likely to occur for genes very close together on a chromosome (Morton 1982). Moreover, genes on different chromosomes will be transmitted independently of each other.

While there are a variety of linkage study techniques available, all linkage work basically involves following "marker" genes or regions of known chromosomal location through generations of related persons to see if they are associated with the trait of interest, or noting the degree of correlation between markers and a trait in persons of varying degrees of relatedness (Morton 1982; Botstein et al. 1980). For example, as a marker, a molecular genetic probe could be used to identify the types of polymorphisms in a region of chromosome 6 (e.g., the HLA locus) for a large group of relatives. These relatives could also be tested for evidence of RD, and then examined to see if there is a statistically significant co-occurence between the marker and the presence of RD. If such a linkage is found, it suggests that at least one of the genes involved in the etiology of RD in these relatives is located somewhere near the marker region or gene on chromosome 6, or, that the chromosome 6 marker is itself somehow involved in the etiology of RD.

Preliminary linkage analyses of siblings and extended pedigrees are consistent with the idea that RD may fit a QTL model. The data that bear on this issue are from some reports by Smith and colleagues (Cardon et al. 1994; Fulker et al. 1991; Smith, Kimberling, and Pennington 1991; Smith et al. 1983). Specifically, in their early papers on families and twins with RD, they reported a number of significant, or near significant, genetic linkages on chromosomes 6 and 15 to a qualitative RD diagnosis as well as the same quantitative reading phenotype used in the segregation and twin analyses reported on above.

The next step after finding genes linked to RD would be to see if the same genes contribute to normal variation in reading as well. If they do, the linked genes are probably part of a QTL system for the entire range of reading skill. A simple extension of the DeFries-Fulker regression model can in fact be used to detect multiple genes linked to variance in a quantitative trait like reading (Fulker et al. 1991).

Briefly, the approach analyzes how the number of genetic markers held in common by relatives affects their degree of similarity for reading scores. But more significantly, this model can be applied to selected samples: in this case, the idea again being that the more similar the twins are in terms of their genes and genetic markers, the less likely co-twins are to regress to the unselected population mean (see above discussion of twin studies). This approach to QTL analysis is quite useful in terms of the distinct etiology question in that it can identify the genes most responsible for liability to RD. Because the comparison of interest is how within-pair variability in genes is related to within-pair variability in reading performance, only DZ twins are used. MZ twins would not be informative in this situation since there is no within-pair genetic variation.

When the twin regression model was applied to data from the Colorado twins it yielded results similar to those of earlier reports using different statistical techniques (Smith, Kimberling, and Pennington 1991; Fulker et al. 1991). More interesting however, was that *the more the sample was selected to represent extremes of low reading ability, the more significant some of these linkages became* (Fulker et al. 1991). In the most recent report, Cardon et al. (1994) show that in two independent samples, a QTL for reading disability (ability) was located within the human leukocyte antigen (HLA) complex of chromosome 6. Although these data are quite preliminary, they suggest that certain quantitative trait loci contribute to reading variance, with some alleles at these loci being significant for extremes in low reading ability. It is also possible, though it has yet to be shown, that other alleles at this particular locus may have neutral or even positive effects on reading skill. Research is in fact in progress testing normal reading twins for evidence of the chromosome 6 QTL. Furthermore, it is important to note that so far, only the HLA linkage has been replicated and appears statistically robust across two different samples, and other preliminary linkages on chromosome 15 do not appear reliable.

The molecular research of Smith and colleagues suggests that allelic differences among people are in part responsible for where they lie on the reading continuum. It is of more than passing interest that the power calculations and statistical methods provided by these authors (e.g., Cardon et al. 1994; Fulker et al. 1991) suggest that the application of their approach to the study of linkage in selected samples holds much promise in the future detection of QTL for a variety of human phenotypes. It is possible that in the future the human genome could be screened for QTL relevant to continous and complex human cognitive traits using a battery of molecular markers.

GENERAL DISCUSSION

Methodological and theoretical issues pertaining to the distinct etiology issue have been the focus of this paper. Using RD as an example, we proposed that the simple epidemiologic techniques previously applied to this problem should be supplemented with the potentially more informative and powerful methodologies found in genetics—especially since it has long been known that RD has some degree of familiality.

Theories and methods of genetic epidemiology have been used to highlight the potential weaknesses in simply using frequency data to look for an excess in the extremes of complex trait distributions (i.e., the simple distribution or "hump" approach). Specifically, we need to be aware of the possible confusion between *distributional versus etiologic uniqueness*, and the potential difficulties in simply assuming that if a disease is pathologically unique there should be evidence of a distinct collection of individuals in the population at large.

While genetic analyses can supplement (and perhaps replace) more conventional methods used to address the unique etiology issue, they are, of course, more time consuming and require data on relatives to address genetic hypotheses. Moreover, while quantitative analyses using segregation, commingling (which does not require data on relatives), and twin methods are quite useful, advances in molecular genetics may ultimately render many of these techniques obsolete. Linkage analysis is in fact the only method that, by itself, can locate the genes responsible for a trait and address the distinct etiology question directly. Another molecular genetic technique, typically called "association," is able to examine large populations of unrelated people for correlations among traits and markers. This allows a test of whether certain alleles are more frequent in one group relative to another, and therefore, if the trait of interest might be related to the location or function of these alleles. With the increasing number of markers becoming available this may now be a reasonable approach to looking for potential QTL for complex human traits (Plomin et al. 1994). Markers may be molecular or biological probes (e.g., restriction fragment length polymorphisms or RFLPs, dopamine 2 receptor clones) or more easily observable phenotypes (e.g., ABO blood groupings). Finding significant correlations between a trait of interest (e.g., low reading ability) and a marker can suggest possible gene locations and/or candidate QTL. This approach has not been applied to the study of RD, but has, to a limited extent to other complex human traits (e.g., alcoholism and schizophrenia, see Devor 1993; Plomin, DeFries, and McClearn 1990; Plomin et al. 1994).

Even if molecular methods yield important discoveries, classic quantitative methods like twin, family, and adoption studies will be needed to characterize the inheritance of the trait and how genetic and nongenetic factors interact in the course of development. Using a variety of different methods can help us define the phenotype of interest and identify the environmental variables that can be later manipulated as part of treatment and prevention (e.g., Pennington 1991; Pennington et al. 1992; Kendler and Eaves 1986; DeFries et al. 1991).

While there is still much to be understood about RD, results of several genetic analyses of reading performance have already been reported. We were therefore able to compare and contrast admixture, segregation, linkage, and twin studies, as they pertain to the distinct etiology question. In fact we discovered that all four types of studies essentially suggested the same conclusion: That RD is probably *not* etiologically distinct from normal reading variation in the *classic sense* (e.g., Yule et al. 1974; Shaywitz et al. 1992; Pennington and Gilger 1992). While we put forth this conclusion, we have noted throughout this paper that more research is still needed—power problems and issues pertaining to statistical decisions are of some concern. The strength of the conclusions we suggest, however, lies primarily with the relative consistency of results across different samples and methods.

To reiterate, if RD was clearly genetically distinct from general reading ability, we should have found differences in the heritability of RD and normal reading in twins (DeFries and Fulker 1988; DeFries et al. 1991) and would have expected differences in the segregation patterns in control versus RD families. Yet no such differences were *statistically* evident. Of course, twin and family analyses are not able to detect genetic heterogeneity in the transmission or heritability of RD and general reading ability, and failure to find different patterns of transmission does not prove the null hypothesis. But the linkage data also support the idea that a number of genes (at different loci) may contribute to the range of reading ability, and that a simple single disease locus, distinct etiology concept of RD, is not as tenable as was once thought. Different loci may contribute, more or less, to reading skills, with some loci having major effects.[2] Which loci have the greatest effects on one or the other extremes of reading (i.e., very high or very low skills), may change with increasing selection on the extremes. This is suggested by the preliminary linkage work where the significant contribution of some loci increases (or decreases) as more severe RD probands are identified. Of course, deleterious environmental factors also contribute to an individual's proclivity to dyslexia. In a sense this proposal is a compromise between prior hypotheses of the etiology of pathology and etiological factors in normal variation. Moreover, other authors have suggested a similar compromise and rethinking for complex traits, such as IQ, open field behavior in mice, schizophrenia, and alcoholism (McClearn et al. 1991; Plomin and Rende 1991; Plomin

---

[2]As mentioned earlier, the distinctions between MFP, Mendelian, QTL, major gene, disease gene, and susceptibility gene, become blurred in some circumstances. The chromosome 6 quantitative trait locus for RD, for instance, has a moderate to large effect on reading scores. In this case some may refer to the gene at this locus as a major gene, although QTLs were not originally conceptualized in this manner.

1990; DeFries and Hegman 1970; Johnson, DeFries, and Markel 1992; Greenberg 1993; Devor 1993).

Future research, in particular molecular genetic analyses, may eventually identify the specific genes for RD and resolve the remaining ambiguities concerning this issue. However, the process of resolution will be complicated and the power of molecular analyses to detect QTL is an issue. Nonetheless, a combination of classic MFP and single gene models may be required to assess more fully the etiology of complex characters such as reading disability, speech and language disorders, and psychiatric illness.

ACKNOWLEDGEMENTS

Portions of the research reported herein were supported by an NICHD Learning Disability Research Center grant (HD 27802) to Drs. J. C. DeFries, R. K. Olson, B. F. Pennington, and S. D. Smith, as well as NIMH grants MH0049 (RSDA) and MH38870 (Merit) to Dr. Pennington. Dr. Borecki was supported in part by NIH GM28719 during preparation of this manuscript. Portions of this paper were presented at the International Neuropsychology Society meeting, San Diego, CA, February, 1992, and the Behavior Genetics Association meeting, Boulder, CO, June, 1992.

REFERENCES

Achenbach, T.M. 1982. *Developmental Psychopathology* (2nd ed.). New York: John Wiley and Sons, Inc.

Botstein, D. R., White, L., Skolnick, M., and Davis, R. W. 1980. Construction of a genetic linkage map in man using restriction fragment length polymorphisms. *American Journal of Human Genetics* 32:314–31.

Cardon, L. R., Smith, S. D., Fulker, D. W., Kimberling, W. J., Pennington, B. F., and DeFries, J. C. 1994. Quantitative Trait Locus for Reading Disability on Chromosome 6. *Science* 266:276–79.

Cohen, J., and Cohen, P. 1983. *Applied Multiple Regression/Correlation Analysis for the Behavioral Sciences* (2nd ed.). Hillsdale, NJ: Lawrence Erlbaum Associates.

DeFries, J. C., and Fulker, D. W. 1985. Multiple regression analysis of twin data. *Behavior Genetics* 15:467–73.

DeFries, J. C., and Fulker, D. W. 1988. Multiple regression analysis of twin data: Etiology of deviant scores versus individual differences. *Acta Geneticae Medicae et Gemellologiae* 37:205–16.

DeFries, J. C., and Gillis, J. J. 1993. Genetics of reading disability. In *Nature, Nurture and Psychology*, eds. R. Plomin and G. McClearn. Washington, DC: APA Press.

DeFries, J. C., and Hegman, J. P. 1970. Genetic analysis of open-field behavior. In *Contributions to Behavior-Genetic Analysis—the Mouse as a Prototype*, eds. G. Lindaey and D. D. Thiessen. New York: Meridith Corp.

DeFries, J. C., Olson, R. K., Pennington, B. F., and Smith, S. D. 1991. Colorado Reading Project: An update. In *The Reading Brain: The Biological Basis of Dyslexia*, eds. D. D. Duane and D. B. Gray. Parkton, MD: York Press.

Devor, E. J. 1993. Why there is no gene for alcoholism. *Behavior Genetics* 23:145–52.

Eaves, L. J., Eysenck, H. J., and Martin, N. G. 1989. *Genes, Culture and Personality: An Empirical Approach*. San Diego, CA: Academic Press.

Eysenck, H. J. 1952. *The Scientific Study of Personality*. London: Routledge & Kegan Paul.

Fain, P. R., Spuhler, K. P., and Kimberling, W. J. 1986. Quantitative genetics and learning disabilities. In *Genetics and Learning Disabilities*, ed. S. Smith. San Diego, CA: College Hill Press.

Falconer, D. S. 1981. *Introduction to Quantitative Genetics* (2nd ed.). London: Longman House.

Fletcher, J. M. 1992. The validity of distinguishing children with language and learning disabilities according to discrepancies with IQ: Introduction to the special series. *Journal of Learning Disabilities* 25(9):546–48.

Fulker, D. W., Cardon, L. R., DeFries, J. C., Kimberling, W. J., Pennington, B. F., and Smith, S. D. 1991. Multiple regression analysis of sib-pair data on reading to detect quantitative trait loci. *Reading and Writing: An Interdisciplinary Journal* 3:299–313.

Fulker, D. W., and Eysenck, H. J. 1979. Nature and nurture: Heredity. In *The Structure and Measurement of Intelligence*, ed. H. J. Eysenck. Berlin: Springer-Verlag.

Gelderman, H. 1975. Investigations on inheritance of quantitative characters in animals by gene markers. I. Methods. *Theoretical and Applied Genetics* 46:319–30.

Gilger, J. W., Borecki, I. B., DeFries, J. C., and Pennington, J. C. 1994. Commingling and segregation analysis of reading performance in families of normal reading probands. *Behavior Genetics* 24:345–55.

Greenberg, D. A. 1993. Linkage analysis of "necessary" disease loci versus "susceptibility" loci. *American Journal of Human Genetics* 52:135–43.

Johnson, T. E., DeFries, J. C., and Markel, P. D. 1992. Mapping Quantitative Trait Loci for behavioral traits in the mouse. *Behavior Genetics* 22(6):635–53.

Kendler, K. S., and Eaves, L. J. 1986. Models for the joint effects of genotype and environment on liability to psychiatric illness. *American Journal of Psychiatry* 143:279–89.

Lalouel, J. M., Rao, D. C., Morton, N. E., and Elston, R. C. 1984. A unified model for complex segregation analysis. *American Journal of Human Genetics* 35:816–26.

Lander, E. S., and Botstein, D. 1989. Mapping Mendelian factors underlying quantitative traits using RFLP linkage maps. *Genetics* 121:185–99.

Leonard, L. 1991. Specific language impairment as a clinical category. *Language, Speech, and Hearing Services in the Schools* 22:66–68.

MacLean, C. J., Morton, N. E., Elston, R. C., and Yee, S. 1976. Skewness in commingled distributions. *Biometrics* 32:694–99.

McClearn, G. E., Plomin, R., Gora-Maslak, G., and Crabbe, J. C. 1991. The gene chase in behavioral science. *Psychological Science* 2(4):222–29.

Matarazzo, J. D., and Pankeratz, L. D. 1980. Intelligence. In *Encyclopedia of Clinical Assessment*, ed. R. H. Woody. San Francisco: Jossey-Bass.

Minton, H., and Schneider, F. 1985. *Differential Psychology.* Prospect Heights, IL: Waveland Press.

Morton, N. E. 1982. *Outline of Genetic Epidemiology.* London: S. Karger.

Morton, N. E., and MacLean, C. J. 1974. Analysis of family resemblance. III. Complex segregation of quantitative traits. *American Journal of Human Genetics* 26:489–503.

Olson, R. K., Gillis, J. J., Rack, J. P., DeFries, J. C., and Fulker, D. W. 1991. Confirmatory factor analysis of word recognition and process measures in the Colorado Reading Project. *Reading and Writing: An Interdisciplinary Journal* 3:235–48.

Pennington, B. F. 1990. The genetics of dyslexia. *Journal of the American Association of Child and Adolescent Psychiatry* 31:193–201.

Pennington, B. F. 1991. *Reading Disabilities: Genetic and Neurological Influences.* Netherlands: Kluwer Academic Press.

Pennington, B. F., and Gilger, J. W. 1992. The relation between normal reading skill and developmental dyslexia: A comment on Shaywitz, et al. *New England Journal of Medicine* 327:280.

Pennington, B. F., Gilger, J. W., Olson, R., and DeFries, J. 1992. External validity of age versus IQ discrepant diagnoses in reading disability: Lessons from a twin study. *Journal of Learning Disabilities* 25:562–73.

Pennington, B. F., Gilger, J. W., Pauls, D., Smith, S. A., Smith, S., and DeFries, J. C. 1991. Evidence for major gene transmission of developmental dyslexia. *Journal of the American Medical Association* 266(11):1527–34.

Penrose, L. S. 1963. *The Biology of Mental Defect* (3rd ed.). London: Sidgwick & Jackson.

Plomin, R. 1990. The role of inheritance in behavior. *Science* 248:183–248.

Plomin, R., DeFries, J. C., and McClearn, G. E. 1990. *Behavioral Genetics: A Primer* (2nd ed.). New York: W.H. Freeman.

Plomin, R., McClearn, G. E., Smith, D., Vignetti, S., Chorney, M. J., Chorney, K., et al. 1994. DNA markers associated with high versus low IQ: The IQ Quantitative Trait Loci (QTL) Project. *Behavior Genetics* 24(2):107–18.

Plomin, R., Owen, M., and McGuffin, P. 1994. The genetic basis of complex behaviors. *Science* 264:1733–39.

Plomin, R., and Rende, R. 1991. Human behavioral genetics. *Annual Review of Psychology* 42:1–66.

Rodgers, B. 1983. The identification and prevalence of specific reading retardation. *British Journal of Educational Psychology* 53:369–73.

Share, D. L., McGee, R., McKenzie, D., Williams, S., and Silva, P. 1987. Further evidence relating to the distinction between specific reading retardation and general reading backwardness. *British Journal of Developmental Psychology* 5:35–44.

Shaywitz, S. E., Escobar, M. D., Shaywitz, B. A., Fletcher, J. M., and Makuch, R. 1992. Evidence that dyslexia may represent the lower tail of a normal distribution of reading ability. *New England Journal of Medicine* 326:145–50.

Silva, P. A, McGee, R., and Williams, S. 1985. Some characteristics of 9 year old boys with general reading backwardness or specific reading retardation. *Journal of Child Psychology, Psychiatry and Allied Disciplines* 26:407–21.

Smith, S. D. 1986. *Genetics and Learning Disabilities.* San Diego, CA: College-Hill Press.

Smith, S. D., Kimberling, W. J., and Pennington, B. F. 1991. Screening for multiple genes influencing dyslexia. *Reading and Writing: An Interdisciplinary Journal* 3:285–98.

Smith, S. D., Kimberling, W. J., Pennington, B., and Lubs, H. A. 1983. Specific reading disability: Identification of an inherited form through linkage analysis. *Science* 219:1345–47.

Stevenson, J. 1988. Which aspects of reading ability show a hump in their distribution? *Applied Cognitive Psychology* 2:77–85.

Tomblin, B. 1991. Examining the cause of specific language impairment. *Language, Speech, and Hearing Services in the Schools* 22:69–74.

van der Wissel, A., and Zegers, F. E. 1985. Reading retardation revisited. *British Journal of Developmental Psychology* 3:3–9.

Yule, W., Rutter, M., Berger, M., and Thompson, J. 1974. Over and under achievement in reading: Distribution in the general Population. *British Journal of Educational Psychology* 44:1–12.

Part • **III**

Visual Cognitive Mechanisms

Reading begins as a visual task, and many researchers have proposed dyslexic models that involve problems of oculomotor control, visual attention, perceptual span, processing speed, visual persistence, or contrast sensitivity. This work has been controversial for several reasons. Some studies of dyslexic visual deficits have not been replicated; some visual perceptual problems could better be viewed as a symptom rather than cause of reading impairments; or experimental tasks have not been conducted under conditions that approximate normal reading. Furthermore, the importance of phonemic awareness as a prerequisite skill for normal reading development has been widely accepted, thus defining dyslexia as a language-based, not a perceptually based, disorder. Nevertheless, behavioral evidence continues to accumulate that demonstrates visual impairments for a subgroup of dyslexics, work which is now inspired in part by the recent report of neurological abnormalities found in a portion of the visual sensory system of five dyslexics. The functional significance of such neurological abnormalities is under study in several labs, but we do not know yet whether they directly interfere with normal reading development.

The following three chapters present interesting arguments on both sides of this debate. Rayner describes what we have learned about reading from the study of eye movements, and makes the case that erratic movements are a symptom rather than a cause of dyslexia. In contrast, Stein summarizes results from several studies that report a much higher incidence of unstable binocular fixations among dyslexic children. He also reports that treatment for instability by means of monocular occlusion in one group of children doubled their reading scores in a year's time compared to a placebo treatment group. Chase describes a new visual deficit model for dyslexia based on a slower processing of low spatial frequencies (the shape of letters and words) and provides evidence from several studies of slower dyslexic performance. Together these chapters renew interest in the exploration of dyslexic subtypes and challenge definitions that propose a unitary language-based etiology.

Chapter • 5

What We Can Learn About Reading Processes From Eye Movements

Keith Rayner

What can we learn about reading from studying eye movements? The simple answer to this question is: quite a lot. In fact, I begin with the bold assertion that we have learned more about reading from eye movement studies than from any other source of data. The vast array of studies dealing with word recognition are all potentially informative concerning processes that may occur in reading; but, one is never really sure of the extent to which findings obtained in word recognition studies (in which single words are responded to) generalize to the more complex process of reading. For virtually any type of task that has been used ostensibly to study some aspect of reading, one can likewise raise questions about the generalizability of the findings since there is almost always a mismatch between what subjects are asked to do in the task and what they do when they read. When people are asked to read text and then recall what they read, the task is ecologically valid, but the research findings really deal with the product of the reading process, rather than with the process per se.

Eye movements, on the other hand, are a normal part of reading, so there is no question about the ecological validity of results obtained via examinations of eye movements. When we read, our eyes do not move smoothly across the page of text as our phenomenological impressions imply. Rather, we make a series of eye movements (called *saccades*) separated by periods of time when the eyes are relatively still (called *fixations*). About 10% to 15% of the time, we move our eyes back in the text to look at material our eyes have already passed over; these backwards movements are called *regressions*.

The earliest research endeavors investigating the reading process (summarized by Huey 1908 and Woodworth 1938) relied heavily on eye movement data. More recent endeavors (see Just and Carpenter 1987 and Rayner and Pollatsek 1989) have likewise relied heavily on eye movement data. Indeed, it is my impression that eye movement data often become the final source in adjudicating between alternative empirical findings obtained via different methods typically used to infer something about the reading process.

There are at least four reasons researchers have been interested in eye movements during reading. First, eye movements per se are an interesting topic of investigation. If we can understand eye movement control in reading, we will have learned something important about motor control processes. Second, there are important questions about perceptual processes during reading that can best be examined via investigations using eye movements. For example, how much information do readers acquire during each eye fixation? What kind of information is integrated across eye movements? Third, eye movement data can be used to investigate cognitive processes in reading: fixation times on words and phrases and the pattern of eye movements can be very informative in terms of understanding moment-to-moment comprehension processes. Finally, eye movements may inform us regarding the difficulties encountered by dyslexic readers. Each of these four issues will be discussed in this chapter. I first discuss perceptual processes in reading, then eye movement control, then cognitive processes reflected in eye movements, and conclude by discussing the issue of dyslexia. I begin by describing some additional facts about eye movements in reading.

BASIC FACTS ABOUT EYE MOVEMENTS IN READING

The reason we move our eyes so frequently during reading is directly related to the acuity limitations of the visual system. A line of text falling on the retina of a reader can be divided into three regions. The *foveal* region, in the center of vision, typically extends one degree of visual angle (or three-or four letter spaces) to the left and right of fixation. The *parafoveal* region extends from the foveal region to about five degrees of visual angle from the fixation point. Beyond the parafoveal region, the remainder of the line consists of the *peripheral* region. Although acuity is good in the center of vision, our ability to resolve or discriminate letters deteriorates rapidly from the foveal region to the parafoveal and peripheral regions. Therefore, in order to clearly see the letters and words we wish to process next, we move our eyes so as to place the fovea over the next unprocessed region of the text.

The average fixation duration in reading is 200-250 ms and the average saccade length is roughly eight letter spaces. With respect to the latter average, letter spaces (and not visual angle) is the appropriate metric since the distance the eyes move remains fairly constant despite variations in the number of letters falling within a degree of visual angle (Morrison and Rayner 1981) as long as the size of the print is fairly normal.

It is important to note that the values just cited are averages; if 15 skilled readers' eye movements were recorded as they read text, the average fixation would be between 200 and 250 ms and the average saccade length would be about eight letter spaces. However, there is considerable between subject variability in these measures: some readers' average fixation duration would be around 200 ms, some around 250, and some around 300; some readers' average saccade length would be around six letter spaces, some around eight, and some around ten (as well as seven and nine). Reading rate is a combination of the average fixation time and the number of fixations (which is also reflected by the average saccade length), as well as the frequency of regressions. Obviously then, someone with average fixations of 200 ms and average saccades of ten letter spaces is going to read at a faster rate than someone with an average fixation of 300 ms and average saccade length of seven letter spaces. The more skilled the reader, the shorter the average fixation time, the longer the average saccade length, and the smaller percentage of regressions in comparison to less skilled readers.

While the variability in eye movement measures between readers is interesting, even more interesting is the variability within readers. That is, for any given reader reading a single passage of text, there is considerable variability in fixation durations and saccade lengths: fixation durations will range from under 100 ms to over 500 ms and saccade lengths will range from one letter space to over 15 letter spaces (though long saccades are typically movements following regressions to get the reader back to the original place in the text).

A final point that needs to be made in this section is that text difficulty has a powerful influence on eye movement measures. As the text gets more difficult, fixations get longer, saccades get shorter, and regressions increase.

PERCEPTUAL PROCESSES IN READING

In this section, I will discuss research relevant to two issues. First, I will discuss research dealing with the size of the effective visual field, or perceptual span, in reading. Second, I will discuss research dealing with the type of information that is integrated across successive eye movements in reading.

The Perceptual Span

During each eye fixation, how much useful information are we able to obtain from the text? This question has intrigued researchers interested in reading since the time of Huey (1908). Numerous experimental paradigms have been used to address this issue, but they all either are unlike normal reading or make overly simple assumptions (see Rayner 1978 for greater discussion of these criticisms). A number of years ago, we (McConkie and Rayner 1975; Rayner 1975) developed the eye-contingent display change technique to determine how much useful information is acquired during eye fixations while reading normally. With this technique, readers' eye movements are monitored every millisecond via an accurate eyetracking system that is interfaced with a computer, which in turn is interfaced with a display monitor (with a rapidly decaying phosphor) from which the reader reads. Changes in the text are made at precise times contingent on the location of the reader's eye.

The first type of eye-contingent display technique developed to study the size of the effective visual field was the *moving window* technique (McConkie and Rayner 1975). With this technique, on each fixation, a portion of the text around the reader's fixation is available for processing. However, outside of this window area, the text is replaced by other letters or by x's, for example, as in figure 1. When the reader moves his or her eyes, the window moves with the eyes. Thus, wherever the reader looks, there is readable text within the window; outside of the window, the text is mutilated in some way. The rationale is that when the window is as large as the region from which a reader

What can we learn about reading from studying
                      *
XXXX Xan we learn about XXXXXXX XXXX XXXXXXXX
                      *
XXXX XXX XX learn about readiXX XXXX XXXXXXXX
                           *

Figure 1. Example of the moving window paradigm. The first line shows a normal line of text with the fixation location marked by an asterisk. The next two lines show an example of two successive fixations with a window of 17 letter spaces. In this example, the letters outside of the window are replaced by X's. Letters outside of the window can also be replaced by other letters, and the spaces between words can also be filled in.

can normally obtain information, reading will not differ from when there is no window present.

A number of studies using the moving window technique have led to the conclusion that the span of effective vision extends to about 14-15 letter spaces to the right of fixation for readers of English text (McConkie and Rayner 1975; Rayner 1986; Rayner and Bertera 1979; Rayner et al. 1981; Rayner et al. 1982). Similar results have been obtained with French (O'Regan 1979) and Dutch readers (DenBuurman, Boersema, and Gerrisen 1981). However, the span is asymmetric in that information is obtained from the currently fixated word, but no more than four letter spaces to the left of fixation (McConkie and Rayner 1976; Rayner, Well, and Pollatsek 1980). For readers of right-to-left orthographies, such as Hebrew, the span is asymmetric in the opposite direction extending further to the left than to the right of fixation (Pollatsek et al. 1981). Characteristics of the orthography also influence the size of the span in that more densely packed orthographies, like Chinese and Japanese, yield smaller spans (Ikeda and Saida 1978; Osaka 1992) than English. Likewise, Hebrew, which is more densely packed than English yields a smaller span (Pollatsek et al. 1981). Finally, reading ability affects the size of the span: beginning readers have a smaller span than skilled readers. The span extends to about 11 letter spaces to the right of fixation for children at the end of the first grade, but is asymmetric (Rayner 1986).

All of the research described in the preceding paragraph dealt with the horizontal span of effective vision. Do readers acquire useful information from below the line they are reading? The answer to this question is that they do not (Inhoff and Briihl 1991; Inhoff and Topolski 1992; Pollatsek et al. 1993). If anything, information below the line of fixation potentially interferes with reading so that readers focus their attention on the fixated line and attempt to ignore information below the line. If the task is changed from reading to visual search (using text, with the task to locate a specific target word), it appears that subjects can obtain information from below the fixated line (Pollatsek et al. 1993).

While research utilizing the moving window technique has provided important information concerning the total size of the span of effective vision, it has not been diagnostic of what type of information is obtained within the span. A second technique, referred to as the *boundary* technique (Rayner 1975), has been much more diagnostic about what type of information is acquired within the span. With this technique, a boundary location is specified in the computer and when the reader's eye movement crosses the invisible boundary, an initially displayed word or letter string is replaced by a target word (see figure 2). The amount of time that the reader looks at the target word is then computed as a function of the relationship between the initially displayed stimulus and the target word and as a function of the distance

What can we happy about reading from studying
  *
What can we learn about reading from studying
                *

Figure 2.   An example of the boundary paradigm. The first line shows text prior to a display change with fixation location marked by an asterisk. When the reader's eye movement crosses an invisible boundary (the letter *e* in *we*), an initially displayed word (*happy*) is replaced by the target word (*learn*). The change occurs during the saccade so that the reader does not see the change.

that the reader was from the target word prior to launching the saccade that crossed the boundary.

Research using this paradigm has demonstrated that the span of word identification is smaller than the span of effective vision: readers acquire information used to identify words from the fixated word and sometimes the word to the right of fixation. If three short words occur in succession, readers can identify all three on the current fixation. In general, it appears that the span of word identification extends to about eight letter spaces to the right of fixation (Underwood and McConkie 1985; Rayner and Pollatsek 1987), though this value is somewhat variable depending on the length of the fixated word and the next word.

A variation of the moving window paradigm in which a mask moves with the eyes (see figure 3) has also yielded important information about the type of information obtained within the perceptual span region (Rayner and Bertera 1979; Rayner et al. 1981; Slowiaczek and Rayner 1987). When the mask is larger than seven letters, this situation results in an artificial foveal scotoma for normal readers. Results from these experiments demonstrated that skilled readers find it very difficult, if not impossible, to read when foveal vision is masked. More interestingly, when the mask was 13 letters or larger (so that it extended six letter spaces to the right of fixation), readers made many errors as they tried to read; these errors suggest that readers obtain only

What can we learn about reading from studying
                *
What can weXXXXXXXabout reading from studying
                *
What can we learn XXXXXXXreading from studying
                        *

Figure 3.   An example of the foveal mask paradigm. The first line shows a normal line of text with the fixation location marked by an asterisk. The lower two lines show two successive fixations with a mask of seven letter spaces. As in the moving window paradigm, the mask moves in synchrony with the eyes.

partial information about words in parafoveal vision. The errors are also informative about the type of information that is acquired. For example, the sentence "The pretty bracelet attracted much attention" was read as "The priest brought much ammunition." Clearly, the reader was obtaining information about the beginning and ending letters of words and trying to construct a meaningful representation on the basis of the information acquired.

Integration of Information Across Fixations

Experiments using both the moving window and the boundary paradigms have demonstrated a *preview benefit* from the word to the right of fixation: information obtained about the parafoveal word on fixation *n* is combined with information on fixation *n+1* to speed the identification of the word when it is subsequently fixated. In a number of different experiments, orthographic, phonological, and semantic similarity between the initially displayed stimulus and the target word have been varied to determine the basis of the preview effect.

The results of a number of experiments (Balota, Pollatsek, and Rayner 1985; Rayner 1975; Rayner, McConkie, and Ehrlich 1978; Rayner, McConkie, and Zola 1980) have indicated that the facilitation in processing is due to orthographic similarity: *chest* facilitates the processing of *chart*. However, the facilitation is not due to strictly visual similarity since the case of letters can change from fixation to fixation (so that *ChArT* on one fixation would be *cHaRt* on the next) with little effect on reading behavior (McConkie and Zola 1979; Raynor, McConkie, and Zola 1980). Thus, the facilitation appears to be due to some type of abstract letter code associated with the first few letters of word *n+1* (Rayner et al. 1982). A number of experiments by Inhoff and colleagues (Inhoff 1989, 1990; Inhoff and Tousman 1990) have demonstrated that some information is obtained from other parts of word *n+1* besides beginning letter information. However, it is clear that the bulk of the preview effect comes from the beginning letters. Inhoff's research also shows that the effect is not simply due to spatial proximity since there is facilitation from the beginning letters of words when readers are asked to read sentences from right-to-left, but with the letters within words printed from left-to-right.

Pollatsek at al. (1992) demonstrated that there is facilitation due to phonological similarity so that *beach* facilitates *beech* and *chute* facilitates *shoot* in a boundary experiment. However, there is less facilitation in the latter case than in the former case (though the latter case does result in facilitation in comparison to an unrelated initial stimulus). Finally, there is no facilitation due to semantic similarity, since Rayner, Balota, and Pollatsek (1986) found that *song* as the initial stimulus did not facilitate the processing of *tune* during reading even though the semantically related pairs of words yielded facilitation under typical priming conditions.

In summary, research dealing with the size of the perceptual span and the type of information integrated across fixations has yielded some important conclusions about perceptual processes during reading. First, the perceptual span is quite limited on each fixation: readers acquire information to about 14-15 character spaces to the right of fixation, with the area from which words are identified being even more limited. Second, while readers obtain preview information about to-be-fixated words, the information is not semantic, but appears to consist of abstract letter codes associated with the first few letters of the next word and phonological information.

EYE MOVEMENT CONTROL

What determines where we look next and what determines when we move our eyes? The evidence is now fairly clear that the decision about *where* to move next and the decision about *when* to move are independent processes (Rayner and McConkie 1976). Most of the literature indicates that fixation locations within words in text are determined by low-level visual information obtained in parafoveal vision: the length of a yet-to-be fixated word in parafoveal vision strongly influences where a reader initially fixates in that word (Blanchard, Pollatsek, and Rayner 1989; O'Regan 1979, 1980, 1981; Rayner and Morris 1992) and perturbing word-boundary information (using the eye-contingent technique) also has a major effect on eye movement patterns (Morris, Rayner, and Pollatsek 1990; Pollatsek and Rayner 1982).

Where readers fixate in individual words is somewhat systematic; that is, the initial fixation on a word tends to be about halfway between the beginning and middle of a word (McConkie et al. 1988; McConkie et al. 1989; O'Regan 1981; Rayner 1979). This phenomenon was labeled the *preferred viewing location* by Rayner (1979). More recently, O'Regan and Levy-Schoen (1987) made a distinction between the preferred viewing location and what O'Regan (1981) originally termed the *convenient viewing location* when describing the same phenomenon. The distinction that has been made is that the preferred viewing location is where the eyes land in the word, whereas the convenient viewing location or *optimal viewing location* (as O'Regan and colleagues now refer to it) is the location in the word where readers can obtain maximal information about the word. Thus, the optimal viewing location is a bit to the right of the preferred viewing location and closer to the center of the word. The reason for this could be due to some inherent property of the oculomotor system (such that the eye typically undershoots targets) or it could be due to the preview effect discussed above. That is, readers may often move their eyes to a position in a word that coincides with the point at which they need to get further information about the word given that they have already processed the first few letters of the word on the prior fixation. Thus, if the first two letters of a seven-letter word were identified parafoveally on fixation n, the reader would move to the third or fourth letter of the word on fixation $n+1$ to obtain the maximal amount of information. The position the eye lands on would not strictly coincide with the point at which new information is needed because readers can acquire information to the left of fixation (Rayner, Well, and Pollatsek 1980).

The type of model of eye movement control consistent with most of the data is one in which parafoveally obtained word length information is the primary determinant of where to look next. In essence, the critical information obtained parafoveally is sublexical and presemantic. However, lexical and semantic information are clearly involved in eye movement control during reading. According to a model proposed by Morrison (1984) and subsequently amplified by Rayner and Balota (1989) and Pollatsek and Rayner (1990), lexical access of the fixated word serves as the trigger for an eye movement. In this type of model, when the fixated word is identified, attention shifts to the next word, and a saccade follows in a time-locked fashion to a fixation location based on word-length cues. However, words can occasionally be identified without direct fixation (they are identified parafoveally), and when they are, the fixation prior to skipping the word is inflated (Hogaboam 1983; Pollatsek, Rayner, and Balota 1986). In addition, factors such as contextual constraint can influence the process because more parafoveal preview is obtained from parafoveal words that are highly predictable (Balota, Pollatsek, and Rayner 1985). Finally, when the fixated word is difficult to process, little or no preview benefit is obtained because foveal processing takes precedence over parafoveal processing (Henderson and Ferreira 1990; Inhoff et al. 1989; Rayner 1986).

Morrison's model has the interesting feature of being able to account for short fixations in text during reading. Given what is known about the reaction time of the eyes (see Rayner et al. 1983), fixations under 140 ms should not occur in reading. However, fixations as short as 50 ms are occasionally noted in eye movement records of reading behavior. Morrison's model accounts for these short fixations by assuming that sometimes the reader identifies word $n+1$ while still fixating on word n but that he or she is so far into the program of the next saccade that it cannot be aborted. In such instances, the program for a second saccade is initiated to word $n+2$ while the reader is still fixated on word n. This concept of parallel programming of saccades thus accounts for short fixations.

While there are other extant models of eye movement control (see O'Regan 1990), the emerging view is one in which the decision about where to fixate next is largely made on the basis of low-level visual cues obtained parafoveally, and the decision about when to move the eyes is based primarily on cognitive processes associated with comprehending the fixated word. However, the decision about where to fixate next can be influenced by lexical processing if the parafoveal word to the right of fixation is identified and skipped by the ensuing saccade. As noted earlier, if two (or three) short words are in the center of fixation, they may all be identified on the current fixation. In such a situation, word length information about the next unidentified parafoveal word would be the basis for deciding where to fixate next. With respect to the decision about when to move the eyes, processes that are higher level than lexical access can also influence the decision of when to move (see Pollatsek and Rayner 1990, for further discussion).

COGNITIVE PROCESSES ARE REFLECTED IN EYE FIXATIONS

A topic of considerable debate involves the extent to which eye movements reflect cognitive processes in reading. According to some views (Bouma and deVoogd 1974; Kolers 1976), there is a significant *eye-mind span* so that information obtained on a given eye fixation would not be available for higher level cognitive processing until the eyes had moved on to another location. However, a considerable amount of research (Just and Carpenter 1980; Rayner and Pollatsek 1981; see Rayner and Pollatsek 1989, for further details) now suggests that the link between the eye and the mind is fairly tight.

The reason the link is fairly tight is that (1) readers typically have a preview of word $n+1$ prior to fixating it (as discussed earlier in this chapter), and (2) readers can extract information from text quickly during each eye fixation. With respect to the latter point, Rayner et al. 1981; (see also Slowiaczek and Rayner 1987; Ishida and Ikeda 1989) presented a visual mask at various points after the onset of a fixation. They found that if the reader had 50 ms to process the text prior to the onset of the mask, reading proceeded quite normally. If the text was masked earlier than that, reading was disturbed. While readers may typically acquire the visual information needed for reading during the first 50 ms of a fixation, it is also clear that they can obtain information at other times during the fixation as needed (Blanchard et al. 1984). But, the fact that information needed for reading is obtained so early in a fixation means that there is time left over during a fixation for cognitive processes to influence the fixation time (since the reader also programs where to move next in parallel with comprehending the fixated word).

Other research demonstrates more directly that the lag between what the eye is fixating and what the mind is processing is quite tight.

For example, effects due to eye-contingent display changes show up immediately on the fixation following a display change, and are not delayed for a couple of fixations. It has also been demonstrated that, with word length controlled, low frequency words yield longer fixation times than high frequency words (Just and Carpenter 1980; Inhoff and Rayner 1986; Rayner and Duffy 1986; Rayner, Sereno, Morris, Schmauder, and Clifton 1989). Furthermore, words that are highly constrained or predictable, given the context, are fixated for less time than words that are not so constrained or predictable (Balota, Pollatsek, and Rayner 1985; Ehrlich and Rayner 1981; Schustack, Ehrlich, and Rayner 1987; Zola 1984). If there were an appreciable eye-mind lag, effects such as these would not show up on the current fixation, but would be delayed for a couple of fixations.

The general finding (noted above) that the area of effective vision and the word identification span are small (so that readers typically identify only the fixated word) coupled with the conclusion that there is no appreciable eye-mind span has led to considerable optimism concerning the use of eye movement data to investigate cognitive processes during reading. Indeed, during the past few years, there has been considerable research using eye movement data to investigate (1) how readers parse sentences containing temporary syntactic ambiguities, (2) the processing of lexically ambiguous words, and (3) inferences during reading. It is beyond the scope of the present chapter to review all of these lines of research (see Rayner and Sereno 1994 for further discussion). The point is that eye movement data have revealed a great deal of important information about moment-to-moment cognitive processes during the reading process. Variations in how long readers look at certain target words or phrases in text have been shown to be due to the ease or difficulty associated with processing those words.

EYE MOVEMENTS AND DYSLEXIA

Can eye movements tell us anything about developmental dyslexia? Dyslexic readers' eye movements differ from those of skilled readers in that they make many more fixations per line, have longer fixations, shorter saccades, and a higher frequency of regressions than skilled readers (Rayner 1978). Are eye movements a contributing causative factor in developmental dyslexia?

From a practical standpoint, if an eye movement control deficit were at the root of the dyslexic's problem, the disability could be diagnosed via simple oculomotor tests. In addition, perhaps dyslexics could be helped by training programs designed to improve their reading by focusing on eye movement control exercises. Related to this, it has often been assumed that skilled readers and dyslexic readers differ in that the former execute smooth, efficient eye movements whereas the latter have highly erratic and unpredictable eye movement patterns. However, the suggestion that good readers execute regular eye movement patterns, and that therefore poor readers can be trained to be better readers by teaching them to make smooth consistent eye movements is not supported by the data. As noted earlier, good readers are highly variable in both how long the fixation lasts and how far they move their eyes.

While readers with some type of oculomotor disturbance such as saccade intrusion (Ciuffreda, Kenyon, and Stark 1983) or congenital jerk nystagmus (Ciuffreda 1979) will have difficulty reading, most of the data currently available suggest that eye movements are a reflection of the processing activities associated with reading and not a cause of reading problems. In contrast to this conclusion, Pavlidis (1981, 1985, 1991) has reported a number of studies demonstrating that dyslexic readers exhibit abnormal eye movement patterns in non-reading tasks. In particular, he found that when dyslexic and normal readers were asked to fixate sequentially on targets that step across a display screen, the dyslexics have much more difficulty doing so than normal readers (particularly when the target moves from left-to-right). However, it is important to note that a number of attempts to replicate Pavlidis' findings have been unsuccessful (see Olson, Conners, and Rack 1991; and Rayner 1985 for summaries). While there have been case studies reported (Zangwill and Blakemore 1972; Pirozzolo and Rayner 1978) in which dyslexic readers manifest erratic eye movements like those reported by Pavlidis' subjects, the evidence does not suggest that eye movements per se are the problem. Rather, the data in these case studies suggest that the eye movements reflect a serious spatial orientation problem.

It has also been suggested that a difference between skilled and dyslexic readers is that the latter have a smaller perceptual span, and that this is a cause of their reading deficiency. However, the available evidence (Rayner 1986; Rayner, Murphy, Henderson, and Pollatsek 1989) suggests that the smaller perceptual span in dyslexic readers is due to difficulty processing the text. That is, so much of their attention is taken up processing the fixated word that they obtain little parafoveal information. Thus, it seems safe to conclude that the smaller perceptual span and erratic eye movements are symptoms, rather than causes, of developmental dyslexia.

CONCLUSIONS

I began this chapter by asserting that we have learned more about reading from studies of eye movements than any other source of data. Although numerous techniques have been used to study the reading process, for the most part one has to question the extent to which results obtained from tasks that differ from normal silent reading are generalizable to the reading process. Eye movements, on the other hand, are a normal part of silent (and oral) reading. When eye movement data represent the dependent variable in a reading study, readers presumably read in the same manner as they would normally do outside of the laboratory. Indeed, data collected by Tinker (1939) many years ago show quite clearly that reading rate and comprehension are the same when subjects' eye movements are recorded in an eye movement laboratory and when they read in a soft easy chair outside of the laboratory.

Eye movement data can be obtained in relatively unobtrusive ways and one need not rely on secondary tasks (which may lead to unusual processing strategies) nor make questionable generalizations from tasks (such as lexical decision, naming, categorization, and tachistoscopic identification) which may or may not resemble reading. Eye movement data also provide for finer resolutions than can be obtained from more gross measures (such as reading time or question answering): specific effects can be localized at precise points in the text.

In this chapter, I have sketched some of the findings that have been obtained recently from studies of eye movements and reading. As I hope the present chapter makes clear, we have learned a lot about issues such as (1) the size of the effective visual field in reading, (2) where readers fixate in words, (3) what kind of information is integrated across fixations, and (4) eye movement control in reading. As important as the findings concerning these issues are, perhaps even more important is the fact that eye movement data are being used successfully to examine a number of issues related to cognitive and perceptual processes during reading. Since the (1) size of the effective visual field is small and (2) the eye-mind span is quite tight, it has become apparent that eye movement data can be used in a number of ways to examine important issues concerning moment-to-moment processes in reading.

While there is, therefore, considerable optimism concerning the use of eye movement data to study reading processes, I am considerably less optimistic about using eye movement data to infer something important about developmental dyslexia. As I have noted in a number of places in this chapter, eye movement patterns (where readers look and how long they look at particular words) primarily reflect the processes associated with comprehending the fixated words. Although dyslexic readers tend to have longer fixations and more forward and regressive fixations, the eye movements per se are not the problem. Rather, eye movements reflect the problems that dyslexic readers have comprehending text. To the extent that eye movements are used to infer processing difficulties of dyslexic readers (see Rayner, Murphy, Henderson, and Pollatsek 1989), they are useful measures. But, erratic eye movements in reading and non-reading situations do not seem to characterize most dyslexic readers.

ACKNOWLEDGEMENTS

The author's research is supported by Grant HD26765 from the National Institute of Child Health and Human Development and Grant DBS-9121375 from the National Science Foundation.

REFERENCES

Balota, D. A., Pollatsek, A., and Rayner, K. 1985. The interaction of contextual constraints and parafoveal visual information in reading. *Cognitive Psychology* 17:364–90.

Blanchard, H. E., McConkie, G. W., Zola, D., and Wolverton, G. S. 1984. Time course of visual information utilization during fixations in reading. *Perception & Psychophysics* 10:75–89.

Blanchard, H. E., Pollatsek, A., and Rayner, K. 1989. The acquisition of para-foveal word information in reading. *Perception & Psychophysics* 46:85–94.

Bouma, H., and deVoogd, A. H. 1974. On the control of eye saccades in reading. *Vision Research* 14:273–84.

Ciuffreda, K. J. 1979. Jerk nystagmus: Some new findings. *American Journal of Optometry and Physiological Optics* 53:389–95.

Ciuffreda, K. J., Kenyon, R. W., and Stark, L. 1983. Saccadic intrusions contributing to reading difficulty: A case report. *American Journal of Optometry and Physiological Optics* 60:242–49.

DenBuurman, R., Boersema, T., and Gerrisen, J. F. 1981. Eye movements and the perceptual span in reading. *Reading Research Quarterly* 16:227–35.

Ehrlich, S. F., and Rayner, K. 1981. Contextual effects on word perception and eye movements during reading. *Journal of Verbal Learning and Verbal Behavior* 20:641–55.

Henderson, J. M., and Ferreira, F. 1990. Effects of foveal processing difficulty on the perceptual span in reading: Implications for attention and eye movement control. *Journal of Experimental Psychology: Learning, Memory, and Cognition* 16:417–29.

Hogaboam, T. W. 1983. Reading patterns in eye movement data. In *Eye Movements in Reading: Perceptual and Language Processes*, ed. K. Rayner. New York: Academic Press.

Huey, E. B. 1908. *The Psychology and Pedagogy of Reading.* New York: Macmillan.

Ikeda, M., and Saida, S. 1978. Span of recognition in reading. *Vision Research* 18:83–88.

Inhoff, A. W. 1989. Lexical access during eye fixations in reading: Are word codes used to integrate lexical information across interword fixations? *Journal of Memory and Language* 28:444–61.

Inhoff, A. W. 1990. Integrating information across eye fixations in reading: The role of letter and word units. *Acta Psychologica* 73:281–97.

Inhoff, A. W., and Briihl, D. 1991. Semantic processing of unattended text during selective reading: How the eyes see it. *Perception & Psychophysics* 49:289–94.

Inhoff, A. W., Pollatsek, A., Posner, M. I., and Rayner, K. 1989. Covert attention and eye movements during reading. *Quarterly Journal of Experimental Psychology* 41A:63–89.

Inhoff, A. W., and Rayner, K. 1986. Parafoveal word processing during eye fixations in reading: Effects of word frequency. *Perception and Psychophysics* 40:431–39.

Inhoff, A. W., and Topolski, R. 1992. Lack of semantic activation from unattended text during passage reading. *Bulletin of the Psychonomic Society* 30:365–66.

Inhoff, A. W., and Tousman, S. 1990. Lexical priming from partial-word previews. *Journal of Experimental Psychology: Learning, Memory, and Cognition* 16:825–36.

Ishida, T., and Ikeda, M. 1989. Temporal properties of information extraction in reading studied by a text-mask replacement technique. *Journal of the Optical Society of America A* 6:1624–32.

Just, M. A., and Carpenter, P. A. 1980. A theory of reading: From eye fixations to comprehension. *Psychological Review* 87:329–54.

Just, M. A., and Carpenter, P. A. 1987. *The Psychology of Reading and Language Processing*. Newton, MA: Allyn and Bacon.

Kolers, P. A. 1976. Buswell's discoveries. In *Eye Movements and Psychological Processes*, eds. R. A. Monty and J. W. Senders. Hillsdale, NJ: Lawrence Erlbaum Associates.

McConkie, G. W., Kerr, P. W., Reddix, M. D., and Zola, D. 1988. Eye movement control during reading: I. The location of initial eye fixations on words. *Vision Research* 28:1107–18.

McConkie, G. W., Kerr, P. W., Reddix, M. D., Zola, D., and Jacobs, A. M. 1989. Eye movement control during reading: II. Frequency of refixating a word. *Perception & Psychophysics* 46:245–53.

McConkie, G. W., and Rayner, K. 1975. The span of the effective stimulus during a fixation in reading. *Perception & Psychophysics* 17:578–86.

McConkie, G. W., and Rayner, K. 1976. Asymmetry of the perceptual span in reading. *Bulletin of the Psychonomic Society* 8:365–68.

McConkie, G. W., and Zola, D. 1979. Is visual information integrated across successive fixations in reading? *Perception & Psychophysics* 25:221–24.

Morris, R. K., Rayner, K., and Pollatsek, A. 1990. Eye movement guidance in reading: The role of parafoveal letter and space information. *Journal of Experimental Psychology: Human Perception and Performance* 16:268–81.

Morrison, R. E. 1984. Manipulation of stimulus onset delay in reading: Evidence for parallel programming of saccades. *Journal of Experimental Psychology: Human Perception and Performance* 10:667–82.

Morrison, R. E., and Rayner, K. 1981. Saccade size in reading depends upon character spaces and not visual angle. *Perception & Psychophysics* 30:395–96.

Olson, R. K., Conners, F. A., and Rack, J. P. 1991. Eye movements in dyslexia and normal readers. In *Vision and Visual Dyslexia*, ed. J. F. Stein. London: Macmillan.

O'Regan, J. K. 1979. Eye guidance in reading: Evidence for the linguistic control hypothesis. *Perception & Psychophysics* 25:501–09.

O'Regan, J. K. 1980. The control of saccade size and fixation duration in reading. *Perception & Psychophysics* 28:112–17.

O'Regan, J. K. 1981. The convenient viewing hypothesis. In *Eye Movements: Cognition and Visual Perception*, eds. D. F. Fisher, R. A. Monty, and J. W. Senders. Hillsdale, NJ: Lawrence Erlbaum Associates.

O'Regan, J. K. 1990. Eye Movements and Reading. In *Eye Movements and Their Role in Visual and Cognitive Processes*, ed. E. Kowler. Amsterdam: Elsevier.

O'Regan, J. K., and Levy-Schoen, A. 1987. Eye movement strategy and tactics in word recognition and reading. In *Attention and Performance 12*, ed. M. Coltheart. London: Erlbaum.

Osaka, N. 1992. Size of saccade and fixation duration of eye movements during reading: Psychophysics of Japanese text processing. *Journal of the Optical Society of America A* 9:5–13.

Pavlidis, G. T. 1981. Do eye movements hold the key to dyslexia? *Neuropsychologia* 19:57–64.

Pavlidis, G. T. 1985. Eye movement differences between dyslexics, normal and slow readers while sequentially fixating digits. *American Journal of Optometry and Physiological Optics* 62:820–22.

Pavlidis, G. T. 1991. Diagnostic significance and relationship between dyslexia and erratic eye movements. In *Vision and Visual Dyslexia*, ed. J. F. Stein. London: Macmillan.

Pirozzolo, F. J., and Rayner, K. 1978. The normal control of eye movements in acquired and developmental reading disorders. In *Advances in Neurolinguistics and Psycholinguistics*, eds. H. Avakian-Whitaker and H. A. Whitaker. New York: Academic Press.

Pollatsek, A., Bolozky, S., Well, A. D., and Rayner, K. 1981. Asymmetries in the perceptual span for Israeli readers. *Brain and Language* 14:174–80.

Pollatsek, A., Lesch, M., Morris, R. K., and Rayner, K. 1992. Phonological codes are used in integrating information across saccides in word identification and reading. *Journal of Experimental Psychology: Human Perception and Performance* 18:148–62.

Pollatsek, A., and Rayner, K. 1982. Eye movement control in reading: The role of word boundaries. *Journal of Experimental Psychology: Human Perception and Performance* 8:817–33.

Pollatsek, A., and Rayner, K. 1990. Eye movements and lexical access in reading. In *Comprehension Processes in Reading*, eds. D. A. Balota, G. B. Flores d'Arcais, and K. Rayner. Hillsdale, NJ: Lawrence Erlbaum Associates.

Pollatsek, A., Rayner, K., and Balota, D. A. 1986. Inferences about eye movement control from the perceptual span in reading. *Perception & Psychophysics* 40:123–30.

Pollatsek, A., Raney, G. E., LaGasse, L., and Rayner, K. 1993. The use of information below fixation in reading and in visual search. *Canadian Journal of Experimental Psychology* 47:179–200.

Rayner, K. 1975. The perceptual span and peripheral cues in reading. *Cognitive Psychology* 7:65–81.

Rayner, K. 1978. Eye movements in reading and information processing. *Psychological Bulletin* 85:618–60.

Rayner, K. 1979. Eye guidance in reading: Fixation locations within words. *Perception* 8:21–30.

Rayner, K. 1985. Do faulty eye movements cause dyslexia? *Developmental Neuropsychology* 1:3–15.

Rayner, K. 1986. Eye movements and the perceptual span in beginning and skilled readers. *Journal of Experimental Child Psychology* 41:211–36.

Rayner, K., and Balota, D. A. 1989. Parafoveal preview effects and lexical access during eye fixations in reading. In *Lexical Representation and Process*, ed. W. Marlsen-Wilson. Cambridge, MA: MIT Press.

Rayner, K., Balota, D. A., and Pollatsek, A. 1986. Against parafoveal semantic preprocessing during eye fixations in reading. *Canadian Journal of Psychology* 40:473–78.

Rayner, K., and Bertera, J. H. 1979. Reading without a fovea. *Science* 206:468–69.

Rayner, K., and Duffy, S. A. 1986. Lexical complexity and fixation times in reading: Effects of word frequency, verb complexity, and lexical ambiguity. *Memory & Cognition* 14:191–201.

Rayner, K., Inhoff, A. W., Morrison, R. E., Slowiaczek, M. L., and Bertera, J. H. 1981. Masking of foveal and parafoveal vision during eye fixations in reading. *Journal of Experimental Psychology: Human Perception and Performance* 7:169–79.

Rayner, K., and McConkie, G. W. 1976. What guides a reader's eye movements? *Vision Research* 16:829–37.

Rayner, K., McConkie, G. W., and Ehrlich, S. F. 1978. Eye movements and integrating information across fixations. *Journal of Experimental Psychology: Human Perception and Performance* 4:529–44.

Rayner, K., McConkie, G. W., and Zola, D. 1980. Integrating information across eye movements. *Cognitive Psychology* 12: 206–26.

Rayner, K., and Morris, R. K. 1992. Eye movement control in reading: Evidence against semantic preprocessing. *Journal of Experimental Psychology: Human Perception and Performance* 18:163–72.

Rayner, K., Murphy, L. A., Henderson, J. M., and Pollatsek, A. 1989. Selective attentional dyslexia. *Cognitive Neuropsychology* 6:357–78.

Rayner, K., and Pollatsek, A. 1981. Eye movement control during reading: Evidence for direct control. *Quarterly Journal of Experimental Psychology* 33A:351–73.

Rayner, K., and Pollatsek, A. 1987. Eye movements in reading: A tutorial review. In *Attention and Performance 12*, ed. M. Coltheart. London: Erlbaum.

Rayner, K., and Pollatsek, A. 1989. *The Psychology of Reading.* Englewood Cliffs, NJ: Prentice Hall.

Rayner, K., and Sereno, S. C. 1994. Eye movements in reading: Psycholinguistic studies. In *Handbook of Psycholinguistics*, ed. M. A. Gernsbacher. San Diego, CA: Academic Press.

Rayner, K., Sereno, S. C., Morris, R. K., Schmauder, A. R., and Clifton, C. 1989. Eye movements and on-line language comprehension processes. *Language and Cognitive Processes* 4 (Special Issue):21–50.

Rayner, K., Slowiaczek, M. L., Clifton, C., and Bertera, J. H. 1983. Latency of sequential eye movements: Implications for reading. *Journal of Experimental Psychology: Human Perception and Performance* 9:912–22.

Rayner, K., Well, A. D., and Pollatsek, A. 1980. Asymmetry of the effective visual field in reading. *Perception & Psychophysics* 27:537–44.

Rayner, K., Well, A. D., Pollatsek, A., and Bertera, J. H. 1982. The availability of useful information to the right of fixation in reading. *Perception and Psychophysics* 31:537–50.

Schustack, M. W., Ehrlich, S. F., and Rayner, K. 1987. The complexity of contextual facilitation in reading: Local and global influences. *Journal of Memory and Language* 26:322–40.

Slowiaczek, M. L., and Rayner, K. 1987. Sequential masking during eye fixations in reading. *Bulletin of the Psychonomic Society* 25:175–78.

Tinker, M. A. 1939. Reliability and validity of eye-movement measures of reading. *Journal of Experimental Psychology* 19:732–46.

Underwood, N. R., and McConkie, G. W. 1985. Perceptual span for letter distinctions during reading. *Reading Research Quarterly* 20:153–62.

Woodworth, R. S. 1938. *Experimental Psychology*. New York: Holt.

Zangwill, O. L., and Blakemore, C. 1972. Dyslexia: Reversal of eye movements during reading. *Neuropsychologia* 10:117–26.

Zola, D. 1984. Redundancy and word perception during reading. *Perception & Psychophysics* 36:277–84.

Chapter • 6

Visual System and Reading

John F. Stein

Until 20 years ago it was generally agreed that some kind of defect of visual processing was likely to underlie most children's reading difficulties. Morgan used the term "word blindness" and Orton, "strephosymbolia" to emphasize this point. More recently this view has come under attack however, and now most people believe that visual perceptual deficits seldom, if ever, cause children's reading problems (Vellutino 1987).

There were two main reasons for the change of opinion. First the evidence became overwhelming that development of phonological skill is a most important prerequisite of learning to read (Liberman et al. 1977; Bradley and Bryant 1983). Of course, this finding did not by itself rule out the possibility that a child's visual processing skills may contribute to his reading progress. But additional evidence accumulated that seemed to show that children's visual skills did not correlate at all with reading ability (Olson et al. 1989). Hence it was reasonable to conclude that visual skills do not set any limits on children's reading. Nevertheless, in this chapter I want to try to put the clock back to show that aquisition of visual perceptual skill does, after all, play a major part in learning to read.

To preview my argument briefly: Many children with reading problems complain that words and letters appear to move around when they try to read; in other words, they seem to experience mild oscillopsia. We, and others, have shown that when viewing small tar-

gets such as letters their binocular fixation is less stable than that of
normal children (Fowler and Stein 1980; Bishop, Jancey, and Steel 1979;
Masters 1988; Bigelow and McKenzie 1985; Evans, Drasdo, and
Richards 1994; Stein and Fowler 1993). These uncontrolled eye movements cause words and letters to appear to move around and blur.
Children with such unstable binocular fixation experience visual confusion. Therefore, they tend to make visual reading and spelling errors
(Stein and Fowler 1985; Cornelissen et al. 1991, 1992, 1994). This suggests that visual skills do, after all, play an important part in learning
to read. Accordingly, I will demonstrate that, contrary to strongly held
opinions, visual perceptual abilities do, in fact, correlate very well with
reading performance in both good and bad readers (Eden, Stein, and
Wood 1993; Eden et al. 1994). Unstable visuomotor control may be a
consequence of an abnormality of the magnocellular, "transient," component of the visual processing system (Lovegrove 1991; Livingstone
et al. 1991; Mason et al. 1993). Since the visual abnormalities of dyslexics are normally accompanied by phonological abnormalities, it is a
false antithesis to present phonological and visual problems as necessarily mutually exclusive. Normally, dyslexics suffer both kinds of
problems (Stein and Fowler 1985; Eden, Stein, and Wood 1993). These
considerations lead me to my final speculation, namely that funda-
mentally both the phonological and visual difficulties of dyslexics may
result from a generalized abnormality of the magnocellular system of
neurons in their central nervous systems (CNS).

DYSLEXICS' OSCILLOPSIA

"The letters move around on the page, so I can't tell what they're
meant to look like or what order they're in." "The letters hover over
the page." "The 'e' moves over the 'c' so that it looks like an 'r'." These
are all remarks made to me by children with reading problems.
Listening to them I was reminded of the symptoms of oscillopsia, of
which many patients with uncontrolled eye movements complain. In
gross form oscillopsia causes the whole world to appear to be in continuous motion. But in mild form small involuntary eye movements may
give rise to the apparent motion of small targets only, perhaps because
larger targets are more easily stabilized in the "mind's eye" by cognitive
processes.

The symptoms described by these children invite the question;
how do we normally manage to keep our perceptual view of the world
stationary despite the frequent eye movements that we make? Each
time we move our eyes, images smear across the retina; yet most of
the time the world does not appear to move around. A century of
experiments in this field has shown that we use every cue available to

decide whether it is our own eyes or objects in the outside world that are moving (Grusser 1982). In essence however, the problem reduces to one of being able to associate correctly the retinal images with which vision supplies us, with eye movement signals provided by the oculomotor system. Before the eyes move, these are provided by corollary discharges that inform the visual system, probably at the level of the posterior parietal cortex (Stein 1992), that the eyes are about to move (Duhamel, Colby, and Goldberg 1992). Once the movement has commenced, feedback from orbital proprioceptors reports back on its progress (Anderson, Essick, and Siegel, 1985). During development, retinal and oculomotor signals must therefore come to be correctly associated with each other, so that under most circumstances we do not see objects appear to move around when our eyes do; only when these associations are correctly made are we able to locate objects accurately and stably with respect to ourselves.

Correct association of retinal and oculomotor signals poses particularly difficult problems when the eyes are converged on a small target as when reading, because under these conditions the angles of the eyes with respect to the head give potentially different indications of its location. Only when the angles of the eyes have been calibrated in terms of their distance apart can the direction and distance of the target be correctly computed. Again, it seems that the posterior parietal cortex, particularly that in the right hemisphere in humans, plays a central role in these calculations (Fowler et al. 1989).

These considerations make it clear that perceptual stability of the visual world, hence our ability to localize targets accurately, depends greatly upon proper functioning of the binocular vergence control system; this provides stable eye fixation, hence accurate eye position signals. We therefore wondered whether the visual symptoms of children with reading problems, which I describe earlier, might be the result of a defect of their binocular control. So in 1978 Sue Fowler and I began looking for instability of eye fixation in these children (Fowler and Stein 1979, 1980; Stein and Fowler 1982). We have been comparing the binocular fixation stability and vergence control of children with dyslexia with that of normal-reading children and correlating our findings with measurements of the accuracy of their visual direction sense and the nature of their visual errors when reading. We have also been searching for techniques that might improve children's oculomotor control to see whether improving this motor function might help them to learn to read (Stein and Fowler 1985).

SUBJECTS

Most of our subjects are referred to us because they have serious reading problems. Our clinic is well known in the area; it is situated in the Royal

Berks Eye Hospital, Reading, U.K. We receive referrals from general practitioners, school medical officers, local educational psychologists, and so forth. Initially we used the Neal Analysis of reading to define a group of children whom we could describe as "dyslexic." If their reading was more than 18 months behind their chronological age and they had IQs above 90 they were so termed. We now use the British Ability Scales (BAS) IQ test; and we classify children on the basis of discrepancy between their reading and IQ. Following Thompson (1982), we define children as dyslexic if their reading ability is more than 2 standard deviations behind that expected from their scores in the similarities or matrice subtests of the BAS.

We have also studied unselected groups of primary school children between the ages of 7–11. As control groups to compare with the dyslexics we have used either normal readers matched on chronological age, sex, and IQ; or younger normal readers, matched for reading age, sex, and IQ. The latter were recruited on the advice of Lynette Bradley (1983) in order to refute the argument that dyslexics may have more unstable ocular motor control simply because they have less reading experience. Normal readers will have had much more reading experience than dyslexics of the same age, so any visual superiority the normal readers show might well be the result, rather than the cause, of their reading superiority. However, younger normal readers with the same reading age as the dyslexics will have had the same reading experience; so any visual superiority they show is likely to be primary, and thus probably a cause of their reading superiority rather than merely a result of it.

BINOCULAR INSTABILITY

We adapted a test developed by Patricia Dunlop (1972) for determining the "dominant," "leading," or "reference" eye in a binocular situation in order to assess the binocular stability of our subjects. In our version of the test, two fusion slides depicting a central front door are presented separately to the two eyes in a synoptophore. This is a stereoscope with adjustable eye tubes, also known as a *major amblyoscope*. The child fuses the slides, and the synoptophore tubes are then slowly diverged. The slide seen by the left eye has a post to the right of the door, and that seen by the right eye a different post to the left of the door. Just before fusion breaks, most subjects see one of the posts appear to move towards the door; and when the test is repeated ten times it is always the post on the same side that appears to move. That on the other side never does so. Such subjects are said to have stable or fixed reference. However, if a subject reports that both posts move or different ones appear to move on more than two occasions out of the ten he or she is said to have unfixed reference. Thus the test indicates how consistently a child is able to associate monocular retinal and oculomotor cues during vergence stress. As mentioned earlier, such binocular conditions are particularly relevant to reading because when reading, small letters are viewed at about 25 cms with the eyes converged and they have to be accurately located and reliably sequenced. Moreover when reading, the vergence angle has to be altered slightly with each fixation.

We found that a very high proportion of dyslexic children had unstable binocular control using this test (52–69% in different studies [Stein, Riddell, and Fowler 1987; Fowler 1991]); whereas a far smaller proportion of normal readers, whether matched for chronological or reading age, showed such instability. These results suggest not just that there is an association, but a clear causal connection between unstable binocular control and poor reading. The younger reading-age-matched normal readers had better binocular control; and this enabled them to read as well as the older dyslexics even though their reading experience was just as limited.

It has been argued that our findings are unreliable because the dyslexics were referrals to an eye hospital and therefore might have been selected to have visual problems, whereas our normal controls were recruited from local primary schools. We therefore carried out a large scale study of unselected primary school children (Stein, Riddell, and Fowler 1986). We assessed the binocular stability of nearly 1000 children in local primary schools (both good and bad readers aged from 6–12 years) and we compared their binocular control with their reading. This study taught us two important things. First, the binocular stability of all the children improved as they grew older; thus only 54% of 6 year olds had achieved stability, but 70% of 7 year olds and 85% of 9 year olds had done so. This normal developmental trend must always be taken into account when interpreting the results of ocular motor tests.

Our second important result confirmed our previous finding in the clinic sample that instability in the Dunlop Test is indeed associated with reading problems. Comparing children of similar ages showed that those who had stable binocular control were on average 6.3 months better at reading than those with unstable control. This difference remained significant even after the effects of age and IQ had been allowed for. Thus, we could generalize our finding from our clinic sample, that a high proportion of dyslexics have unstable binocular control, to an unselected population of primary school children. Those who had worse binocular control were likely to be worse readers.

We have recently confirmed this result in another way by following a cohort of children from their entry into primary school for three years. Those who started with stable binocular control were significantly better readers at the end of the first, second, and third years than those who did not; and the rate at which children developed stable control was a strong predictor of their reading progress.

It must be admitted, however, that our ideas are considered highly controversial. Although our major result has been confirmed by a number of other groups (Bishop, Jancey, and Steel 1979; Masters 1988; Bigelow and McKenzie 1985; Dunlop 1979), it has also been heavily criticized (Newman et al. 1985; Bishop 1989; Evans and Drasdo 1990). The main reason for this is that the Dunlop Test is not an easy test to use, especially in inexperienced hands. It requires a child to report accurately his perceptions in a complex situation; and the experimenter has to be alert to the common tendency of children to attempt to second guess what they think the tester wants to hear. The random results of these attempts give rise to the possibility of a high proportion of false positives (Newman et al. 1985; Evans and Drasdo 1990). Therefore, we have been trying to find a more objective test for binocular instability. Using infrared eye movement recording we have measured children's fixation stability when reading and when attempting to fixate small targets at the reading distance; and we have tried to quantify children's vergence stability under different conditions.

FIXATION INSTABILITY

Figure 1a shows recordings (Eden, Stein, and Wood 1993) of the positions of the two eyes when two children were attempting to keep their eyes fixed for 5 seconds on a small (0.5 degree) target at a viewing distance of 30 cms. It is easy to see that the child with unstable binocular control in the Dunlop Test showed considerably larger unwanted eye movements than the normal-reading child. We were able to confirm

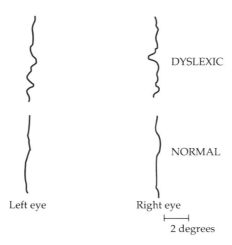

Figure 1a.   Five second recordings of a dyslexic and a non-dyslexic subject fixating on a small target at the reading distance.

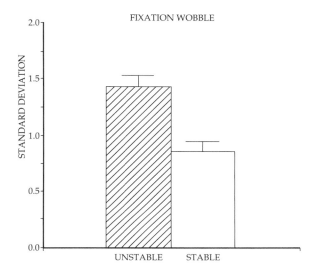

Figure 1b. Standard deviation from the mean fixation point of 30 dyslexic and 30 non-dyslexic subjects when fixating on a small target at the reading distance for five seconds.

that dyslexics as a group have more unstable fixation than normal controls, and that this correlates with their Dunlop Test responses (figure 1b). However, the amplitude of the unwanted eye movements that these children make during attempted fixation is never larger than one degree; so measuring them routinely in dyslexic children is not a viable proposition.

Another approach we have taken is to measure the vergence movements made during the Dunlop Test to see whether there are any clear differences between those of children who pass or fail it (Stein, Riddell, and Fowler 1988). We were able to show that those who failed the test had a more limited vergence range, particularly in divergence, than normals. This result has been confirmed by others (Evans, Drasdo, and Richards 1993). However, because children may be differently motivated to perform this time-consuming and not very exciting test, again it has not proved suitable for routine testing. So far, therefore, we have not been able to develop an eye movement recording method that is a notable improvement on the Dunlop Test, despite its clear shortcomings.

An important prediction of our hypothesis that many dyslexic children suffer visual confusion because of binocular instability is that their confusion should not occur only when they are attempting to read; but whenever they are required to localize any small target accurately. We have, therefore, compared the precision of the visual direction sense of children who failed the Dunlop Test with those who passed it, by means of a computer game (Stein, Riddell, and Fowler 1988). A small target subtending 0.25 degrees was displayed on the screen for 2 sec (long enough for any fixation instability to manifest itself). After a delay of 0.5 secs, a second test spot was then displayed slightly to the left or right of the first for 200 msecs. The child's task was to indicate, by pointing, the direction in which the spot had appeared to move. The distance between target and test spot was adjusted so that the child made approximately 75% correct responses (halfway between random and perfect scores in this 2 alternative forced choice paradigm). The results were clear and consistent. Children with unstable binocular control made many more errors than either age or reading-age-matched controls. Interestingly, while normal-reading children made slightly more errors when the test spot moved to the right of the target, the children with unstable binocular control made many more errors on the left.

NON WORD READING ERRORS

In order to make sure that the disorder of binocular control that we were finding was, in fact, the cause of their visual reading problems as we were claiming, and not merely an unrelated epiphenomenon, we needed to be able to show that children with unstable binocular control make characteristically "visual" kinds of reading errors. Piers Cornelissen, therefore, classified the errors made by dyslexics in the BAS single word reading test; he found that the children who failed the Dunlop Test tended to produce more nonsense (non-word) than real word errors. We thought that these might be the result of the children sounding out the confused visual images with which their visual system was presenting them. But, there is, of course, a well known phonological mechanism that can generate non-word reading errors; children with higher phonological ability tend to produce more nonsense words because they mistakenly try to apply the phonological rules that they have successfully learned to unfamiliar irregular words. So we needed to find out whether children with unstable binocular control made more non-word errors than children of the same reading age with stable control, even when we kept the phonological load on the two groups identical and made allowances for differences in the children's phonological ability. Results still showed that children with unstable binocular control made more non-word errors. Moreover we found that if print size were increased to reduce the chances of visual confusion, these children with unstable control decreased their non-word error rate considerably, whereas children with stable responses in the Dunlop Test did not change their proportion of non-word errors (Cornelissen et al. 1991). These results demonstrate clearly that visual confusion is a significant cause of these children's reading errors.

Despite all this evidence, however, some people still argue vehemently that there is no causal relationship between unstable binocular fixation and reading problems. Two alternative possibilities have been put forward. The first is that poor reading is what causes poor binocular stability rather than the other way round; the second is that some other neurological abnormality causes both. The first possibility is refuted by our evidence that younger normal children reading at the same level as older dyslexics have better ocular motor control (Stein, Riddell, and Fowler 1987). If their ocular motor stability were dependent upon their reading, it should have been no better than that of the dyslexics.

We also believe the second possibility to be unlikely, namely that some third independent neurological factor may blight both ocular motor stability and reading, and that binocular stability and reading skill are independent. First, the association between non-word errors and binocular instability, together with their improvement when print size was increased, strongly suggest a causal relationship between the two. Second, we discovered another intervention that significantly reduced the proportion of non-word and other errors made by children with unstable binocular fixation, namely having them read using only one eye (Cornelissen et al. 1992).

Our rationale for treating these problems by means of monocular occlusion was that, if the binocular fixation of a child is unstable, he may be confused by the competing views provided by each eye, hence occluding one might alleviate the confusion. Reading with one eye turned out not only to reduce, as expected, the non-word errors made by these children; but, we also found that if these children wore monocularly occluding spectacles for all reading and close work for 6 months, this permanently stabilized the binocular control of over half the children with unstable control. From our studies of normal primary school children, we knew that approximately 20% of children of this age with unstable control would stabilize spontaneously in the 6 months we were studying them (Stein, Riddell, and Fowler 1986); but, with the help of occlusion (Stein and Fowler 1985) 54% of dyslexics with unstable control became stable, a highly significant advantage to occlusion (Stein and Fowler 1985).

In addition, achieving binocular stability had a dramatic effect on the children's reading. In a pilot study we compared 15 dyslexic children with unstable controls treated by means of monocular occlusion with 15 who were not so treated (Stein and Fowler 1981). The 15 who received the occlusion increased their reading age by 12.3 months in the 6 months of observation, whereas those not so treated, who did not gain stable fixation, increased their reading age by only 5.3 months; in other words, their reading regressed in relation to their age (figure 2). In a later placebo controlled trial (Stein and Fowler 1985), we found that 48 dyslexics with unstable control, who gained stable oculomotor control

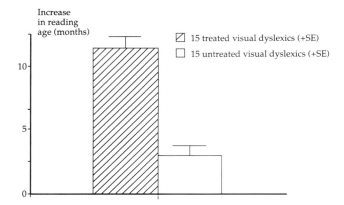

Figure 2. Increase in reading age in 15 dyslexics with unstable binocular control whose control improved following six months occlusion of the left eye for close work, compared with 15 who were not occluded.

with the help of monocularly occluding spectacles, increased their reading age by 12.6 months in the first 6 months and 20.3 months in a full year. In contrast those treated with placebo plain spectacles who did not gain stable binocular control did much worse, gaining only 5.6 months in reading age in the first 6 months and 11.3 months in the whole year. These results strongly imply that correcting children's binocular instability helps them to learn to read. So we believe we can safety conclude that unstable fixation is indeed a potent cause of visual confusion, hence, of reading problems.

CORRELATION BETWEEN VISUAL AND PHONOLOGICAL IMPAIRMENTS

One reason people have found this idea hard to accept is that the evidence is very strong that most dyslexics have major problems with phonological segmentation; tests of this ability not only predict reading difficulties extremely well, but they also correlate highly with reading skill in unselected groups of normal primary school children. Contrary to strongly held opinions, however, these facts do not rule out the possibility that many of these children suffer visual problems as well. In most of our studies, we have used Bradley and Bryant's rhyming test to assess the phonological skills of our subjects; more recently, we have been fortunate enough to be given access to Dr. Frank Wood's large Orton Dyslexia Study data base at Bowman Gray Medical School, Winston-Salem, North Carolina. Studying two very different groups, one from Berkshire U.K. (Stein and Fowler 1985), the other from Winston-Salem, U.S.A. (Eden, Stein, and Wood 1993) we have confirmed the strong correlation between phonological and reading abilities. In our Bowman Gray group of dyslexics and matched controls, a test of auditory analysis skills alone accounted for over 37% of the variance in the children's reading ability.

In addition, however, we have been able to show that there is a strong correlation between visual and phonological tests in both populations. In the Bowman Gray group, the correlation between some of our visual and phonological tests reached 0.4 and this was highly significant. This finding not only implies that both phonological and visual skills may share a common neurobiological mechanism, but they also confirm that, often, dyslexics suffer both phonological and visual deficits. In addition, however, a substantial proportion of the variance in reading ability could only be accounted for by a particular visual skill that did not covary with phonological ability, namely binocular stability. In the Winston-Salem group, we found that a highly significant 15% of reading variance was independently predicted by recording binocular stability. Thus, in most dyslexics, visual and phonological disabilities seem to coexist; but beyond this, stable binocular fixation is probably a significant independent contributor to reading skill.

VISUAL MAGNOCELLULAR DEFICIT

Clearly the question that immediately arises is whether a common neurological mechanism might underlie the impairment of both phonological and visual skills in dyslexics. A number of different lines of inquiry have now converged to suggest that the magnocellular, transient, division of the CNS may play a crucial role. Throughout the 1980s, Bill Lovegrove and his colleagues published studies that show that dyslexics have slightly reduced performance of the "transient" component of their visual processing system (Lovegrove 1991). I believe that this abnormality is the basic cause of the binocular instability and visual confusion I have been describing.

The visual transient systems begins with the large "parasol" ganglion cells in the retina. These project to the magnocellular layers of the lateral geniculate nucleus (LGN) and to the superior colliculus. Thence, they provide the dominant input to the dorsomedial pathway through the striate and prestriate cortices, which culminates in the posterior parietal cortex (Merrigan and Maunsell 1993). This is widely known as the "where" pathway. Neurons along it respond preferentially to large contour, low contrast moving targets. It has high contrast sensitivity at low spatial and high temporal frequencies and it is achromatic, not differentiating between colors. It thus helps to determine the location and motion of targets with respect to the observer. Therefore, it plays a particularly important role in the control of eye and limb movements. In contrast, the parvocellular, "what" pathway has high spatial and low temporal sensitivity combined with color selectivity. Its projection route is mainly via the ventrolateral visual cortical pathway into the inferotemporal cortex. It is believed to help identify objects from the details of their contours and colors.

Measurement of contrast sensitivity has become a standard method of assessing the function of the whole visual system (Campbell 1974). Whereas tests of visual acuity indicate the performance of only the high resolution, high spatial frequency part of visual processing that is dominated by the parvocellular system, the contrast sensitivity function gives an indication of performance across the whole range of spatial scales. In particular by using low spatial frequency, low contrast stimuli rapidly changing in time, the specific functions of the magnocellular system may be studied in humans. In a series of studies, Lovegrove and his colleagues were able to show that many dyslexics exhibit a slight reduction in contrast sensitivity at low spatial and high temporal frequencies (Lovegrove 1991). These differences from normal are consistent with the hypothesis that they have a mild abnormality of the transient, magnocellular system. We have confirmed Lovegrove's results and added the finding that unstable binocular control is associated with these reductions in contrast sensitivity (Mason et al. 1993).

The magnocellular system is believed to provide the main input to the cortical system responsible for visual motion detection. We have, therefore, measured the motion sensitivity of dyslexics by determining the proportion of dots that need to move coherently in one direction in a random dot display in order for the subject to see global motion. Consistent with the idea that their magnocellular system is slightly impaired we found that the dyslexics required a significantly higher proportion to move together in order to perceive the motion (Cornelissen et al. 1994).

Another way of demonstrating an abnormality of the magnocellular system is to measure averaged EEG potentials in the visual cortex (visual evoked potentials—VEPs) evoked by visual stimuli of low spatial frequency and low contrast. We (Maddock, Richardson, and Stein 1992; Lehmkuhle and Williams 1993; and Livingstone et al. 1991) have all confirmed that many dyslexics show reduced and abnormal visual evoked potentials under these conditions (figure 3).

Livingstone et al. also examined histologically the brains of five known dyslexics post mortem and found that neurons in the magnocellular layers of the LGN in these brains appeared shrunken and less numerous than normal. This adds to other evidence of Galaburda, Rosen, and Sherman (1985) that there are structural neuroanatomical differences distinguishing the brains of dyslexic from non-dyslexic individuals; and again it focuses on the possibility that the magnocellular system is particularly vulnerable.

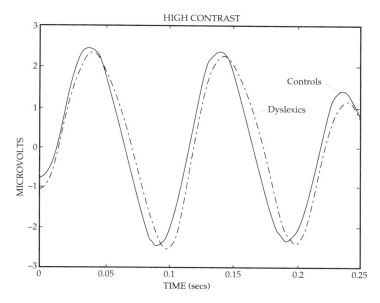

Figure 3. Delayed averaged evoked potential in 15 dyslexics in response to black and white checker board stimulus reversing 10 times a second presented in one half field, compared with 15 non dyslexics.

The highest level of the magnocellular "where" system is the posterior parietal cortex. In humans, the right posterior parietal cortex is more important for visual localization, whereas the left probably plays a more important part in temporal processing, for example, for phonological discriminations. When the right posterior parietal cortex is damaged by disease in adults, a characteristic set of symptoms ensues. The most prominent is left "neglect," the inability to direct attention to the left hand side of space or to the left hand side of objects. This leads to misjudgements of the direction, distance, and the spatial relations of objects, particularly on the left. These are all symptoms that remind us of the visual confusions reported by dyslexic children.

We therefore began looking for more signs that dyslexics may exhibit "right parietal" abnormalities. Their greater error rates in dot localization on the left are suggestive. We have now found many more indications of this (Eden, Stein, and Wood 1993). Dyslexics make more errors on the left than normals when copying the Rey figure. They also make more errors on the left when judging the angle of lines. Furthermore, they make more errors on the left in cancellation tasks; in these the subject has to strike out, with a pencil, all targets of a certain type amidst a jumble of others. Finally many dyslexics tend to draw clocks like those in figure 4, cramming all the figures into the right hand side and leaving the left empty. This is a classic sign of

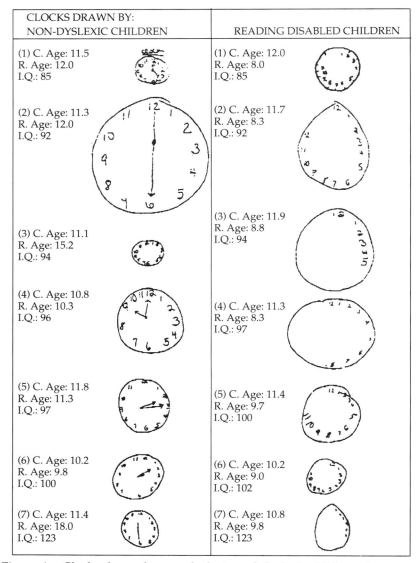

CLOCKS DRAWN BY: NON-DYSLEXIC CHILDREN	READING DISABLED CHILDREN
(1) C. Age: 11.5 R. Age: 12.0 I.Q.: 85	(1) C. Age: 12.0 R. Age: 8.0 I.Q.: 85
(2) C. Age: 11.3 R. Age: 12.0 I.Q.: 92	(2) C. Age: 11.7 R. Age: 8.3 I.Q.: 92
(3) C. Age: 11.1 R. Age: 15.2 I.Q.: 94	(3) C. Age: 11.9 R. Age: 8.8 I.Q.: 94
(4) C. Age: 10.8 R. Age: 10.3 I.Q.: 96	(4) C. Age: 11.3 R. Age: 8.3 I.Q.: 97
(5) C. Age: 11.8 R. Age: 11.3 I.Q.: 97	(5) C. Age: 11.4 R. Age: 9.7 I.Q.: 100
(6) C. Age: 10.2 R. Age: 9.8 I.Q.: 100	(6) C. Age: 10.2 R. Age: 9.0 I.Q.: 102
(7) C. Age: 11.4 R. Age: 18.0 I.Q.: 123	(7) C. Age: 10.8 R. Age: 9.8 I.Q.: 123

Figure 4. Clocks drawn by non-dyslexic and dyslexic children show tendency for left neglect.

neglect in patients with right parietal lesions. These high-left-sided error rates in dyslexic children combine to suggest that there may indeed be something abnormal about the development of their right posterior parietal cortices.

Of course, it should not be forgotten that there is equally strong evidence that most dyslexics have left sided, linguistic problems as well. Paula Tallal and colleagues have published a series of studies over the last 20 years showing that, like the visual problems of dyslexics described in this chapter, in developmental dysphasics, phonological difficulties are not confined to the linguistic domain, but form part of a more generalized defect of auditory analysis (Tallal and Schwartz 1980). She has shown that dysphasics take longer than normals to be able to distinguish two tones presented in rapid sequence. Likewise, their voice onset time is prolonged, compared with normals. Interestingly, from our point of view, she has also found that visual discrimination of small symbols (not letters) presented in rapid sequence is also defective in these dysphasics. Many such dysphasics go on to become dyslexics and many dyslexics turn out to have had mild problems with learning to speak (Stein and Fowler 1985). Hence, Tallal has found that many dyslexics have problems discriminating rapid auditory transients similar to those of dysphasics.

We have, therefore, been analyzing the basic auditory processing of dyslexics using tests analogous to those that we have used to assess rapid temporal processing in the visual system. In the auditory system, the main way in which the timing of acoustic events is signaled is by neurons that lock on to the peaks of sound waves, known as *phase locking*. These neurons tend to be large, heavily myelinated magnocellular types, analogous to the magnocells, which are so much better characterized in the visual system. We have, therefore, used tasks that require phase locking to solve, such as low frequency discrimination, detection of frequency modulations, and binaural masking level differences (BMLD) when the phase of the sound in one ear is reversed. We found that dyslexics are significantly worse than normal controls in all these tests (McAnally and Stein 1994) which suggests that their auditory magnocellular system may also be compromised (figure 5). It was, therefore,

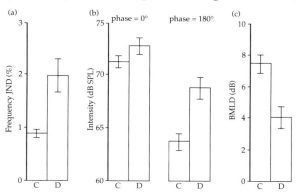

Figure 5.   (a) Just noticeable difference in tone around 1 KHz in controls (C) and dyslexics (D). (b) Intensity of 1 KHz tone required to hear above dB noise when interaural phase of the tone was the same (0°) or inverted (180°). (c) Difference between the phase conditions in Figure 5b is the binaural masking level difference (BMLD). Binaural unmasking when interaural phase is inverted was significantly smaller in the dyslexics.

particularly exciting for us when Galaburda and colleagues published their results of examining the auditory thalamic relay nucleus, the medial geniculate, in dyslexic brains (Galaburda, Rosen, and Menard 1994). They confirmed that the magnocellular division of the dyslexic medial geniculate nucleus was disorganized, and the neurons smaller than in control brains. An impairment of their auditory magnocellular system, which is responsible for phase locking, hence the processing of auditory transients, would obviously begin to explain why dyslexics have such problems with phonological discrimination, since this task depends heavily on the analysis of rapid acoustic changes.

CONGENITAL MAGNOCELLULAR IMPAIRMENT

Angela Fawcett and colleagues have found that dyslexics show signs of impaired rapid signal processing in several other sensory and motor domains as well (Fawcett and Nicolson 1992). They have a longer latency P300 auditory evoked potential in an auditory "oddball" paradigm; dyslexics have slower choice reaction times, despite normal simple reaction times; they have higher two-point touch thresholds but normal sensitivity to a single point; and they have a tendency to fall over when balancing on a beam if blindfolded or given a secondary cognitive task to perform. All these findings can be interpreted in terms of impairment of rapid signal processing in the auditory, somaesthetic, and motor systems, not in their peripheral pathways, but in the centers responsible for stimulus and response categorization.

The parallels between the signal processing deficits of dyslexics in different sensory and motor domains are clearly striking. Paula Tallal, Angela Fawcett and we have all found that dyslexics display a wide variety of auditory, visual, and motor deficits. Their ubiquity prompts us to speculate that they may all share a common origin. The very different techniques of genetic analysis suggest the same thing. Dyslexia is strongly heritable, as are reading and its component skills, visual and phonological analysis (Olson et al. 1989). The heritability of somaesthetic and motor skills has not been studied in the same way. Nevertheless, a plausible hypothesis is that what is inherited in non-dyslexic as well as dyslexic individuals are not specific visual, auditory, or other skills but the general ability to perform rapid neuronal processing operations. These are required for all the rapid visual, auditory, and articulatory sequencing tasks that are important for reading.

My final speculation is, therefore, that a genetically based defect of rapid signal processing is the fundamental cause of dyslexic problems. So far, such a defect has been most clearly shown for the visual magnocellular system. But magnocellular neurons contribute not only to visual processing, but also to every other function of the nervous system: auditory, somaesthetic, and motor. The development of magnocullular systems probably involves the expression of a common surface-action molecule. It has recently been shown that dyslexia may cosegregate with a gene that is located among the histocompatibility loci on chromosome 6.5. Clearly, if immunological action in utero attacked this surface active molecule, which is specific to large neurons, this would damage magnocellular systems throughout the brain, and give rise to just such a combination of visual, auditory, and motor disorders as we see in dyslexics. The multidimensional nature of dyslexics' problems could thus be explained by a single underlying molecular mechanism occurring during development.

REFERENCES

Anderson, R. A., Essick, G. E., and Siegel, R. M. 1985. Encoding spatial location by posterior parietal neurones. *Science* 230:456–58.

Bigelow, E. R., and McKenzie, B. E. 1985. Unstable ocular dominance and reading ability. *Perception* 14:329–35.

Bishop, D. V. M. 1989. Unstable vergence control and dyslexia—a critique. *British Journal of Ophthalmology* 73:223–45.

Bishop, D. V. M., Jancey, C., and Steel, A. McP. 1979. Orthoptic status and reading disability. *Cortex* 15:659–66.

Bradley, L., and Bryant, P. 1983. Categorising sounds and learning to read—a causal connection. *Nature* 301:419–21.

Campbell, F. W. 1974. The transmission of spatial information through the visual system. In *The Neurosciences 3rd Study Program*, ed. F. O. Schmidt. Cambridge, MA: MIT Press.

Cardon, L. R., Smith, S. D., Fulker, D. W., Kimberling, W. J., Pennington, B. F., and deFries, J. C. 1994. Quantitative trait locus for reading disability on Chromosome 6. *Science* 266: 276–79.

Cornelissen, P., Bradley, L, Fowler, M. A., and Stein, J. F. 1991. What children see affects how they read. *Developmental Medicine and Child Neurology* 33:755–62.

Cornelissen, P., Bradley, L., Fowler, M. S., and Stein, J. F. 1992. Covering one eye affects how some children read. *Developmental Medicine and Child Neurology* 34:296–304.

Cornelissen, P. L., Bradley, L., Fowler, M. S., and Stein, J. F. 1994. What children see affects how they spell. *Developmental Medicine and Child Neurology* 36:716–27.

Cornelissen, P. L., Richardson, A. R., Mason, A., Fowler, M. S., and Stein, J. F. 1994. Contrast sensitivity and coherent motion detection measured at photopic luminance levels in dyslexics and controls. *Vision Research* 35:1483–95.

Duhamel, J. R., Colby, C. L., and Goldberg, M. E. 1992. The updating of the representation of visual space in parietal cortex by intended eye movements. *Science* 255:90–92.

Dunlop, P. 1972. Dyslexia: The orthopic approach. *Australian Journal of Orthoptics* 12:16–20.

Dunlop, P. 1979. Orthoptic management of learning disability. *British Orthoptic Journal* 36:25–35.

Eden, G. F., Stein, J. G., and Wood, F. G. 1993. Visuospatial ability and language processing in reading disabled and normal children. In *Facets of Dyslexia and Its Remediation*, ed S. F. Wright and R. Groner. Oxford: Elsevier.

Eden, G. F., Stein, J. F., Wood, H. M., and Wood, F. B. 1994. Differences in eye movements and reading problems in dyslexic and normal children. *Vision Research* 34:1345–58.

Eden, G., Stein, J. F., and Wood, F. 1993. Dyslexia: Preserved and impaired visuospatial and phonological functions. *Annals of the New York Academy of Sciences* 682:335–39.

Evans, B. J. W., and Drasdo, N. 1990. Ophthalmic factors in dyslexia. *Ophthalmic and Physiological Optics* 10:123–32.

Evans, B. J. W., Drasdo, N., and Richards, I. L. 1993. Optometric aspects of reading disability. In *Transactions of the British College of Optometrists*, 10th Conference. London: Butterworths.

Evans, B. J. W., Drasdo, N., and Richards, I. L. 1994. Investigation of accommodative and binocular function in dyslexia. *Ophthalmic and Physiological Optics* 14:5–20.

Fawcett, A. J., and Nicolson, R. I. 1992. Automatisation deficits in balance in dyslexic children. *Perceptual and Motor Skills* 75:507–29.

Fowler, M. S. 1991. Binocular instability in dyslexics. In *Visual Dyslexia, Vol. 13. Vision and Visual Dysfunction*, ed. J. F. Stein. London: Macmillan Press.

Fowler, M. S., Munro, N., Richardson A., and Stein, J. F. 1989. Vergence control in patients with posterior parietal lesions. *Journal of Physiology* 417:92.

Fowler, S., and Stein, J. 1980. Visual dyslexia. *British Orthoptic Journal* 37:11.

Fowler, S., and Stein, J. 1979. New evidence for ambilaterality in visual dyslexia. *Neuroscience Letters*. Supplements 3:214.

Galaburda, A., Rosen, G., and Sherman, G. P. 1985. Developmental dyslexia: Four consecutive cases with cortical anomalies. *Annals of Neurology* 18:222–33.

Galaburda, A., Rosen, G. D., and Menard, M. T. 1994. Aberrant auditory anatomy in developmental dyslexics. *Proceedings of the New York Academy of Science* 91:8010–13.

Grusser, O.-J. 1982. Space perception and the gaze motor system. *Human Neurobiology* 1:73–76.

Lehmkuhle, K., and Williams, M. 1993. Defective visual pathway in children with reading disability. *New England Journal of Medicine* 328:989–95.

Liberman, I. Y., Shankweiler, D., Liberman, A. A., Fowler, C., and Fischer, F. W. 1977. Phonetic segmentation and recoding in the beginning reader. In *Reading: Theory and Practice*, eds. A. S. Reber and D. Scarborough. Hillsdale, NJ: Lawrence Erlbaum Associates.

Livingstone, M. S., Rosen, G. D., Drisland, F. W., and Galaburda, A. M. 1991. Physiological and anatomical evidence for a magnocellular defect in developmental dyslexia. *Proceedings of the National Academy of Science* 88:7943–47.

Lovegrove, W. 1991. Spatial frequency processing in normal and dyslexic readers. In *Visual Dyslexia, Vol 13. Vision and Visual Dysfunction*, ed. J Stein. London: Macmillan Press.

McAnally, K., and Stein, J. F. 1994. Reduced auditory temporal resolution in dyslexic subjects? 23rd Rodin Academy International Conference, Malta.

Maddock, H., Richardson, A., and Stein, J. F. 1992. Reduced and delayed visual evoked potentials in dyslexics. *Journal of Physiology* 459:130.

Mason, A., Cornelissen, P., Fowler, M. S., and Stein, J. F. 1993. Contrast sensitivity, ocular dominance and reading disability. *Clinical Visual Science* 8:345–53.

Masters, M. D. 1988. Orthoptic management of visual dyslexia. *British Orthoptic Journal* 45:40–48.

Merrigan, W. H., and Maunsell, J. R. 1993. How parallel are the primate visual pathways? *Annual Review of Neuroscience* 16:369–402.

Newman, S. P., Karle, H., Wadsworth, J. F., Archer, R., Hockly, R., and Rogers, P. 1985. Ocular dominance, reading and spelling: A reassessment of a measure associated with specific reading difficulties. *Journal of Research in Reading* 8:127–38.

Olson, R. K., Wise, B., Conners, F., Rack, J., and Fulker, D. 1989. Specific deficits in component reading and language skills: Genetic and environmental influences. *Journal of Learning Disabilities* 22:339–48.

Riddell, P., Fowler, M. S., and Stein, J. F. 1990. Spatial discrimination in children with poor vergence control. *Perceptual and Motor Skills.* 70:707–18.

Stein, J. F. 1992. The representation of space in the posterior parietal cortex. *Behavior and Brain Science* 15:691–700.

Stein, J. F., and Fowler, M. S. 1981. Visual dyslexia. *Trends in Neuroscience* 4:77–80.

Stein, J. F., and Fowler, M. S. 1985. Effect of monocular occlusion on visuomotor perception and reading in dyslexic children. *Lancet* (13 July) 69–73.

Stein, J. F., and Fowler, M. S. 1993. Unstable binocular control in dyslexic children. *Journal of Research in Reading* 19:30–45.

Stein, J. F., and Fowler, S. 1982. Diagnosis of dyslexia by means of a new indicator of eye dominance. *British Journal of Ophthalmology* 66:332–36.

Stein, J. F., Riddell, P., and Fowler, M. S. 1986. The Dunlop Test and reading in primary school children. *British Journal of Ophthalmology* 70:317.

Stein, J. F., Riddell, P., and Fowler, M. S. 1987. Fine binocular control in dyslexic children. *Eye* 1:433–38.

Stein, J. F., Riddell, P., and Fowler, M. S. 1988. Disordered vergence eye movement control in dyslexic children. *British Journal of Ophthalmology* 72:162–66.

Tallal, P., and Schwartz, J. 1980. Temporal processing, speech perception and hemispheric asymmetry. *Trends in Neuroscience* 3:309–11.

Thompson, M. E. 1982. The assessment of children with specific reading difficulties using the British Ability Scales. *British Journal of Psychology* 73:461–78.

Vellutino, F. R. 1987. Dyslexia. *Scientific American* 256:20–27.

Chapter • 7

A Visual Deficit Model of Developmental Dyslexia

Christopher H. Chase

To understand the etiology of developmental reading disorders (dyslexia), many researchers stress the importance of identifying and describing the cognitive and perceptual prerequisites that are necessary to develop normal reading skills (Johnson 1988; Stanovich 1988). Such an approach assumes that dyslexic children have trouble learning to read because they suffer from a specific impairment that affects one or more of these prerequisite abilities. Such deficits are specific to the reading task; otherwise the designation of dyslexia would be superfluous, and other educational terms, such as underachiever or slow learner, would more aptly apply. Knowing which skills have been impaired will provide information critical for designing remediation strategies and organizing effective early screening and intervention programs.

Considerable progress has been made in the study of auditory and linguistic prerequisites for reading, and some have suggested that impairments in the phonological analysis of language is the primary cognitive deficit underlying dyslexia (Liberman 1983). However, other studies have reported visual perceptual deficits for many dyslexic children (Williams and Lecluyse 1990; Lovegrove, Martin, and Slaghuis 1986). Because the processing of text starts in the visual system (for most individuals except the blind), it is important to know the prevalence and developmental course of these visual deficits, particularly as they pertain to dyslexia. This chapter reviews the evidence for visual dyslexic impairments and presents a working model for dyslexia that explains these cognitive deficits in the context of known neuroanatomical and physiological abnormalities.

A THEORETICAL PERSPECTIVE ON NEURODEVELOPMENTAL PATHOLOGY

Dyslexia is an example of a disorder in which specific brain abnormalities affect the normal course of neural development, producing damage that is broadly distributed across different cortical and subcortical regions and that is quite variable from one individual to another (see below for details). The structural damage produced is unlike anything seen in acquired dyslexia—both in regard to the site and particular type of abnormality; in fact, if an adult were to suffer brain lesions as extensive as those seen in developmental dyslexia, such damage would most likely produce symptoms of global aphasia. The reason for such functional differences can be understood only from a developmental perspective.

When studying developmental neuropathology, it is important to make the distinction between the *form* and *function* of neurological processes. Brain damage has a different effect on children than on adults, particularly when the childhood damage has occurred during fetal development. In a mature adult brain there is considerable evidence to suggest that many cognitive functions (particularly linguistic ones) are localized to specific neural pathways and cortical regions. For example, using PET technology, Petersen et al. (1990) demonstrated that words and pronounceable non-words (pseudowords) selectively activated a discrete area in left medial extrastriatal cortex, but that random strings of letters or non-letter symbols did not stimulate this region. This area could be viewed as a visual feature extraction system, specialized for processing familiar stimuli, or as a storage area for visual word forms or letter clusters. When an adult suffers brain damage that affects reading ability, the acquired dyslexic impairment in some cases can produce very specific types of reading errors, suggestive of damage to a particular functional module, such as the one found by Petersen et al. 1990.

A study of cortical representation in an *adult* brain may be best understood from a *functional* perspective. Through a detailed study of a behavioral task, models of complex functions such as reading can be analyzed into components. The cortical representations of such subprocesses can be located either by studying patients with focalized acquired brain damage or by the use of experimental PET procedures.

Neurodevelopmental pathology, however, has a very different effect on the organization of cortical representational maps. Since mental representations for linguistic functions develop after birth and over a period of several years, any anatomical abnormalities acquired during fetal development will affect the course of this development. Simply put, the brain of a developmental dyslexic child may be damaged in ways that primarily affect the *form* of sensory signals, which compromises the subsequent development of reading *functions*. Analyzing a child's reading errors by employing the research approach used to study acquired adult dyslexia will not lead to an understanding of how fetal damage affects the formation of cortical linguistic and visual word-form representations because different types of impairments can, over the course of development, produce similar behavioral outcomes, even at the level of reading errors. Seidenberg (1993), for example, has recently shown that his connectionist developmental model of reading learned to produce the same patterns of reading errors regardless of where the damage had been placed in the system prior to training. Identifying and describing developmental dyslexic functional errors does not lead to a deeper understanding of their neurobiological origin. Rather than working from the top-down, the study of neurodevelopmental pathology must proceed from the bottom-up, beginning with an analysis of the pathology found at the neuroanatomical and neurophysiological level. From these data one can proceed to build a bridge toward an understanding of how such neuropathology has disrupted the development of psychological functions.

DEFINITIONS AND BACKGROUND

Developmental dyslexia is a neurobiological disorder that affects the development of reading and written language expression. Some dyslexic children may also have delays in their language development (dysphasia); over 80% of children with developmental dysphasia also develop academic problems when they reach school age (Tallal 1988). Some researchers have suggested that all dyslexic children have some degree of language impairment, although this depends upon the way linguistic skills are measured and the criteria used (Liberman 1983).

Learning to read is sensitive to many developmental factors. To make a diagnosis of dyslexia, exclusionary criteria are used. Even though dyslexia can co-occur with other handicapping conditions, such as sensory impairment, mental retardation, or poor social, emotional, or environmental factors, dyslexia is thought to be the result of intrinsic neurological factors and not of these other conditions. As a result of the use of such exclusionary criteria, dyslexic children form quite a heterogeneous group that varies in severity, concomitant neuropsychological dysfunction, and probably etiology.

Dyslexia is quite common with prevalence estimates as high as 10–15% of the population (Johnson 1988). The incidence varies depending upon the availability of special educational services and diagnostic criteria used. For example, 40% of the children who receive special educational services in this country are considered to have a learning disability, of which dyslexia is the most common (Office of Special Education 1984); however, this average varies considerably from state to state with a high of 63% in Rhode Island and a low of 26% in Alabama (Keogh 1986). Although it may be possible that more children with learning disabilities live in the Northeast, a more likely explanation is that different diagnostic criteria lead to different prevalence estimates.

ANATOMICAL ABNORMALITIES

Reading disorders were first noticed in adults with acquired left hemisphere parietal and posterior temporal lesions, and early reports of children with developmental reading disorders were thought to have similar cortical lesions (Morgan 1896; Hinshelwood 1917). More recently, anatomical studies of the brains of seven dyslexic individuals have shown cortical and subcortical pathology, involving bilateral damage affecting both the auditory and visual systems (Galaburda, Rosen, and Sherman 1989). At cortical levels these abnormalities appear as focal dysplasias and ectopias, small areas less than a millimeter in size where neurons are dislocated and the normal layered structure of cortex has been disorganized. These ectopic collections of neurons usually appear in the molecular region of the cortex (layer I), and recent animal studies suggest that such cortical abnormalities occur early during fetal development, possibly as a result of ruptures in the glial limiting membrane, which limits the outward migration of neurons during gestation (Caviness, Misson, and Gadisseux 1989). From an analysis of Galaburda et al.'s (1985) data, Hynd and Semrud-Clikeman (1989) reported 23% of the ectopias occurred in the right hemisphere versus 77% in the left hemisphere. Most of the abnormalities appeared in the frontal and temporal lobes (52% and 37%, respectively.)

In addition to these cortical abnormalities, a region of the temporal lobe known as the planum temporale, which lies along the posterior portion of Heschl's gyrus, was symmetrically sized in the two hemispheres. Such hemispheric symmetry is not unusual, although 65% of a normal sample showed a left asymmetry, 11% had a right asymmetry, and 24% were symmetric (Geschwind and Levitsky 1968). Since rupture of the cortically asymmetrical regions appears to occur early in fetal development, probably before the birth of the first neuron, these dyslexic cortical abnormalities are probably produced early in the first trimester (Rosen, Sherman, and Galaburda 1991). More callosal fibers also may be present in symmetric regions. Abnormalities in the left hemisphere may reduce competition during post-migrational stages of pruning and neuronal death, enlarging the right hemisphere by allowing it to compete more successfully for additional callosal projections.

Subcortical abnormalities also have been observed in dyslexic brains. Galaburda and Eidelberg (1982) reported cellular disorganization in the medial geniculate nucleus of the thalamus, part of the auditory sensory system, in three of their four cases. Recently, Livingstone et al. (1991) reported abnormalities in magnocellular region of the lateral geniculate nucleus (LGN) of the thalamus, part of the visual sensory system, in five dyslexic cases. The magno layers were disorganized and cell bodies were 27% smaller than those measured in a control sample. Livingstone et al. (1991) speculated that smaller magno-cells would have smaller axons and that these abnormalities may affect the speed with which information is processed in the magnocellular pathway. Using evoked potential techniques to record visual signals processed in cortex, they provided some neurophysiological support for this hypothesis.

AUDITORY PROCESSING DEFICITS

Many efforts have been made to identify concomitant neuropsychological conditions that may provide clues to diagnostic subtypes (Malatesha and Dougan 1982). Over the years several different classification schemes have been proposed for developmental dyslexia, based upon patterns of associated test scores that are correlated with reading performance. Verbal impairments have been consistently reported, but many studies also have found visual deficits, depending upon the type of task used.

Auditory Processing Speed Deficits

Several studies have reported that dyslexic and language impaired (LI) children have perceptual deficits that affect the ability to process certain types of auditory information rapidly (Tallal and Piercy 1973; Tallal 1980). Tallal has reported that a very high proportion of dysphasic children are unable to process non-verbal auditory stimuli rapidly (Tallal 1988; also see Chapter 8). This deficit is quite severe in young children (approximately 4 years old) but also can be found in LI adolescents and some dyslexics with oral language impairments (Tallal 1980). For example, in a task where 2 tones of different pitches are rapidly presented in sequence, young children require only an 8 millisecond (ms) inter-stimulus interval to discriminate and identify correctly the sounds; however, LI children of the same age require, on average, almost 300 ms to perform successfully the same task. This temporal processing deficit has been observed with visual, tactile, and cross-modal stimuli also (Tallal, Stark, and Mellits 1985).

Impaired Phonological Awareness

Liberman and her colleagues (1983) were among the first to show that dyslexics are impaired in their phonological analysis of language.

Most dyslexic children have difficulty sounding out words and are less aware of the phonological structure in words than other children their age (Johnson 1988); they have difficulty organizing phonological information in short-term memory and recalling it; and they suffer from auditory perceptual impairments that make it difficult to discriminate between speech sounds (Tallal 1980). Measurements of phonological awareness in pre-readers has been shown to be predictive of later reading performance (Stanovich, Cunningham, and Cramer 1984). Early training in phonological awareness also appears to facilitate reading acquisition (Bradley and Bryant 1983).

Goswami and her colleagues (Goswami and Bryant 1990) have proposed that beginning readers who are phonologically able use their awareness of spoken syllables to analyze text into subcomponents that are segmented into the initial consonant/s (onset) and the vowel and final consonant/s (rime). For a word, such as "break," the onset corresponds to the grapheme cluster "br" and the rime to the cluster "eak." In a series of studies, Goswami (1986; 1988; 1991) has shown that novice readers (reading age 6-5) correctly learn to pronounce more words when a clue word, which they are taught to use, shares the onset (e.g., *trim-trot*) or rime (e.g., *beak-weak*) with the unknown words. When clue words share a grapheme cluster that does not correspond to onsets and rimes (e.g., *beak-bean*), learning does not transfer as easily at this early age. However, with just a little more experience, children (reading age 6-10) have refined their awareness to include onset-vowel grapheme clusters (e.g., *beak-bean*). At this age they still do not recognize individual phonemes and so fail to transfer learning between *beak* and *bank*.

Goswami's work suggests that children's awareness of phonology is not only a precursor for reading but also improves as a consequence of better reading skills. Children initially decode words at the onset-rime level, but as their reading skills improve their decoding skills are refined to include other grapheme clusters and eventually knowledge of individual grapheme-phoneme correspondences. Dyslexic children, who have little phonological awareness, do not form analogies sponta-neously between words that share grapheme clusters (Lovett et al. 1989) and may learn to read primarily by memorizing each word individually, in the same way that normally developing readers learn to pronounce highly irregular words, such as *colonel* or *yacht*.

Phonological awareness, however, is not the only factor to consider. Reading begins as a visual task. If the quality of visual information has been compromised by processing impairments in the visual system, subsequent linguistic analysis may be affected by the poverty of the internal visual representation. Goswami and Bryant's (1990) model for decoding unfamiliar words presupposes that children can parse at the onset-rime level because they have sufficiently mastered individ-ual letter perception and are reliably able to recognize, retain, and, with experience, reorganize the word into different grapheme clusters. Such parsing depends upon the ability to recall other words and their constituent parts in ways that orthographically match the new word, thus facilitating its pronunciation. If the quality of the visual input is weakened, then the degraded signal may be insufficient to establish and then activate selectively the matching grapheme clusters within the child's lexicon.

VISUAL PROCESSING DEFICITS

Temporal processing deficits also have been found in the visual system of dyslexic children (Williams and Lecluyse 1990; Lovegrove, Martin, and Slaghuis 1986). Many studies have suggested that dyslexics have impaired temporal resolution in the early stages of processing that can impair the speed of their visual perception (e.g., DiLollo, Hanson, and McIntyre 1983; Brannan and Williams 1988). A brief summary of the neurophysiology of vision is in order to familiarize the reader with basic concepts supporting this work.

Neurophysiology of the Visual System

The primate visual system has two parallel pathways that conduct information from the retina to the occipital lobe of the cortex (Livingstone and Hubel 1987). The two channels are most clearly distinguished in the LGN of the thalamus, where cell-body stains show 6 layers of cells organized into 4 bands of small cells (parvo) and 2 bands of large cells (magno). Extensive psychophysical studies (see Bassi and Lehmkuhle 1990 or Shapley 1990 for recent reviews) have shown these two pathways to be sensitive to different spatial and temporal characteristics of the visual display. The parvocellular channel of primates responds to color, transmits information more slowly, and is more sensitive to fine visual details (high spatial frequencies of the visual spectra), whereas the magnocellular channel is color-blind, faster, and more sensitive to the global shape (or low spatial frequencies), and the perception of movement and depth of stimuli. The magno system also has greater contrast sensitivity than the parvo system, enabling better discrimination of fine shades of gray.

Visual perception is not instantaneous but results from the integration of information as it is processed through the parvo and magno channels at different rates. Flavell and Draguns (1957), in a review of visual perceptual literature, proposed that processing begins initially with the global shape of the display and then slowly discriminates the finer details that require higher acuity. Legge (1978) showed that the low spatial frequencies (0.375-1.5 cycles/degree), which define the shapes of objects, are extracted rapidly in 60-80 ms; higher spatial frequencies

(6.0-12.0 cycles/degree) are processed more slowly, requiring 150-200 ms. Increases in the exposure duration, contrast, or luminance intensity of a display clarify perception. In the early stages of visual processing, perceptual information is diffuse, primarily made up of low spatial frequency components. In the later stages, higher spatial frequencies are added, providing finer details. Perceptual identification begins immediately with the first available information (e.g., low frequency spectra), integrating the higher frequency information within the context of mental representations already formed (Eriksen and Schultz 1979; McClelland 1979). Thus the processing speed efficiency depends upon the acuity requirements of the task. Global shape discrimination can be made more rapidly (Navon 1977; Badcock et al. 1990), based on an analysis of low spatial frequency spectra carried in the faster magno pathway, whereas perception of details requires the better acuity and higher spatial frequency information provided by the slower parvo pathway.

Transient and Sustained Theory of Visual Processing

The magno- and parvocellular pathways are closely analogous to the transient and sustained visual systems (Breitmeyer and Ganz 1976). In this model the 2 channels also have separate but overlapping responses that are differentially selective to spatial and temporal characteristics of the display. The transient system, like the magno channel, responds early in visual analysis to provide information about the global shape, location, movement, and depth of objects; whereas the sustained system, which corresponds to the parvo channel, responds more slowly and provides a more detailed analysis of patterns and color. Transient/sustained theory also acknowledges the importance of how the 2 systems work together, proposing that saccadic eye movements trigger an inhibitory response from the transient channel, which suppresses activation in the sustained channel. According to Breitmeyer's reading model (1980), this transient-on-sustained inhibition serves a very important function for normal vision and reading because without it, the sustained system would summate the new visual display brought into focus by the saccade with the previous image that still persists due to the relatively longer response (several hundred milliseconds) of the sustained channel. The resulting composite image would be blurred and disrupt normal visual functions. Consequently, the timing and coordination of the two channels is essential for normal visual perception.

Dyslexic Transient System Deficits

Several researchers have reported that the speed of processing in the transient or magno channel is impaired for dyslexics. Using measures of visible persistence and contrast sensitivity, several studies have shown dyslexic children to have longer persistence and to be less sensitive with low spatial frequency displays than normal readers, but to be comparable or more sensitive with high spatial frequencies (e.g., Lovegrove, Garzia and Nicholson 1990). These visual processing deficits are reported to occur with high frequency among dyslexic readers. Pooling results from five studies, Lovegrove, Martin, and Slaghuis (1986) reported that 46 out of 61 dyslexic children (75%) showed longer visual persistence at low spatial frequencies compared to only 5 of 61 controls (8%) with this same deficit. According to Breitmeyer's theory of transient-on-sustained inhibition, these results can be explained by hypothesizing that the transient system, which is activated by the low spatial frequencies, has a slow or weakened inhibitory response on the sustained channel, allowing longer sustained responses that increase visual persistence (Williams and Lecluyse 1990; Breitmeyer 1989). Weaker contrast sensitivity at low spatial frequencies also is consistent with a dysfunction in the transient system.

Critique of the Transient Deficit Model of Dyslexia

Breitmeyer's model (1984) for transient/sustained visual function has been broadly successful in accounting for a wide variety of visual data; however, the application of this model for dyslexic performance (Breitmeyer 1989) has a few problems. First, reading is assumed to be performed only in the sustained system. This premise is based on old and erroneous neurophysiological data and on a misunderstanding of what degree of detail is needed for accurate perception of text. Early versions of this model (Breitmeyer and Ganz 1976) were based in part on neurophysiological evidence that showed two types of ganglion cells (X and Y) in the retina of cats. These cells had different sized receptive fields, Y being larger (Enroth-Cugell and Robson 1966). They had different response properties to the stimulus at onset and offset, Y responding in a rapid and transient fashion, X responding more slowly to stimulus onset and sustaining a response longer after offset (Saito, Shimahara, and Fukada 1970). Retinal distributions also were reported to differ, with X–cells concentrated in the fovea and Y–cells more evenly distributed (Fukuda 1971). Although there are differences of opinion about what is the homology of X– and Y–cells for primates, for purposes of spatial and temporal processing, many neurophysiologists have considered the parvo- and magnocellular pathways, and the retinal ganglion cells P- and M- (which project to these respective layers of the LGN) to be the equivalent of cat X– and Y–cells, respectively. Since reading can only occur when the text is focused on the fovea (Rayner and Pollatsek 1989), Breitmeyer assumed that processing of text must take place through the P-cells, which correspond to the transient or parvocellular channel.

Recent research (Livingstone and Hubel 1988), however, has shown that the magno- and parvocellular projections from the retina maintain a constant ratio across the retina. P-cells, which project to the parvocellular layer, comprise about 80% of the ganglion cells, M-cells represent 10% of retinal projections, and the remaining 10% are composed of W-cells, which project to the superior colliculus and other subcortical structures. This 8:1 ratio remains constant even though there is a higher concentration of all ganglion cell types in the fovea. Better visual acuity, which is provided by the higher concentration of cells found in the fovea, is required for reading. Nevertheless, relative to the parvo system, the magno pathway contributes just as much information about a foveal display as one presented peripherally.

Another erroneous argument for the parvo channel's unique contribution to reading involves its greater sensitivity to high spatial frequency (SF) information. Since text is usually small, some have wrongly assumed this means that only high spatial frequency information is used for reading. However, Legge and his colleagues (1985) have shown that the critical spatial frequency bandwidth for reading is about two cycles per character. Adding higher frequencies provides more visual detail but does not significantly improve reading performance. Two cycles/character represents a fairly low bandwidth, primarily within the sensitivity range of the magno pathway. Furthermore, a recent study by Legge et al. (1990) found that with high contrast (0.2–0.4 or better Michelson contrast) normal subjects read at the same rate using either the magno or parvo systems. With lower contrasts subjects read faster using the magno system.

A second problem for Breitmeyer's reading model concerns the necessity for well-timed transient-on-sustained inhibition to prevent the merging of retinal images in the sustained channel, which would produce blurred text. Unfortunately there is no direct evidence that such blurring occurs without transient inhibition. There is, however, some evidence that it may not occur. First, in the Rapid Sequential Visual Presentation (RSVP) experimental procedure, words are presented at a fixed point at rates equal to or greater than normal reading (Chen 1986). Under such circumstances, reading occurs without saccadic eye movement or the peripheral movement of images reported to be necessary to trigger the transient-on-sustained inhibition (Breitmeyer 1984). Yet RSVP does not produce a blurred image between successively read words. Second, if the transient-on-sustained inhibition is slower in the visual system of developmental dyslexics, then not only should words be blurred between successive saccades but all other visual images should blur as well. However, there is no evidence that dyslexics suffer from such general visual impairments; in fact, many studies have failed to find dyslexic impairments on a wide range of visual tasks (Vellutino 1979).

In summary, the transient processing deficit model of dyslexia is both too general and too specific. It is too specific in the sense that reading is assumed to occur only through the sustained or parvocellular pathway when recent evidence shows that reading also can occur through the magnocellular channel. The model is too general because it postulates that delayed transient-on-sustained inhibition during reading blurs dyslexic vision but does not explain why such blurring is specific for reading and does not affect visual perception in general. These arguments do not discount the considerable experimental evidence in support of a visual processing speed deficit for dyslexic readers but do raise questions about how such an impairment specifically affects reading development.

The transient processing deficit model of dyslexia can be modified to accommodate these criticisms by assuming that the magnocellular system provides information, in the form of low spatial frequency components, that directly facilitates normal reading development. When low spatial frequencies are processed too slowly, a child's ability to make rapid visual discriminations and to establish internal representations of letters and grapheme clusters in lexical memory is critically affected. This hypothesis is consistent with current neurophysiological (Livingstone et al. 1991) and psychophysical (Legge et al. 1985; Legge et al. 1990) reading research. This low spatial frequency deficit hypothesis will be explained in more detail below, after presenting supporting evidence from preliminary studies.

PROCESSING SPEED IN THE MAGNO- AND PARVOCELLULAR SYSTEMS

Many studies that have measured the rate of processing in the transient channel have found slower dyslexic performance (Brannan and Williams 1988; Lovegrove, Garzia, and Nicholson 1990; Lehmkuhle et al. 1993). However, none has used the same task to compare directly processing speed in the magno- and parvocellular systems of the same individual. The results of previous studies that have reported normal parvocellular or sustained function in dyslexics (Lovegrove et al. 1982) could be due to the different tasks used to activate selectively the 2 channels or due to subject differences. Consequently, we undertook a study that would directly compare processing speed in both channels of the same subject using a flicker fusion procedure (Chase and Jenner 1993).

Flicker fusion thresholds for dyslexic adults and matched controls were compared using a random, 2-stair procedure. Thresholds were measured individually for different tasks that examined the perception of shape, apparent movement, and equiluminant color. With black and white displays, subjects judged a point at which the display no longer appeared to flicker—a luminance flicker threshold. With colored displays, however, variation in the flicker rate can produce two thresholds: at a slower rate, subjects report a fusion of the red and green to a flickering brownish yellow; at higher rates, the luminance flicker disappears to produce a steady brownish yellow square. Researchers (Livingstone and Hubel 1987; Schiller, and Logothetis 1990) have presumed that the color fusion threshold corresponds to the speed of processing in the parvocellular channel, whereas the luminance threshold reflects the processing speed in the magnocellular channel. Using equiluminant stimuli reduced the sensation of a luminance flicker, making it easier for subjects to perceive the color threshold and minimizing the processing that might occur in the magno system.

Results showed that flicker thresholds for shape or movement were higher than for color (32 Hz versus 16.7 Hz, respectively), but a significant interaction between grouping and task effects (p=.008) revealed the dyslexics to have lower thresholds than controls when processing shape or movement (26 Hz versus 38 Hz, respectively) but not when processing color. These results (see figure 1) suggest that dyslexics are slower to process information in their magnocellular pathways but have normal processing speed in the parvo channel.

THE MAGNOCELLULAR ROLE IN VISUAL PERCEPTION

How would slower magnocellular processing affect visual perception? In a recent study (Chase, Heuer, and Blake, in preparation), we found the magno channel's relatively greater sensitivity for low SF information plays an important role in object perception and affects the speed with which individual features of an object can be extracted from a display.

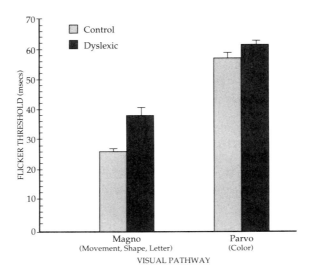

Figure 1. Flicker fusion thresholds of dyslexics and controls for magno- and parvocellular tasks.

Many studies (Weisstein, and Harris 1974; McClelland 1978; Williams and Weisstein 1978; Lanze, Weisstein, and Harris 1982) have shown that under tachistoscopic conditions, a single feature, such as a line, can be more easily identified in the context of a three-dimensional object than by itself (see figure 2).

This phenomenon, termed the object-superiority effect (OSE), is highly correlated with the perceived depth of the contextual pattern (Lanze et al. 1982), and depth perception has been suggested to be based primarily on information carried by the magno system (Livingstone and Hubel 1987). Consequently, we reasoned that the object superiority effect also may be dependent upon low SF information, which is more selectively processed in the magno pathway. We tested this hypothesis by filtering displays to create conditions with only high (greater than 11 cycles/degree) SF spectra and then compared performance accuracy on filtered display to a full spectra display with a matched Michelson contrast (.33). High and low SF targets, which were either alone or in the three-dimensional figure context, were displayed on a computer screen with exposure durations of 29, 57, 86, 100, 128, 157, and 257 ms, using a backward masking, forced-choice paradigm (McClelland 1978).

We have completed several preliminary studies with normal and dyslexic adults as well as dyslexic and normal-reading children. Data from all 6 exposure durations were averaged for each subject. Results confirmed our hypothesis (see figure 3). For normal and dyslexic adult readers, accuracy dropped 20% when the low spatial frequencies were removed from the displays, but only in the figure context, demonstrating that low SF information is necessary to produce the object superiority effect. Similar results were found for normal and dyslexic children using a slightly different paradigm (see figure 5). Low frequency spectra, however, are not sufficient for this effect since the 2 unfiltered displays (target in object and target alone) contain about the same proportion of low and high SF spectra. Consequently, perceptual judgments about visual features are not based solely upon low SF information, but do depend upon the magno channel to process global information about the display rapidly. This global percept sets up an initial representation that is available early in perceptual analysis from which partial information about individual features can be extracted for better accuracy under short exposure durations.

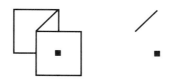

Figure 2.   Sample Target Stimuli from the study of the object-superiority effect.

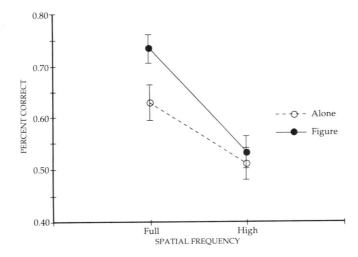

Figure 3. Accuracy on the object superiority task for normal adults on full spatial frequency displays and displays with only high spatial frequencies in the figure or single line context.

LOW SF PROCESSING DEFICIT FOR DYSLEXICS

In addition to the interaction between context and the SF of the displays, we also have found differences between groups in the way SF information is processed. All the adult controls ($N=12$) were significantly better at processing the full SF displays compared to the high SF displays, whereas the performances of the dyslexics ($N=15$) were mixed. Some dyslexic individuals were better with full SF displays, however, many processed the full and high SF stimuli at the same rate. We suspected that individual dyslexic differences might be related to reading ability, and so divided the dyslexic group into two groups based on current reading skills (Compensated, $N=9$ and Decompensated, $N=6$). Both groups have well documented histories of reading disabilities and each received comparable private and public remediation. Both groups also were recruited from among college students, and therefore have achieved some degree of reading and academic proficiency. Current reading ability was measured by the Woodcock Reading Mastery Test–Revised (WRMT-R) and IQ was assessed using the Kaufmann Brief Intelligence Test (KBIT). Reading Quotients (RQ) were calculated for each individual using the formula:

$$RQ = \frac{RQ = 2 * \text{Reading Age (WRMT-R)}}{\text{Chronological Age} + \text{Mental Age (KBIT)}}$$

Dyslexic adults who achieved RQ < .90 were considered decompensated, whereas those with RQs >=.90 were classified as compensated. Comparisons of the two dyslexic groups and controls are shown in figure 4.

Analysis of variance revealed a significant interaction between SF and grouping factors ($F(1,23)=4.57$, $p =.04$). Planned t-test comparisons showed that the decompensated dyslexic group was slower than both the compensated dyslexics and controls under the full SF condition, but both dyslexic groups were better at processing high SF displays than controls. The controls and compensated dyslexics did significantly better with full SF displays as compared to high SF displays, but the decompensated dyslexic group was about the same under both conditions.

To further test the visual processing abilities of children, we have gathered some pilot data measuring the OSE with dyslexic and normally developing readers. The dyslexic children were recruited from the Curtis Blake Day School, a private school for children with severe learning disabilities. Children ranged in age from 8 to 14 with an average age of 11.5. In this task, subjects viewed tachistoscopically displayed stimuli as shown in figure 2, using a forced-choice, backward masking paradigm in which the duration of the display was varied between trial blocks to maintain performance near 75%. As found with the adults, both child groups performed better with the figure context (see figure 5) and showed no OSE with high SF displays. However, the groups differed in their response to the SF condition. The dyslexic subjects performed equally well with the full and high SF displays, whereas the controls were significantly worse with the high SF displays.

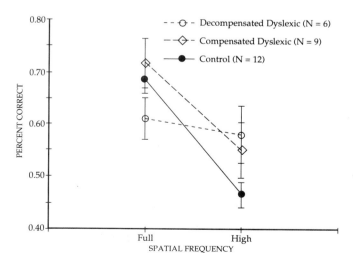

Figure 4.   Comparison of adult dyslexics and controls on the Object Superiority task under high and full SF display conditions. See text for a description of differences between compensated and decompensated dyslexics.

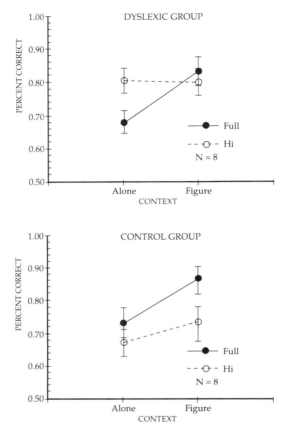

Figure 5.   Dyslexic and control children's performance on an Object Superiority task with full and high SF displays.

Furthermore, the dyslexic children needed longer exposure durations to perform at a comparable level with controls (167 ms vs. 113 ms, p = .12), indicating a slower rate of visual processing. Although the number of subjects is small and some p values only approach significance, these results are quite similar to the decompensated dyslexic adult data and support the feasibility of using these tasks with developing readers.

To summarize, these studies have produced three significant results: first, adult dyslexics do better than controls with high SF displays (e.g., a display which only contains SF above 10 c/d). Second, accuracy in the context of the three-dimensional figure is better than in the target alone context (the OSE) but only with the full SF displays (e.g., the original unfiltered). This was true for all subject groups. Third, the proficient adult dyslexic readers and adult controls are more accurate with full SF displays than the impaired dyslexic adults.

The first result suggests that dyslexic adults process high SF information faster than controls. There are three possible explanations: (1) the magno systems are tuned to a broader-band of SF, resulting in high SF information being more rapidly processed in the magno system (presuming that the processing speed in the dyslexic magno system—though impaired—is not worse than the speed of the parvo system in controls); (2) their parvo systems are working more proficiently; or (3) the magno channel does a more effective job of inhibiting processing in the parvo channel in controls. The first alternative is unlikely because: (1) dyslexics do not show an OSE with high SF displays, something that should happen if the high SF components are being rapidly processed in their magno channels; and (2) retuning the SF sensitivities would require rewiring connections between retinal ganglion cells and the LGN or changing the sizes of the ganglion cells' receptive fields. We have no evidence to support such a radical change in dyslexic visual neurophysiology, and suspect such changes would have a more dramatic effect on other aspects of visual perception. The second alternative has some merit. Some studies have found that reading disabled children have better contrast sensitivity in the high spatial frequency range (12-16 c/d; Lovegrove et al. 1982). Greater sensitivity would account for their improved accuracy under the high SF condition. The third alternative also has been proposed in several studies that report dyslexics to have a weak magno->parvo inhibition (Lovegrove, Martin, and Slaghuis 1986; Williams and Lecluyse 1990). This interpretation suggests that weak inhibition also may have the effect of improving the speed of processing of high SF components in the parvo channel. Future studies are needed to resolve these two alternative explanations.

The second result showed that an OSE was found only when low SF components were present, either as a broad bandwidth display (full) or as just a low SF display. This effect could be produced either by the rapid processing of the low SF components in the magno channel, which then sets up a cortical template prime providing global shape information to facilitate visual processing of details, or by low SF components facilitating the cortical processing of details in some other (unknown) way. Like controls, dyslexics produced an OSE only with full SF displays, suggesting they can process low SF rapidly enough to facilitate the global priming effect; however, the decompensated adult dyslexics were not as accurate with the full SF displays as the compensated dyslexics and controls, suggesting some processing speed deficiency remains.

Our third finding showed that the dyslexic processing speed deficiency can be most clearly seen with full SF displays. The controls and compensated dyslexic adults were more accurate than the decompensated dyslexic adults under this condition. Using a slightly different paradigm, the children's data produced a similar result, showing that the dyslexic children needed longer exposure durations to produce the same accuracy as the control group. Since reading occurs under normal, full SF conditions, this result confirms that visual processing speed will be impaired for many dyslexics while they are reading.

There is considerable interest in understanding why some people are able to compensate for dyslexia but others are not (Lefly and Pennington 1991). Although there is widespread consensus that given similar educational backgrounds, decompensated adult dyslexics have more severe processing deficits, there is little agreement about how to characterize these impairments. Recent work combining data from two longitudinal studies has introduced the hypothesis of a double-deficit (Bowers and Wolf 1993). Dyslexic children were subgrouped according to phonological or lexical access impairments. The very worst readers were deficient in both cognitive domains, but even children with good phonological skills and slow lexical access were impaired readers. These results suggest that perceptual factors that affect the development of and access to orthographic representations play a critical role in reading development. Based on modeling work described below, we believe that slow processing of low SF components can impair the development of lexical memory and slow down lexical access. We suspect that compensated dyslexic adults may not suffer from visual processing speed deficits, allowing them to develop a lexical system without the benefit of phonologically based information. However, decompensated adult dyslexics may suffer from a double-deficit affecting both phonology and orthography. These ideas will be discussed further in the section on the magnocellular deficit model of dyslexia.

These preliminary results are particularly relevant for understanding which visual physical attributes play a critical role in text perception and the development of fluent reading skills. The object-superiority task requires the ability to analyze the constituent features of a visual display in the same way that letter and word recognition requires a reader to distinguish the features that make up the alphabetic font of the text. Rapid identification was shown to be dependent upon the processing of low SF spectra in the display. Impaired dyslexic performance resulted from an inability to utilize low SF information, presumably because the magno pathway is processing this information too slowly to be of full benefit. Low SF spectra may play a critical role in letter perception as well, and the slow dyslexic processing speed of low SF information may interfere with their ability to identify text rapidly and accurately.

SPATIAL FREQUENCY MODEL OF LETTER PERCEPTION

Additional support for this hypothesis can be found in studies that have developed SF models for letter perception. Gervais, Harvey, and Roberts (1984) have shown that SF models performed better than template matching or geometric feature models in their predictions of how readers identify letters of the alphabet. Template models conceive of letter perception as a comparison process between the displayed image and an internal representation stored in memory (Neisser 1967). Feature models make a different comparison based on an analysis of the features found in the letter display with a list of features associated in memory with different letters. SF models make comparisons that are similar to template models but are based upon a Fourier analysis of the visual display. In a Fourier transform, an image of various luminance intensities displayed on spatial coordinates is converted to amplitude spectra mapped on SF coordinates. Both representations are mathematically equivalent (Brigham 1974), and there is evidence to suggest that cortical cells have the requisite properties to perform a SF analysis (DeValois, Albrecht, and Thorell 1982; Robson et al. 1988). SF models also have advantages over template and feature models. Template models are too rigid to adapt to variations in size, shape, or letter orientation (Neisser 1967), and feature models have difficulty accounting for variation in size and font between alphabets and letter case. SF models are not restricted to a particular font and are resilient to variations in orientation or shape.

In a test of these models the highest correlation (.70) between actual and predicted performance on a tachistoscopic letter identification task and the resulting letter confusion matrix data was achieved by a SF model in which the Fourier transform was filtered by the human contrast sensitivity function (Gervais, Harvey, and Roberts 1984). This filter takes into account the actual performance of the human optical system, accounting for the system's relative sensitivity to different SF components. The filter had a peak sensitivity at 5 cycles/degree, functioning to boost the contribution made by low SF information (2-5 cycles/degree) and attenuating high (above 10 cycles/degree) and low (below 1.5 cycles/degree) SF components. The unfiltered SF model more poorly predicted actual data ($r=.45$), suggesting that low SF components provide essential information for letter identification.

Developmental studies of children's letter perception skills, which could provide comparable information about which letters are easily confused with each other, are rare. Eleanor Gibson and her colleagues (Gibson, Shapiro, and Yonas 1968) completed one such study comparing the RT latencies for letter pair judgments made by 7 year olds. Their results showed the 7 year olds judged letters by feature sets that were quite similar to those of adults. The few differences suggested that adults based early judgments predominantly on global features, whereas the children tended to combine some global and local features. Further study would provide invaluable information about how internal representations of graphemes are acquired and what types of representational mappings exist at different stages of reading development.

SPATIAL FREQUENCY COMPONENTS AND THE WORD SUPERIORITY EFFECT

We have hypothesized that low SF components are important to the priming of orthographic memory units, rapidly activating the global features of letters and words to facilitate their identification. We directly tested this hypothesis by manipulating SF components of words and random letter strings in a tachistoscopic identification task called the word superiority effect (WSE). In the WSE, letter perception is enhanced by presentation in the context of a word. We have argued elsewhere (Chase and Tallal 1991) that experimental results from the WSE provide an ideal set of data for studying how lexical memory organizes itself during reading development. How lexical representational units are formed and how connections between units develop with experience can be analyzed in detail using a PDP model of the experimental data (Chase and Tallal 1991; Chase and Tallal 1990).

Our research on the OSE suggests that feature perception is better in the context of a three-dimensional object because rapid processing of low spatial frequencies enhances perception. A similar process may be at work in the WSE for young readers. Many studies have shown children's reading to be strongly affected by the manipulation of physical characteristics of the display (Gibson and Levin 1975). Although several adult studies have reported the WSE to be primarily a linguistic phenomenon (Adams 1979; Krueger and Shapiro 1979), manipulations of the physical characteristics in these experiments may have been insufficient to counteract the strong linguistic effects. Young readers show a strong WSE but their linguistic component is weaker (Chase and Tallal 1990), suggesting that physical characteristics may contribute relatively more to the WSE in children than adults.

As a preliminary test, we conducted a pilot study to examine the effect of full and high SF displays on WSE performance. If low SF components contribute to word recognition, then the WSE should be reduced in the high SF condition, as compared to a full SF condition with the same Michelson contrast (.33). We used a forced-choice, backward masking paradigm in which four-letter, high-frequency words or random letter strings were presented tachistoscopically at exposure durations that were adjusted between trial blocks to maintain subject performance at around 75% (see experiment 3 below for details). This procedure limits the time course of processing and controls for response biases, short-term memory factors, and guessing strategies. In addition, fatigue, practice, and floor and ceiling effects were controlled by maintaining performance accuracy at a challenging level within a trial block, allowing a direct comparison of subject performance in each experimental condition (Chase and Tallal 1990). Trial blocks were balanced for word type and target serial position. Each block had the same SF stimuli, and blocks alternated between full and high SF displays.

Results from 9 normal subjects (see figure 6) showed significant SF ($F(1,8)=10.08$, $p=.01$) and word type ($F(1,8)=5.07$, $p=.05$) effects. Letters were more accurately identified in the context of words than random letter strings (the WSE). Letters also were much easier to perceive when the full SFs were present. To examine the importance of low SF components for the WSE, planned comparisons were made between full SF words and nonwords and between high SF words and non-words. T-test comparisons showed the WSE only occurred with full SF displays ($t=3.41$, $p=.009$). Word context did not facilitate performance with high SF displays ($t=1.33$, $p=.22$). As can be seen in figure 6, the lack of a WSE in high SF conditions was not the result of floor effects, since subject performance was well above chance (50%).

This pilot study supports our hypothesis that low spatial frequencies contribute to the early stages of visual processing of orthographic information. First, subjects' accuracy improved by 12% when low SF components were present in the letter display. Other factors that may have differentially affected the visibility of the display, such as Michelson contrast, visual acuity, or luminance energy, were carefully matched between the full and high SF displays. Second, the WSE only occurred with full SF displays, suggesting that low SF components may play an important role in facilitating rapid identification of familiar orthographic information. Additional work is needed to compare dyslexic performance

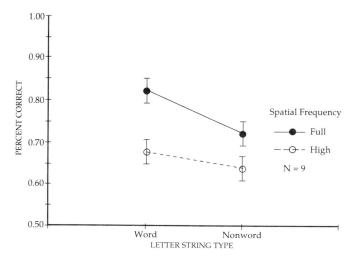

Figure 6.   Spatial Frequency and the Word Superiority Effect. Subjects showed a WSE with Full SF displays, but no WSE with high SF displays.

with controls and also to test the effect of orthographic familiarity on the SF effect.

A MAGNOCELLULAR DEFICIT MODEL OF DYSLEXIA

This review of cognitive and neuroanatomical evidence suggests a model of developmental dyslexia that is based on the slow rate of processing in the magnocellular channel among dyslexics. This delay primarily affects the processing of low SF information. These SF components function to activate cortical representational maps that define the global shape of the letters in the text. In a normal reader the magnocellular pathway processes information more rapidly than the parvocellular route, providing the cortical maps with the global pattern information before information about the finer visual details arrives via the parvo pathway.

From a parallel, distributed processing (PDP) framework (Rumelhart and McClelland 1986), cortical representations of letters or words are broadly distributed across many processing units that mutually excite and inhibit one another. Processing goes on simultaneously, so the system operates in parallel without an executive unit responsible for coordination and routing of processing functions. Representation is a dynamic process in which patterns of activation across units compete with one another. Over time information accumulates, allowing competing units to settle into a stable state. For adults this process takes only tens of ms (Rayner and Duffy 1988) but it can take over 200 ms for young readers (Chase and Tallal 1990). Rapid identification of text can be made with only a partial analysis before a stable state has been reached if sufficient contextual cues constrain the likely alternatives (Rumelhart 1977). These constraints could come from bottom-up (perceptual) or top-down (linguistic comprehension) sources, providing additional information that rapidly increases the activation of unit patterns that are consistent with contextual cues. From this perspective, reading is viewed as a probabilistic interpretation of the letter string that results from the dynamic interactions of units from multiple levels of representation (e.g., features, letters, words, and story schemata).

The time course within which information reaches and activates the distributed memory system is critical not only for recognition but also for learning. Based on studies of the way the somatosensory cortex maps the surface of the body, Merzenich and his colleagues (1987) have proposed that the organization of cortical receptive fields is based on the temporal synchronization of sensory input. The cortex integrates sensory input within a narrow, fixed time window on the order of tens of milliseconds. Cortical representational maps are created by grouping together sensory input that is temporally correlated. These data suggest that the speed with which the visual system processes information plays a critical role in how it is organized and represented. Dyslexic delays in processing low SF components will disrupt temporal synchrony of the signal, making it difficult for cortical maps to organize. As a result, low SF information is likely to be under-utilized in rapid visual perception tasks (see discussion of the object-superiority effect above).

In a study of word recognition development (Chase and Tallal 1990) we found that visual processing speed dramatically improved with age and/or reading skill. On a tachistoscopic word recognition task, 8 year olds required ten times the exposure duration to equal adult performance, whereas some 10 year olds were already performing at adult levels. The dyslexic 10 year olds in our study required exposure durations comparable to their reading-age matched younger readers (8 years old). These results are consistent with a study of visual processing speed in children, using a non-linguistic flicker fusion threshold task (Brannan and Williams 1988). Ten and 12 year olds had threshold sensitivities that were comparable to adults, but 8 year olds were less sensitive at the intermediate frequencies. Poor readers (ages 8-12) were less sensitive at almost all frequencies.

A PDP computer simulation model of our developmental data (Chase and Tallal 1990) suggested that complex changes occur during development, which improve perceptual and lexical memory functioning. Perceptually, adults processed the sensory input more rapidly than children, and they were able to distribute their attention across more of the letter display, enabling more letter information to be extracted in parallel. In their lexical memory, adults produced a more distributed pattern of activation that excited many word units, whereas younger normal readers were more selective and tended to focus activation on specific word units that closely resembled the stimulus. Dyslexic 10-year-old children produced a weakly distributed pattern of activation across many units, which was about half the level of activation produced by adults.

These modeling results suggest a method by which low SF components could facilitate the rapid identification of text. Initial lexical processing is based on the low frequency components. For adults, this information is rapidly conducted along the magno pathway, setting up a distributed pattern of activation that primes orthographic units consistent with the global features in the display. As more detailed information is dynamically accumulated, the primed units consistent with the new information rapidly strengthen, inhibiting competing units. Without the low SF prime, it would take much longer to stabilize a pattern. Many more units would be activated at the same time by the high SF components, prolonging the competition between units, since each started out at comparable strength.

The absence of a low frequency prime not only would slow down the process of identification but also would interfere with the development and organization of grapheme representation. Our computer simulations suggest that connection strengths between representational units in an adult lexical memory system are well organized. Letters that share similar features are mutually activated just as words that share similar letters and grapheme clusters also are activated together. The organization of these grapheme patterns appeared to go through three stages of development. First, novice readers distribute activation broadly and non-selectively. Second, activation patterns become more tightly focused on a few representational units fully consistent with the stimulus input. Third, activation then begins to spread to other grapheme units, creating patterns of grapheme clusters, which share common features or letters. Dyslexic 10 year olds appeared to be operating in the first stage of development, unable to organize a more tightly focused network of units that are specifically responsive to a particular stimulus pattern. The rapid processing of low SF information may be critical for the development of such specific unit networks.

To explore these ideas further, we began exploring recurrent connectionist models, incorporating SF components as the priming input, to learn more about the computational role of low SFs in complex pattern recognition. We studied both an Elman and Jordan 3-layer network consisting of a 121 unit input matrix (an 11x11 retinotopic array), a 25 unit hidden matrix, a 25 unit context matrix, and a 25 unit output matrix using one unit for each letter of the alphabet (excluding Z). The networks are fully interconnected and trained using a back-propagation learning algorithm (Rumelhart and McClelland 1986). Networks were trained to discriminate among 25 letters in both a normal upright and 90 degree rotated form.

We wondered whether a network during training would discover a computational solution that could benefit from a low SF prime. Networks were trained on full SF input patterns. Once trained, letter recognition was staged into two parts using two different input displays: a low or high SF prime and the letter on which the network had been trained. Low Primes were patterns of the target letter constructed to represent the Fourier low SF bandpasses of the training letter. The low SF primes appeared to be blurred versions of the original training letter, but the borders of the prime extended beyond the boundary of the original letter. High SF primes were constructed using Fourier analysis to make high bandpass filters of the training letters.

During recognition testing, primes were presented for a few cycles of recurrent processing, allowing units in the network to update each other gradually. We then recorded the amount of activation produced for the correct output unit and also recorded other output units that might be partially activated by the prime. Then the original letter input pattern was presented and output activation was again recorded.

Results showed that both network architectures produced low SF priming effects but no high SF priming; however, the Elman network appeared to produce a more robust priming effect. Variability could be due to the fact that the SF primes extended beyond the borders of the training letter set, thus activating input units that had not been trained.

These results are important in two respects. First, they show that the global precedence effect from low SF primes may be an innate part of any computational solution to a pattern recognition task. Second, they suggest the possibility that translation invariance, the ability to recognize a pattern regardless of variations in fine details or in spatial location, may be related to the low SF priming effect and be produced from the same computational solution.

BEYOND UNITARY EXPLANATIONS

We believe that unitary explanations for dyslexia based upon phono-logical awareness deficits are premature. As the neuroanatomical data above suggests, dyslexics have multiple sites of neuropathological disorganization, and comparisons between different dyslexic brains show considerable variation. Both visual and auditory systems are involved in learning to read, and so far the neuroanatomical evidence indicates pathological changes in both systems. It also is difficult to identify which subsystem is more "critical" for developing readers. Certainly phonological awareness is essential for sounding out words and developing the strategies necessary to decode new vocabulary. However, the inability to process visual information rapidly can severely handicap perceptual analysis and is likely to interfere with phonemic discrimination, but in exactly what way and to what degree is difficult to determine. While considerable research effort has identified some of the auditory perceptual skills necessary for normal reading development, little work has been done in the visual domain. As yet we still know very little about which visual physical attributes of text are most critical for young readers and what visual perceptual skills are necessary to develop the rapid processing needed for fluent reading.

These arguments apply to a magnocellular deficit model as well. We do not expect to find visual processing speed deficits in all develop-mental dyslexics. However, we do think that those who show such deficits will be among the more severely impaired readers. Impairments that affect the visual perceptibility of text are likely to be quite debili-tating, since such deficits also would disrupt the quality of all subsequent linguistic analysis. Many dyslexic children suffer from phonological impairments, but other strategies besides phonological decoding are available for developing a reading vocabulary, as evidenced by the fact that many dyslexic adults, who are unable to perform phonological decoding tasks, nevertheless have acquired large sight vocabularies (Lefly and Pennington 1991). We suspect that compensated adult dyslexics may not have visual processing speed deficits but that reading-impaired adults, who have failed to develop good sight vocabularies, could suffer from a visual processing deficit.

REFERENCES

Badcock, J. C., Whitworth, F. A., Badcock, D. R., and Lovegrove, W. J. 1990. Low-frequency filtering and the processing of local-global stimuli. *Perception* 19:617–29.

Bassi, C. J., and Lehmkuhle, S. 1990. Clinical implications of parallel visual pathways. *Journal of the American Optometric Association* 61:98–110.

Bowers, P. G., and Wolf, M. 1993, March. A double-deficit hypothesis for developmental reading disorders. Paper presented at the Annual Convention of the Society for Research in Child Development, New Orleans.

Bradley, L., and Bryant, P. 1983. Categorizing sounds and learning to read—A causal connection. *Nature* 301:419–21.

Brannan, J. R., and Williams, M. C. 1988. The effects of age and reading ability on flicker threshold. *Clinical Vision Sciences* 2:137–42.

Breitmeyer, B. 1980. Unmasking visual masking: A look at the "why" behind the veil of the "how." *Psychology Review* 87:52–69.

Breitmeyer, B. 1984. *Visual Masking: An Integrative Approach*. Oxford: Oxford University Press.

Breitmeyer, B. G. 1989. A visual based deficit in Specific Reading Disability. *Irish Journal of Psychology* 10:534–41.

Breitmeyer, B. G., and Ganz, L. 1976. Implications of sustained and transient channels for theories of visual pattern masking, saccadic suppression, and information processing. *Psychological Review* 83:1–36.

Brigham, E. O. 1974. *The Fast Fourier Transform*. Englewood Cliffs, NJ: Prentice-Hall.

Caviness, V. S., Misson, J., and Gadisseux, J. 1989. Abnormal neuronal patterns and disorders of neocortical development. In *From Reading to Neurons*, ed. A. M. Galaburda. Cambridge, MA: MIT Press.

Chase, C. H., and Jenner, A. 1993. Magnocellular processing deficits affect temporal processing of dyslexics. *Annals of the New York Academy of Sciences* 682:326–30.

Chase, C. H., and Tallal, P. 1990. A developmental, interactive activation model of the word superiority effect. *Journal of Experimental Child Psychology* 49:448–87.

Chase, C. H., and Tallal, P. 1991. Cognitive models of developmental reading disorders. In *Neuropsychological Foundations of Learning Disabilities*, eds. J. E. Obrzut and G. W. Hynd. San Diego: Academic Press.

Chase, C. H., Heuer, H., and Blake, D. in preparation. Spatial frequency and the Object-superiority effect. .

Chen, H.-C. 1986. Effects of reading span and textual coherence on rapid-sequential reading. *Memory and Cognition* 14:202–08.

Conners, C. K. 1989. *Conners' Rating Scales*. Austin, TX: PRO-ED.

DeValois, R. L., Albrecht, D. G., and Thorell, L. G. 1982. Spatial frequency selectivity of cells in macaque visual cortex. *Vision Research* 22:545–59.

DiLollo, V., Hanson, D., and McIntyre, J. S. 1983. Initial stages of visual information processing in dyslexia. *Journal of Experimental Psychology: Human Perception and Performance* 9:923–35.

Enroth-Cugell, C., and Robson, J. G. 1966. The contrast sensitivity of retinal ganglion cells of the cat. *Journal of Physiology* 187:517–52.

Eriksen, C. W., and Schultz, D. W. 1979. Information processing and visual search: The continuous flow conception and experimental results. *Perception and Psychophysics* 29:249–63.

Flavell, J. H., and Draguns, J. 1957. A microgenetic approach to perception and thought. *Psychological Bulletin* 54:197–217.

Fukuda, Y. 1971. Receptive field organization of cat optic nerve fibers with special reference to conduction velocity. *Vision Research* 11:209–26.

Galaburda, A. M., and Eidelberg, D. 1982. Symmetry and asymmetry in the human posterior thalamus: II. Thalamic lesions in a case of developmental dyslexia. *Archives of Neurology* 39:333–36.

Galaburda, A. M., Rosen, G. D., and Sherman, G. F. 1989. The neural origin of developmental dyslexia: Implications for medicine, neurology, and cognition. In *From Reading to Neurons*, ed. A. M. Galaburda. Cambridge, MA: MIT Press.

Galaburda, A. M., Sherman, G. F., Rosen, G. D., Aboitiz, F., and Geschwind, N. 1985. Developmental dyslexia: Four consecutive patients with cortical anomalies. *Annals of Neurology* 18:222–33.

Gervais, M. J., Harvey, L. O., and Roberts, J. O. 1984. Identification confusions among letters of the alphabet. *Journal of Experimental Psychology: Human Perception and Performance* 10:655–66.

Geschwind, N., and Levitsky, W. 1968. Left-right asymmetry in temporal speech region. *Science* 161:186–87.

Gibson, E. J., and Levin, H. 1975. *The Psychology of Reading*. Cambridge, MA: MIT Press.

Gibson, E. J., Schapiro, F., and Yonas, A. 1968. Confusion matrices for graphic patterns obtained with a latency measure. In *Perception and Its Development: A Tribute to Eleanor J. Gibson*, ed. A. Pick. Hillsdale, NJ: Lawrence Erlbaum Associates.

Goswami, U. 1986. Children's use of analogy in learning to read: A developmental study. *Journal of Experimental Child Psychology* 42:73–83.

Goswami, U. 1988. Orthographic analogies and reading development. *Quarterly Journal of Experimental Psychology* 40A:239–68.

Goswami, U. 1991. Learning about spelling sequences: The role of onsets and rimes in analogies in reading. *Child Development* 62:1110–23.

Goswami, U., and Bryant, P. E. 1990. *Phonological Skills and Learning to Read*. Hillsdale, N J: Lawrence Erlbaum Associates.

Gregory, R. L. 1978. *Eye and Brain, 3rd Edition*. New York: MaGraw-Hill.

Hinshelwood, J. 1917. *Congenital Word-Blindness*. London: Lewis.

Hynd, G. W., and Semrud-Clikeman, M. (1989). Dyslexia and brain morphology. *Psychological Bulletin* 106:447–82.

Johnson, D. 1988. Specific developmental disabilities of reading, writing and mathematics. In *Learning Disabilities: Proceedings of the National Conference*, eds. J. F. Kavanagh and T. J. Truss, Jr. Parkton, MD: York Press.

Keogh, B. 1986. Future of the LD field: Research and practice. *Journal of Learning Disabilities* 19:455–60.

Krueger, L. E., and Shapiro, R. G. 1979. Letter detection with rapid serial visual presentation: Evidence against word superiority at feature extraction. *Journal of Experimental Psychology: Human Perception and Performance* 5:657–73.

Lanze, M., Weisstein, N., and Harris, J. R. 1982. Perceived depth vs. structural relevance in the object-superiority effect. *Perception and Psychophysics* 31:376–82.

Lefly, D. L., and Pennington, B. F. 1991. Spelling errors and reading fluency in compensated adult dyslexics. *Annals of Dyslexia* 41:143–62.

Legge, G. E. 1978. Sustained and transient mechanisms in human vision: Temporal and spatial properties. *Vision Research* 18:69–81.

Legge, G. E., Parish, D. H., Luebker, A., and Wurm, L. H. 1990. Psychophysics of reading. XI. Comparing color contrast and luminance contrast. *Journal of the Optical Society of America* 7:2002–10.

Legge, G. E., Pelli, D. G., Rubin, G. S., and Schleske, M. M. 1985. Psychophysics of Reading I. Normal Vision. *Vision Research* 25:239–52.

Lehmkuhle, S., Garzia, R. P., Turner, L., Hash, T., and Baro, J. A. 1993. A defective visual pathway in children with reading disability. *New England Journal of Medicine* 328:989–96.

Liberman, I. Y. 1983. A language-oriented view of reading and its disabilities. In *Progress in Learning Disabilities*, ed. H. Mykelburst. New York: Grune and Stratton.

Livingstone, M. S., and Hubel, D. H. 1987. Psychophysical evidence for separate channels for the perception of form, color, movement, and depth. *Journal of Neuroscience* 7:3416–68.

Livingstone, M. S., and Hubel, D. H. 1988. Do the relative mapping densities of the magno- and parvocellular systems vary with eccentricity? *Journal of Neuroscience* 8:4334–39.

Livingstone, M. S., Rosen, G. D., Drislane, F. W., and Galaburda, A. M. 1991. Physiological and anatomical evidence for a magnocellular defect in developmental dyslexia. *Proceedings of the National Academy of Science* 88:7943–47.

Lovegrove, W., Martin, F., and Slaghuis, W. 1986. A theoretical and experimental case for a visual deficit in specific reading disability. *Cognitive Neuropsychology* 3:225–67.

Lovegrove, W. J., Garzia, R. P., and Nicholson, S. B. 1990. Experimental evidence for a transient system deficit in specific reading disability. *Journal of the American Optometric Association* 61:137–46.

Lovegrove, W. J., Martin, F., Bowling, A., Blackwood, M., Badcock, D., and Paxton, S. 1982. Contrast sensitivity functions and specific reading disability. *Neuropsychologia* 20:309–15.

Lovett, M. W., Ransby, M. J., Hardwick, N., Johns, M. S., and Donaldson, S. A. 1989. Can dyslexia be treated? Treatment-specific and generalised treatment effects in dyslexic children's response to remediation. *Brain and Language* 37:90–121.

McClelland, J. L. 1978. Perception and masking of wholes and parts. *Journal of Experimental Psychology: Human Perception and Performance* 4:210–23.

McClelland, J. L. 1979. On time relations of mental processes: An examination of systems of processes in cascade. *Psychological Review* 86:287–330.

Malatesha, R. N., and Dougan, D. R. 1982. Clinical subtypes of developmental dyslexia: Resolution of an irresolute problem. In *Reading Disorders: Varieties and Treatments*, eds. R. N. Malatesha and P. G. Aaron. New York: Academic Press.

Merzenich, M. M. 1987. Dynamic neocortical processes and the origins of higher brain functions. In *The Neural and Molecular Bases of Learning*, eds. J. Changeux and M. Konishi. New York: John Wiley and Sons.

Morgan, W. P. 1896. A case of congenital word-blindness. *British Medical Journal* 2:1378.

Navon, D. 1977. Forest before trees: The precedence of global features in visual perception. *Cognitive Psychology* 9:353–83.

Neisser, U. 1967. *Cognitive Psychology*. New York: Appleton-Century-Crofts.

Office of Special Education 1984. *Sixth Annual Report to Congress on the Implementation of the Education of the Handicapped Act*. U. S. Department of Education.

Petersen, S. E., Fox, P. T., Snyder, A. Z., and Raichle, M. E. 1990. Activation of extrastriate and frontal cortical areas by visual words and work-like stimuli. *Science* 240:1627–31.

Rayner, K., and Duffy, S. A. 1988. On-line comprehension processes and eye movements during reading. In *Reading Research: Advances in Theory and Practice*, eds. M. Daneman, G. E. MacKinnon, and T. G. Waller. San Diego: Academic Press.

Rayner, K., and Pollatsek, A. 1989. *Psychology of Reading*. Englewood Cliffs, N.J: Prentice Hall.

Robson, J. G., Tolhurst, D. J., Freeman, R. D., and Ohzawa, I. 1988. Simple cells in the visual cortex of the cat can be narrowly tuned for spatial frequency. *Visual Neuroscience* 1:415–19.

Rosen, G. D., Sherman, G. F., and Galaburda, A. M. 1991. Ontogenesis of neocortical asymmetry: A [^{3}H] thymidine study. *Neuroscience* 41:779–90.

Rumelhart, D. E. 1977. Toward an interactive model of reading. In *Attention and Performance VI*, ed. S. Dornic. Hillsdale, N J: Lawrence Erlbaum Associates.

Rumelhart, D. E., and McClelland, J. L. ed. 1986. *Parallel Distributed Processing: Explorations in the Microstructures of Cognition*. Cambridge, MA: MIT Press.

Saito, H., Shimahara, T., and Fukada, Y. 1970. Four types of responses to light and dark spot stimuli on the cat optic nerve. *Tohoku Journal of Experimental Medicine* 102:127–33.

Schiller, P. H., and Logothetis, N. K. 1990. The color-opponent and broad-band channels of the primate visual system. *Trends in Neuroscience* 13:392–98.

Seidenberg, M. S. 1993. A connectionist modeling approach to word recognition and dyslexia. *Psychological Science* 4(5):299–304.

Shapley, R. 1990. Visual sensitivity and parallel retinocortical channels. *Annual Review of Psychology* 41:635–58.

Stanovich, K., Cunningham, A., and Cramer, B. 1984. Assessing phonological awareness in kindergarten children: Issues of task comparability. *Journal of Experimental Child Psychology* 38:175–90.

Stanovich, K. E. 1988. The right and wrong places to look for the cognitive locus of reading disability. *Annals of Dyslexia* 38:154–77.

Tallal, P. 1980. Language and reading: Some perceptual prerequisites. *Bulletin of The Orton Dyslexic Society* 30:170–78.

Tallal, P. 1988. Developmental language disorders. In *Learning Disabilities: Proceedings of the National Conference*, eds. J. R. Kavanagh and T. J. Truss, Jr. Parkton, MD: York Press.

Tallal, P., and Piercy, M. 1973. Defects of non-verbal auditory perception in children with developmental aphasia. *Nature* 241:468–69.

Tallal, P., Stark, R., and Mellits, F. 1985. Identification of language-impaired children on the basis of rapid perception and production skills. *Brain and Language* 25:314–22.

Vellutino, F. R. 1979. *Dyslexia: Theory and Research.* Cambridge, MA: MIT Press.

Weisstein, N., and Harris, C. S. 1974. Visual detection of line segments: An object superiority effect. *Science* 186:752–55.

Williams, A., and Weisstein, N. 1978. Line segments are perceived better in a coherent context than alone: An object-line effect in visual perception. *Memory and Cognition* 6:85–90.

Williams, M. C., and Lecluyse, K. 1990. Perceptual consequences of a temporal processing deficit in reading disabled children. *Journal of the American Optometric Association* 61:111–23.

Part • IV

Auditory Cognitive Mechanisms

As stated in the definition of developmental dyslexia recently adopted by The Orton Dyslexia Society (for a discussion of the definition see Lyon 1995), phonological processing is a fundamental deficit in dyslexia and forms the basis for many of the language problems seen in dyslexic individuals. The following two chapters accept the important role of phonological deficits in dyslexia, but attempt to explore and explain its role in different ways. Van Orden and Goldinger hypothesize that accurate and efficient phonological processing is a primary and fundamental process necessary for skilled reading. They discuss a cognitive systems model of reading that may help us understand how neural networks function in skilled reading and how the developmental process may break down in dyslexics.

Tallal, Miller, and Fitch also acknowledge the importance of proper phonological processing for skilled reading. They suggest, however, that language learning impairments and developmental dyslexia result from a primary deficit in temporal processing ability that leads to the phonological processing problems. This intriguing hypothesis states that there is an initial failure of language-disabled children to process correctly components of information that enter the central nervous system in rapid succession. The linguistic/phonological system of the brain initially is normal, but with the improper perception of speech sounds come developmental changes in language-related brain networks resulting in a dysfunction in phonological awareness. Their chapter emphasizes the primary importance of temporal processing deficits in the auditory system, but also suggests that these deficits may be present in other sensory and motor networks. Recently, this group, in a pair of collaborative studies (Tallal et al. 1996; Merzenich et al. 1996) of language-learning impaired children, found that acoustically modifying speech by slowing down and emphasizing rapidly changing speech components in combination with temporal processing training resulted in improved speech perception and language comprehension. This chapter reviews the groundwork upon which these new studies are based.

Lyon, G. R. 1995. Toward a Definition of Dyslexia. *Annals of Dyslexia* 45:3–27.
Merzenich, M. M., Jenkins, W. M., Johnston, P., Schreiner, C., Miller, S. L., and Tallal, P. 1996. Temporal processing deficits of language-learning impaired children ameliorated by training. *Science* 271:77–81.
Tallal, P., Miller, S. L., Bedi, G., Wang, X., Nagarajan, S. S., Schreiner, C., Jenkins, W. M., and Merzenich, M. M. 1996. Language comprehension in language-learning impaired children improved with acoustically modified speech. *Science* 271:81–84.

Chapter • 8

Neurobiological Basics of Speech: A Case for the Preeminence of Temporal Processing

Paula Tallal
Steve Miller
Roslyn Holly Fitch

Epidemiological surveys have reported that somewhere between 3% and 10% of preschool children exhibit some form of developmental speech or language disorder that cannot be attributed to a known cause such as hearing impairment, general mental retardation or frank neurological disorder (e.g., seizures or an acquired brain lesion) (Beitchman, Nair, and Patel 1986). Research is now showing that dysfunction of higher level speech processing, necessary for normal language and reading development, may result from difficulties in the processing of basic sensory information entering the nervous system in rapid succession (within milliseconds). In this paper we present evidence supporting the hypothesis that a basic temporal processing impairment in language impaired children underlies their inability to integrate sensory information that converges in rapid succession in the central nervous system. We provide data showing that this deficit is pansensory, that is, affects processing in multiple sensory modalities, and also affects motor output within the millisecond time frame. We also provide data which links these basic temporal integration deficits to specific patterns of speech perception and speech production deficits

This chapter is reprinted with kind permission of the New York Academy of Sciences. It originally appeared in Volume 682, June 14, 1993, pages 27–47. Minor changes have been made in order to conform to the style of this book.

in language impaired children. We suggest that these basic temporal deficits cause a cascade of effects, starting with disruption of the normal development of an otherwise effective and efficient phonological system. We propose further that these phonological processing deficits result in subsequent failure to learn to speak and to read normally. That is, both the language and reading problems have their basis in deficiently established phonological processing and decoding. Finally, we use data derived from our ongoing behavioral studies with language impaired children to address some fundamental issues pertaining to the neurobiological basis of speech perception and production (e.g., hemispheric specialization) underlying these processes. We suggest that results from magnetic resonance imaging (MRI) and positron emission tomography (PET) studies, as well as studies of behavioral performance in normal adults and adults with acquired lesions, combined with more recent results from animal studies, all support the view that a left-hemispheric specialization for speech initially developed through evolution as a specialization for processing and producing sensory and motor events which occur in rapid succession.

EXPERIMENTAL STUDIES OF SPECIFICALLY LANGUAGE IMPAIRED CHILDREN

The term "specific language impairment" (LI) has come to refer to the diagnostic classification which, for research purposes, is based on quantitative exclusionary and inclusionary criteria. For the purposes of the studies reviewed below, LI refers to children who were developing normally in every respect but failed to develop language at the expected rate. Criteria for inclusion as a LI subject in our research studies began with exclusion of all children with sensory hearing loss, general mental retardation, paralysis or lack of sensation in the oral musculature, or frank neurological or psychiatric disorders (including attention deficit disorder). In addition, potential subjects had to demonstrate a nonverbal performance IQ of 85 or above, and a significant discrepancy between both their chronological and mental age in receptive and/or expressive language development (based on standardized clinical tests). The results of the behavioral experiments reported below have been replicated on three separate samples of LI children meeting these criteria, and control children matched on age, IQ, and socioeconomic status. The sample sizes for these replications included 12 subjects per group, 36 subjects per group, and 100 LI and 60 controls. Details of subject selection, test scores and demographics for these populations are given by Tallal and Piercy (1973b), Stark and Tallal (1981), and Zeigler, Tallal, and Curtiss (1990).

Our studies began in 1970 with an interest in understanding the severe deficits in both phonological perception and production that characterized most LI children. We reasoned that before studying speech per se, it would be important to assess the integrity of the component acoustic processes that are critical to the analysis of the complex acoustic spectra of speech. Put simply, it is clearly important to determine that a child can hear normally before interpreting deficits in their ability to process or produce speech. Similarly, even where it can be shown that the sensory organ is intact, it is still important to assess other central aspects of auditory processing to ensure that the fundamental components of acoustic analysis throughout the nervous system are intact and functioning normally.

With this premise in mind we began by developing a hierarchical battery of subtests for assessing detection, temporal integration, association, discrimination, sequencing, rate processing, and serial memory for acoustic events. In order to avoid verbal instructions or response requirements, Tallal and Piercy (1973a) developed an operant conditioning paradigm in which subjects were trained to detect and discriminate varied sequential presentations of two complex steady-state tones with different fundamental frequencies (100 Hz and 305 Hz), and to respond by pressing panels on a response box.

We used two test methods. In the association method subjects were trained to respond to each tone separately by pushing the top panel to Tone 1 and the bottom to Tone 2. Discrimination training continued until criterion was reached. Subjects were then trained to respond to each of the 4 possible two-tone sequences (1-1, 1-2, 2-1, 2-2) by pushing the panels in the corresponding order. In the first series, the interstimulus interval (ISI) was constant at 428 ms. In the second series, subjects were tested on the same two-tone sequences, but with ISIs ranging from 8 ms to 4,062 ms, presented in random order. A similar procedure was used to test serial memory using the same two tones in sequences of three to seven elements (ISI 428 ms).

Because a subject may have been able to perceive the elements of a temporal sequence but unable to reproduce a corresponding motor pattern, a same-different method was also used. The response panel was turned through 90° to avoid confusion between methods. Subjects were initially presented with the two tones in varied sequences (ISI 428 ms), and were trained to press the right panel if the tones were the same and the left panel if different. Training again continued until criterion was reached. The same series of two-tone sequences, 24 with ISI 428 ms and 48 with ISI varied as above, were then presented, and the subject indicated whether the two tones were the same or different. Half of the subjects in each group performed the association task first; half performed the same-different task first.

In the first series of experiments, twelve 6- through 9-year-old LI children and matched controls were tested on these procedures using a fixed duration (75 ms) for tones 1 and 2 (Tallal and Piercy 1973a). In trials in which more than one tone was presented, the (ISI) was varied between 8 and 4,062 ms. Results showed that there were no significant differences between the performance of LI and control children on the detection, association, or sequencing subtest when the ISI was at 428 ms or longer. As can be seen in figure 1, however, the performance of the LI children deteriorated rapidly with shorter ISIs. No LI subject reached a criteria of 75% correct at a 150 ms ISI or shorter. In contrast, all controls were able to reach 75% correct at ISIs of 8 ms or longer. A similar pattern of results was demonstrated in both the same-different and sequential ordering paradigms. That is, at rapid rates of presentation, LI children were significantly impaired in their ability to both discriminate and sequence auditory stimuli.

Two points should be emphasized regarding the pattern of data presented in figure 1. First, the processing time needed by LI subjects to respond correctly on this basic auditory processing test was *orders of magnitude* greater than that required by matched controls. Second, the perceptual function for the LIs was bimodal rather than linear. That is, at sufficiently slow presentation rates, LI children were unimpaired in their ability to identify, discriminate, and sequence basic acoustic information. But, when the rate of presentation was speeded up by decreasing the interval between stimuli the LIs' performance dropped to chance levels. These data suggest that when given sufficient input time for signal processing, LI children are able to utilize central auditory processes for discrimination and sequencing of sensory information normally. However, they need orders of magnitude

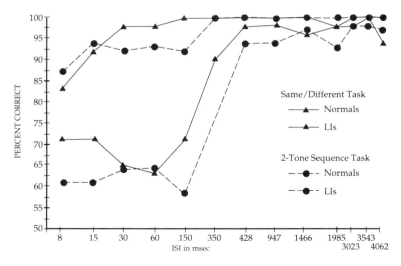

Figure 1. Percent correct for normals and LIs with varied ISIs. Duration of complex tones = 75 ms (tone 1 = 100 Hz, tone 2 = 305 Hz). (Adapted from data presented in Tallal and Piercy 1973.)

more time between the input of basic sensory events in order to access these higher level processes.

In the next set of experiments the role of stimulus duration on auditory perception was examined (Tallal and Piercy 1973b). The most significant findings were on the serial memory task. Whereas all controls (100%) reached criterion on the three-element serial memory task at 75 ms tone durations, only 2 out of 12 LI children (17%) reached this same criterion. When the stimulus duration was lengthened to 250 ms, however, 10 out of 12 LIs reached criterion on this same three element task. It is important to note that control performance did not deteriorate significantly as a function of increasing the number of elements in a sequence (up to five items), even at 75-ms tone durations. However, severe deterioration in the LI subjects' performance was seen at sequence lengths above three elements, even with longer stimulus durations. Thus it is clear from these results that even though increasing the duration of the stimulus improved the serial memory performance of LI children, serial memory remained impaired for LIs in comparison to controls.

In conclusion, the time available for acoustic processing is clearly important for sequential memory performance. However, since increasing stimulus duration did not completely ameliorate deficits in serial memory for tone sequences of greater than three elements for LI children, the impairment of serial memory may be independent of the temporal processing deficit. Conversely, given the developmental nature of language impairment, it is possible that a primary temporal processing deficit may result in a form of auditory deprivation that, in turn, alters neuronal mapping and connections across the auditory system (see Merzenich et al. 1993) with cascading effects on other higher level auditory processes. The effects of this deprivation may result in, among other things, retarded development of complex acoustic processes (e.g., auditory serial memory), as well as deficits in the perception of rapid and sequential transients within speech.

STUDIES OF SPEECH PERCEPTION AND PRODUCTION

The previous nonverbal acoustic studies clearly showed that LI children exhibited a profound deficit in processing rapidly presented acoustic information. How could such a basic temporal integration dysfunction undermine speech and language development? The results of the psychoacoustic studies reviewed pointed to an area of temporal dysfunction within the tens of milliseconds range. This time frame led us, in turn, to focus our attention on the phonemic level of speech processing, as specific temporal elements of the acoustic signal within a phoneme occur within this time frame and are essential for perceptual discrimination of speech. For example, vowels transmit the same acoustic information throughout their spectra and are thus referred to as steady state. Stop consonant syllables (such as /ba/, /da/, /ga/, /pa/, /ta/, and /ka/), on the other hand, have a transitional period between the release of the consonant and the initiation of the vowel, during which the frequencies (called *formants*) change very rapidly over time (see figure 2). Information carried within these brief formant transitions are critical for syllable discrimination. We predicted that LI children would be particularly impaired in discriminating brief-duration temporal cues within speech, such as the brief formant transitions within stop-consonant/ vowel syllables. However, we predicted that they would be unimpaired in discriminating between speech sounds that were characterized by steady-state acoustic spectra, such as vowels.

Figure 2 shows two pairs of computer synthesized speech stimuli used in these initial studies. The first pair shows the spectra of two steady-state vowels, /ɛ/ and /æ/. Note that the acoustic spectra of these speech stimuli are constant (and differ from each other) throughout their entire 250-ms duration. The second pair represent the acoustic spectra of the syllables /ba/ and /da/. Here we see that these syllables differ only over the initial 40 ms, during which the frequencies change very rapidly in time, followed immediately by the vowel /a/, which is steady-state throughout the remainder of both 250 ms syllables. That is, for most of the 250 ms both syllables are composed of identical steady-state formant frequencies of the vowel /a/. Consequently, discrimination of these two syllables critically depends on an accurate analysis of the initial 40-ms formant transitions.

Using the same response paradigm described for the nonverbal acoustic studies reported above, we investigated LI children's ability to detect, associate, and sequence these two pairs of speech sounds. The experimental results were clear. The LI children were unimpaired

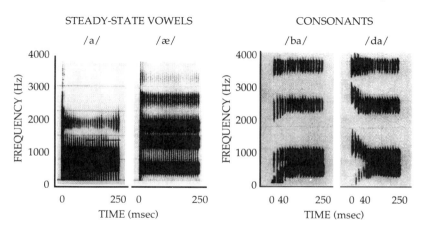

Figure 2.

in performing any of these tasks with the steady-state vowel stimuli. However, when the stop consonant-vowel (CV) syllables, incorporating 40-ms formant transitions, were used as stimuli 10 out of 12 of the LI children were unable even to reach criterion on the association subtest. That is, they were unable even to learn to associate the bottom button on the response panel with the stimulus /ba/ and the top button with the stimulus /da/. The children insisted that they could not hear the difference between the two stimuli being presented (Tallal and Piercy 1974).

In a subsequent experiment, we sought to determine whether the poor performance found on tests with CV syllables derived from an impaired ability to process transitional elements of auditory information per se, or was due to an inability to resolve other brief-duration cues typically found within phonemes as well (Tallal and Piercy 1975). In this experiment the preceding paradigm was modified by using computer-generated speech stimuli whose spectral or temporal characteristics had been systematically manipulated. The first stimulus pair was a set of computer-generated vowel-vowel syllables based on the temporal characteristics of the CV syllables /ba/ and /da/. In the new pair, however, the initial 40-ms segment of each syllable was steady-state rather than transitional, and represented the acoustic spectra for one of the vowels /ɛ/ or /æ/. The remaining portion of the 250 ms in each syllable was composed of the same steady-state vowel, /I/. A second pair of stimuli based on the original /ba, da/ syllables was also generated. In this stimulus pair, however, the initial 40 ms formant transition within each of the CV syllables /ba/ and /da/ was synthetically extended, to approximately 80 ms.

Again, the LI children were tested using the sequential associative response paradigm described earlier, this time using the two new pairs of stimuli. The results were quite intriguing. This time, the LIs were *impaired* in their ability to discriminate the vowel-vowel stimuli (incorporating a critical 40 ms-duration segment), but *unimpaired* in processing the CV syllables where the duration of the critical formant transition had been extended to 80 ms. Subsequent studies asking subjects to discriminate many different speech sounds based on a variety of temporal and/or spectral cues, confirmed the hypothesis that LI children were impaired in their ability to integrate brief acoustic components of information occurring within tens of ms. in the ongoing speech stream, regardless of phonetic classification (Tallal and Stark 1981). Results from other laboratories assessing the perceptual speech abilities of language and/or learning impaired children, as well as adults with a lifelong history of dyslexia, also support this conclusion (Elliot, Hammen, and Scholl 1989; Steffens et al. 1992; and Tomblin, Freese, and Records 1992).

We were interested in determining whether the influence of this temporal integration deficit would extend beyond the domain of speech perception. In a series of studies (Stark and Tallal 1979; Tallal, Stark, and Curtiss 1976) we undertook detailed spectrographic analyses of speech production data from LI and control children, specifically focusing on the temporal aspects of their speech production. We found a remarkable similarity between the pattern of temporal production impairments and temporal perception impairments at the phonetic level in the LI subjects. That is, we demonstrated that language impaired children were not only impaired in their ability to process the temporal components of the acoustic spectra that characterize speech syllables, but were also impaired in their ability to control the *production* of these brief temporal events in their motor output. This remarkable mirroring of specific temporal constraints in both sensory and motor systems subserving speech has important implications for theories that pertain to neural mechanisms underlying speech in humans.

We were also interested in whether the degree of deficit in nonverbal temporal integration would correlate with the degree of language impairment beyond the phoneme level. We hypothesized that the degree of impairment in nonverbal temporal processing would be highly correlated with the overall degree of receptive language delay in LI children. In order to investigate this hypothesis we rank ordered the LI subjects according to which child showed the greatest impairment and which the least on our temporal processing tests. Next, we rank ordered the same children based on their performance on a battery of standardized clinical receptive language tests. The results were clear cut. There was a highly significant multiple correlation ($r = .85$, $p < .001$) between the degree of temporal processing impairment and the degree of receptive language impairment (Tallal, Stark, and Mellits 1985a).

On the basis of the multiple studies reviewed here, we conclude that a primary inability to process acoustic information that enters the nervous system in rapid succession (within a time frame of tens of milliseconds) will serve to disrupt or delay the development of phonological processes, and subsequently lead to more global delayed development of receptive language.

MODALITY SPECIFICITY

The previous experiments clearly support the existence of an auditory temporal processing deficit in LI children which affects their performance in both speech perception and production, as well as the degree of their receptive language impairment. In the next set of experiments we addressed whether this temporal processing deficit is specific to the auditory modality. In this series of studies, we used a comprehensive battery of sensory and motor tests designed to assess visual, tactile, and cross-modal sensory integration, as well as rapid sequential motor output. Studies were well controlled to compare performance in these modalities using verbal and nonverbal stimuli. The hierarchy of processing subtests described earlier for the auditory experiments were employed to assess visual and cross-modal temporal processing. The assessment of tactile processing utilized a modification of these procedures based on discrimination of single, sequential or simultaneous touches to the fingers, hands and/or cheeks. Motor tasks included the ability to make rapid sequential nonverbal finger and mouth movements, as well as the ability to rapidly produce single or sequential speech syllables and words (Johnston et al. 1981; Katz, Curtiss, and Tallal 1992; Tallal et al. 1981; Tallal, Stark, and Mellits 1985b).

The results of this extensive series of studies can be summarized in the following manner. Language impaired children were significantly impaired in comparison to matched controls in their ability to discriminate, sequence or remember any brief stimulus if followed in rapid succession (tens of ms) by another stimulus, regardless of the modality of stimulation. Importantly, LI children were unimpaired on precisely the same tasks when the interval between the offset of one stimulus and the onset of another was extended. A similar pattern was found for the production of rapid, sequential, and fine-grained oral or manual movements. These deficits were found regardless of whether the stimuli were verbal or nonverbal.

The results of these studies demonstrate that LI children have a pervasive pansensory/motor deficit that impedes their ability to perceive or produce information within a tightly delineated time frame of tens of ms. Importantly, in a study of 36 LI and well-matched control children, we found a striking bimodal distribution in the performance of these groups on temporal sensory/motor tasks. Figure 3 shows the results of a discriminate function analysis that incorporated six variables representing auditory, visual, tactile, and cross-modal temporal integration, as well as rapid sequential motor performance obtained from LI versus control children. As can be seen in this figure we found virtually *no overlap* between the ranges in performance for these two groups.

IMPLICATIONS FOR DYSLEXIA

There appears to be a striking convergence of experimental data obtained from language impaired and reading impaired (dyslexic) children. Longitudinal studies have demonstrated that the vast majority of children identified in preschool as developmentally language impaired exhibit inordinate difficulty learning to read when they reach elementary school (see Tallal, Curtiss, and Kaplan 1988, for review). A broad body of research now suggests that phonological awareness and decoding deficits may be at the heart of developmental reading disorders (Liberman and Shankweiler 1985). But, what is the physiological basis of disorders

(a) Discriminant Function Analysis Summary

Variable step number	Variable entered	F value to enter	p
1	Rapid speech production	50.5	.001
2	Finger identification (two touches)	14.6	.001
3	Discriminating /ba/ vs. /da/	10.1	.01
4	Sequencing cross-modal nonverbal stimuli presented rapidly	5.6	.05
5	Sequencing letters presented rapidly	7.2	.01
6	Simultaneous tactile stimulation (face/hand)	8.0	.01

(b) Discriminant Function Equation

Y = −1.684 (Constant) + 0.049 (Variable 1) − 0.401 (Variable 2) − 0.148 (Variable 3) − 0.467 (Variable 4) + 0.242 (Variable 5) − 0.570 (Variable 6).

(c) Histogram of Canonical Variables

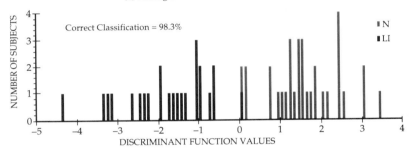

Figure 3. (a) The discriminant analysis summary lists the actual variables entering the discriminant function equation, in the order of their effect on discrimination and the F-test value and appropriate significance level (p) at each step. (b) The discriminant function equation itself is displayed. (c) A discriminant function value is calculated for each subject, based on individual performance on the test variables, and is converted to a probability score as displayed in the histogram of canonical variables. (L = language impaired; N = normal control.) (From Tallal, Stark, and Mellits 1985. Reprinted with permission.)

in phonological awareness and decoding? We have been struck by the considerable overlap between the performance profiles reported in the literature for developmentally language impaired and dyslexic children. Both groups show specific deficits at various levels of temporal integration of basic sensory information, although most of the research with language impaired children focuses on these deficits in the auditory modality, while the research with reading impaired children focuses on similar deficits in the visual modality (see Lovegrove 1993). Similarly, both LI and dyslexic children appear to be plagued by deficits in rapid sequential, fine motor performance (see Wolff 1993; Katz, Curtiss, and Tallal 1993).

In an attempt to investigate the similarities and differences between LI and dyslexic children, the same series of auditory, visual, cross-modal, tactile and motor tasks described above were administered to two groups of dyslexic children (see Stark and Tallal 1988 for review of these studies). One group showed not only a significant discrepancy from normals on standardized reading tests (an expected finding), but also differed from controls on measures of oral language. The other group of dyslexics was impaired in reading, but fell within normal limits on all tests of oral language. In studying these two groups we were specifically interested in identifying a relationship between deficits in phonological decoding (reading nonsense words) and temporal processing abilities, as well as assessing how the dyslexics compared to LI children on these measures. The results were clear. The dyslexic children *with* concomitant oral language disabilities showed, like the LI children, a significant deficit in both nonsense word reading and nonverbal temporal processing. Furthermore, these deficits were highly correlated ($r = .81$; $p<.001$) in this subgroup of dyslexics. This finding replicated results reported previously in Tallal 1980. As can be seen in figure 4, (taken from Tallal 1980) there was a striking correspondence between the degree of deficit in nonverbal auditory temporal processing and the degree of deficit in reading nonsense words (decoding skills). On the other hand, the dyslexics with normal oral language scores had neither phonological decoding nor temporal processing deficits in *any* sensory modality. Their reading difficulties appeared to occur at a higher level of analysis.

CONCLUSIONS OF BEHAVIORAL STUDIES WITH LANGUAGE IMPAIRED AND DYSLEXIC CHILDREN

This large body of data derived over a 20-year period led us to the conclusion that some children have a severe developmental deficit in

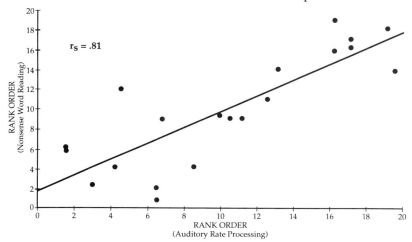

Figure 4. Dyslexics-correlation between nonsense word reading and auditory rate processing. (Adapted from data presented in Tallal 1980.)

processing brief components of information which enter the nervous system in rapid succession, and a concomitant motor deficit in organizing rapid sequential motor output. Importantly, this deficit appears to be highly specific, impinging primarily on neural mechanisms underlying the organization of information within the tens of ms range. The neurobiological basis of this deficit is, as yet, unknown. However, this deficit appears to account for the pattern of abberations in the development of several aspects of higher level cognitive processes that are known to characterize children with developmental language and reading impairment.

One hypothesis about the emergence of the processing deficit described here is provided by Merzenich et al. (1993). Merzenich has suggested that pansensory temporal/motor deficits could emerge through a lack of "sharpening" of temporal processes in a single modality. He theorizes that a lack of critical experience in early development could bias the nervous system, rendering it unable to process rapidly presented information. In addition, because the brain has to assure that it keeps the external world in sync, processing in all modalities would have to adjust to the slowest processing rate of any single modality.

Galaburda and Livingstone (1993) offer another plausible hypothesis. Based on neuroanatomical as well as physiological studies of adult developmental dyslexics, they report differences both in the structure and function of thalamocortical magnocellular systems, but intact parvocellular systems. At the physiological level, the magnocellular system appears to respond most strongly to rapid, transient, or moving stimuli presented in peripheral fields, while the parvocellular system responds most strongly to detailed, static stimuli presented foveally. Importantly, Galaburda and Livingstone report that they have found significant cellular differences at the thalamic level in the magnocellular system, but not in the parvocellular system of dyslexic brains. These cellular differences occur not only in the lateral geniculate nucleus (LGN) of the thalamus, which carries visual information, but also in the medial geniculate nucleus (MGN) of the thalamus, which carries auditory information to the cortex (including language areas). These results are very powerful, as they are the first empirical data that provide a potential direct link between anatomical, physiological, and behavioral data in dyslexia. Importantly, they pinpoint a specific neuroanatomical and physiological deficit that is compatible with the behavioral evidence of a pansensory temporal deficit in phonologically language and reading impaired children.

Llinas (1993) offers still another hypothesis. He suggests that a specific intrinsic "clock" controlling the rate of neuronal firing patterns or oscillations might be impaired in some LI and dyslexic individuals. Interestingly, he reports that an oscillation in neuronal firing rates in the cortex of normal human subjects can be characterized in the 40 (Hz) range (i.e., one cycle every 25 ms). Furthermore, these neuronal oscillations have been hypothesized to be an essential and important component for gating or "binding" sensory information in cortico-thalamo-cortical networks. If these intrinsic oscillation rates of neural firing were "slowed" due to some developmental variation in CNS organization, one of the main functional results would be an inability to process sensory and/or motor information presented in rapid succession within tens of mss - precisely the deficit we have described for language and reading impaired children having concomitant phonological disorders.

The suggestion of deficient cortico-thalamo-cortical networks is intriguing in light of recent data from magnetic resonance imaging (MRI) studies with LI children. Jernigan, Hesselink, and Tallal (1991) report finding significant reduction in gray matter volume in subcortical structures (including striatum and thalamus), as well as in cortical structures known to subserve language. In addition, we reported strikingly aberrant patterns of cerebral lateralization in the brains of LI children as compared to well-matched controls, in both prefrontal and parietal regions. It is compelling to note that highly significant correlations were found between the extent of aberrant hemispheric asymmetry of these cortical regions, and the degree of deficit on our tests of auditory temporal processing for these LI children (Tallal, Sainburg, and Jerigan 1991).

Each of these hypotheses are extremely provocative, and not necessarily mutually exclusive. We are currently investigating several of these hypotheses empirically in studies with language and reading impaired individuals.

One last point needs to be addressed before moving away from our studies with LI and dyslexic children. The question has frequently been asked as to how these children function relatively normally if they have such a severe and basic temporal processing deficit. It must be emphasized that the time frame that we have identified for the temporal processing disorder is in the range of tens of ms. Therefore, it would be expected that only processes critically dependent on information presented (or movements produced) within this time frame would be affected (see Philips 1993). Processing of information presented over longer durations, such as environmental noises, scene analysis, or coordination of gross motor movements, would not be expected to be impaired. However, the phonological processes subserving both speech perception and production would be expected to be particularly vulnerable to this type of temporal dysfunction. This *would* be the case for both oral or written language, although the effect of a temporal processing deficit on written language may be more difficult for the reader to relate to this hypothesis.

While it is true that letters remain static on the page for the reader to observe for any length of time, the visual identification of graphemes is useful only if the visual representation can be associated with a neural representation of the appropriate phoneme. We suggest that language and reading impaired children, due to their basic temporal processing deficit, are unable to establish stable and invariant phonemic representations. As suggested by Isabelle Liberman, these children never become proficient at "phonemic awareness" (Liberman and Shankweiler 1985). Many studies support such an assumption (see Goswami 1993), that deficits in reading may derive from a faulty phonological foundation on which subsequent language processes must be built.

HEMISPHERIC SPECIALIZATION—WHAT IS SPECIALIZED?

Shifting gears, we would like to focus on issues pertaining to hemispheric specialization for speech perception. If there is one tenet in neuropsychology which is consistently supported by numerous and diverse studies, it is that speech is processed and produced preferentially by the left cerebral hemisphere. Support for this important hypothesis derives both from studies of adults who have sustained selective brain damage leading to specific functional disorders, and from studies designed to evaluate differences in information processing within and between the cerebral hemispheres in normal intact subjects. Although there is considerable discussion about the distribution of processing of various components of language between the right and the left hemisphere, there is strong support from craniotomy and split brain studies (Gazzaniga 1970; Ojemann and Mateer 1979) that phonological perception and production is primarily specialized in the left hemisphere. But, what is the neurobiological basis of this specialization? Put simply, how do neural networks or assemblies in the auditory system "know" that certain acoustic events are "speech," leading these acoustic stimuli to be selectively processed and represented in the left hemisphere? And, why did processing of such complex motor and sensory patterns become specialized in a single hemisphere? Finally, are there evolutionary precursors to hemispheric specialization for speech?

Our studies with developmental language and reading impaired children have led us to focus on mechanisms which could subserve rapid temporal integration of ongoing streams of information within a time frame of tens of mss. These data also led us to hypothesize a critical role for these temporal processes in speech perception and production. Indeed, our studies with LI and dyslexic children demonstrate clearly that major deficits in temporal analysis, in the tens of mss range, may preclude the normal development of perceptual and motor phonological systems.

We turn now to a series of studies in which we addressed whether processes that have been interpreted to be hemispherically specialized for speech may in fact be specialized, more generally, for the analysis of rapidly changing acoustic information. The results from four different studies will be reported. The first addresses the interpretation of speech processing studies in adults with acquired brain lesions. The second questions the results derived from speech processing studies using the dichotic listening technique. The third reports very recent data from a PET study with normal adult listeners. The final study questions the notion that hemispheric specialization is specific to humans, by investigating functional hemispheric lateralization for auditory temporal processing in rats.

ADULT ACQUIRED LESION STUDIES

It is well established that damage to the left cerebral hemisphere in humans often results in disruption of speech and language processing, a deficit known as *aphasia*. Receptive and expressive phonological processing disorders are a common sequelae of both Broca's aphasia, which results from damage to the anterior quadrant of the left hemisphere, and Wernicke's aphasia, which results from damage to the posterior quadrant of the left hemisphere. While damage to the left hemisphere is usually associated with impaired phonological processing, damage to the right hemisphere has been associated with impairments in speech prosody and other nonverbal aspects of acoustic analysis (see Blumenstein and Cooper 1974; Milner 1962; Zatorre et al. 1992). If this assumed dissociation between verbal and nonverbal processing of acoustic events is valid, and verbal versus nonverbal acoustic processing functions are in fact subserved by different hemispheres, such a dichotomy would raise grave questions regarding common mechanisms postulated to underlie nonverbal rapid tone processing and perceptual speech processing disorders in LI and dyslexic children.

In order to investigate this paradox, we studied a very well characterized group of men with acquired missile wounds to either the right or left hemisphere of the brain. These subjects had previously been extensively assessed by Dr. Freda Newcombe in Oxford, England. The questions we asked were as follows: (1) Does damage to the left or right cerebral hemisphere disrupt nonverbal rapid temporal processing? (2) Are adult aphasics with acquired left-hemisphere damage impaired in perceiving all speech sound contrasts, or, like language impaired children, selectively impaired in perceiving only those speech sound contrasts that require them to process very rapid acoustic change? (3) Is there a correlation between the degree of temporal processing impairment and receptive language impairment in adult aphasics? The results, reported in Tallal and Newcombe (1978), can be seen in figure 5. Clearly, selective damage to the left, but not the right, cerebral hemisphere disrupted the ability to respond correctly to two tones with short, but not long, interstimulus intervals (ISI). Importantly, neither

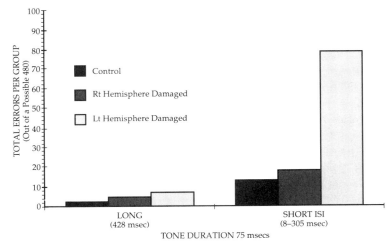

Figure 5. Sequencing nonverbal auditory stimuli presented at various rates. (From Tallal and Newcombe 1978. Reproduced by permission.)

left- nor right-hemisphere damaged subjects differed significantly from controls in processing these nonverbal stimuli when the stimuli had longer duration ISIs. Thus, contrary to expectation, processing of rapidly changing *nonverbal* acoustic information was severely disrupted by *left-* hemisphere, not right-hemisphere, brain damage in adults.

A pattern of results similar to those reported earlier for LI children regarding impaired speech perception were also found for these adult aphasics. That is, adult aphasics only showed deficits in discriminating between speech sound contrasts that incorporated brief, rapidly changing temporal cues. They were completely unimpaired in the discrimination of other speech sounds that had longer duration steady-state, or more slowly changing, acoustic spectra. Finally, as can be seen in figure 6

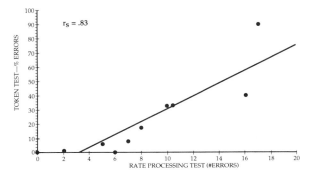

Figure 6. Adult aphasics-Correlation between auditory rate processing and language comprehension. (Adapted from data presented in Tallal and Newcombe 1978.)

there was a highly significant correlation between the degree of receptive language impairment and the number of errors made in processing rapidly presented sequential tones for left-hemisphere damaged, adult aphasic patients.

The result of these studies with adult aphasics showed a pattern identical to results obtained from children with developmental language impairments. Furthermore, the current results demonstrate that damage to the left cerebral hemisphere disrupts the processing of rapidly changing acoustic spectra, regardless of whether stimuli are verbal or nonverbal, while leaving intact the mechanisms underlying the processing of steady-state or slowly changing information, again regardless of whether the stimuli are verbal or nonverbal.

These results support the conclusion that what is selectively damaged by left-hemisphere lesions involves mechanisms critical to the processing of information within a time frame of tens of mss. We suggest that it is a disruption of this mechanism that leads to the phonological disorders so commonly seen in aphasia. We would hypothesize that these mechanisms are common to both the perception and production of speech information within this time range, and point to the work of Kimura and Archibald (1974), and Ojemann and Mateer (1984), in support of this hypothesis.

DICHOTIC LISTENING STUDIES

One technique that has been used extensively to study hemispheric specialization in intact normal subjects is the dichotic listening paradigm (Kimura 1961; see also Hugdahl 1988, for review). This paradigm utilizes the fact that in humans, information from each ear travels primarily via a contralateral (crossed) auditory pathway, and also via an ipsilateral auditory pathway, to respective cerebral hemispheres. Information entering one hemisphere is also transferred across the corpus callosum to the opposite hemisphere. The dichotic listening technique sets up an unusual competition between these pathways by simultaneously presenting different auditory stimuli to the two ears. Myriad studies have shown that when competing *verbal* information is presented to the two ears, subjects more often respond correctly to the information presented to the right, as compared to the left ear. This right ear advantage (REA) has been hypothesized to result from the right ear having primary access, via contralateral pathways, to the left hemisphere. The preferential processing of speech information presented dichotically to the right ear has, historically, been used as strong evidence of left-hemisphere specialization for speech perception.

What is it about speech stimuli that gain them specialized access to left hemisphere processing? Put a different way, what is it about left-hemisphere processing that results in more accurate perception of speech? We (Schwartz and Tallal 1980) hypothesized that the left hemisphere has specialized mechanisms allowing sensory information in the range of tens of ms to be processed more effectively than in the right hemisphere. Since many components of speech fall within this critical temporal range, our hypothesis would predict that speech sounds should be processed preferentially by the left hemisphere. That is, we hypothesized that the left hemisphere is specifically specialized for the processing of information changing rapidly in the temporal dimension. We suggest that it is the temporal requirement, not the requirement for verbal analysis per se, underlying the observed REA for speech.

To address this hypothesis we prepared two sets of computer-generated speech stimuli. Each set derived from the consonant-vowel (CV) syllables /ba/, /da/, /ga/, /pa/, /ta/, /ka/. Recall that each of these syllables is characterized by rapidly changing formant transitions lasting approximately 40 ms. In one set of computer-generated stimuli these CV syllables were synthesized to contain the typical 40-ms-duration formant transitions. For the second set of syllables, however, we extended the duration of the formant transitions to approximately 80 ms. To ensure the "validity" of these computer-generated stimuli, we demonstrated that normal listeners and trained phonetic transcribers were equally proficient at correctly identifying the six CV syllables in both the 40- and 80-ms set. These initial results demonstrated that the temporal manipulation had not distorted phonological perception.

The two sets of CV syllable stimuli were then used to test the ear preference of normal adult listeners in a dichotic listening paradigm. Presentations of all stimuli were counterbalanced across subjects. Figure 7 shows the results of the study. As expected, we found a signifi-

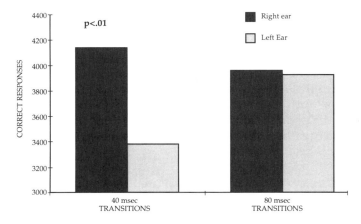

Figure 7.   Dichotically presented CV syllables 40- vs. 80-ms formant transitions. (Adapted from data presented in Schwartz and Tallal 1980.)

cant REA for the dichotically presented syllables with 40-ms-duration formant transitions, replicating the results of numerous other studies performed with similar stimuli. However, when the CV syllables with extended-duration formant transitions were presented dichotically to subjects, the REA was significantly reduced (Schwartz and Tallal 1980).

This critical result prompts a re-evaluation of hypotheses regarding mechanisms underlying hemispheric specialization for speech. These data demonstrate that the left hemisphere may be specialized for processing rapidly changing temporal information, rather than speech per se. Previous studies have shown that speech stimuli that are steady state, or do not incorporate brief or rapidly changing temporal cues, fail to show an REA (Cutting 1974). It could be argued that category differences, or differences between vowels and consonants, may have contributed to these results. In our studies, however, we used an identical set of speech syllables in each condition; these syllables were equally identifiable with respect to the intended syllable, and differed *only* in the duration of critical temporal cues. Thus, these data provide strong support for the hypothesis that, even in normal listeners, what is specialized in the left hemisphere relates to temporal constraints rather than phonological processes per se.

In a recent study, Poizner and Tallal (unpublished data) investigated the modality specificity of this hemispheric specialization for temporal processing. In this study, visual nonsense letters were presented tachistoscopically to either the right or left visual hemifield of normal adults, in the time range of tens of ms. Right-handed adults showed superior performance in responding to the temporal order of two briefly presented visual stimuli when the stimuli were presented to their right visual field (left hemisphere) as compared to when the same stimuli were presented to their left visual field. These data taken in combination with the dichotic listening results support the hypothesis that the left hemisphere is better equipped to process temporal events that converge in the nervous system within tens of ms regardless of sensory modality, and regardless of whether stimuli are verbal or nonverbal.

PET STUDIES

Fiez et al. (in press) reported the results of a study using positron emission tomography (PET) scanning to investigate neural aspects of speech and temporal perception in healthy adult volunteers. Subjects listened to four sets of sounds that were designed to determine which areas of the brain were significantly activated during speech and nonspeech acoustic processing. Speech stimuli that either did (syllables, words) or did not (vowels) incorporate rapidly changing acoustic spectra were used. In addition, complex acoustic stimuli that incorporated temporal changes within the range that occur in speech, but did not have verbal meaning, were used. Significant decreases in activity occurred bilaterally for all 4 sets of stimuli in a number of regions in the parietal lobe. Increases in activity were found in both the left and right temporal and frontal cortex. One area (Brodmann 45) in the left frontal cortex was particularly interesting. This area was near Broca's area, a frontal area that when damaged is known to lead to aphasia. The left frontal area was significantly activated only by the sets of stimuli that incorporated rapid acoustic change (syllables, words and brief tone sequences). Importantly, significant distinctions in activation in the left hemisphere did not occur along verbal versus nonverbal lines, as may have been expected. The vowels, which are verbal, but do not incorporate a rapidly changing acoustic spectrum, did not significantly activate the same left frontal brain region as the three sets of stimuli that did incorporate brief temporal cues (see Fiez, unpublished dissertation).

These PET data, derived from imaging metabolic activity in the brains of healthy adults, are consistent with the findings from studies of children who experience developmental language and reading disorders. These children have great difficulty processing stimuli incorporating brief temporal cues (rapidly presented auditory, visual, or tactual sequences, syllables, and words) but have no problem processing steady-state vowels and other verbal and nonverbal stimuli that do not require the integration of sensory information within the tens of ms range. They are also consistent with the results of a magnetic resonance imaging (MRI) study in which Jernigan and Tallal found that language-impaired children failed to show expected cerebral asymmetry in the frontal and parietal regions (Jernigan, Hesselink, and Tallal 1991). The degree of aberrant cerebral asymmetry in these two brain regions was highly correlated with deficits in processing rapidly presented tone sequences (Tallal, Sainburg, and Jernigan 1991).

ANIMAL STUDIES

The belief has long been held that the ability to perceive and produce human speech represents a unique and special process. Even though the basic mechanisms for encoding speech stimuli are, technically, a form of acoustic information processing, many have held fast to the notion that speech processing is distinct from the discrimination of other complex but nonverbal acoustic sounds. Central to this philosophy is the assumption that key components in speech processing are to be found only in the human brain, and not in any other species (see Liberman 1993). However, accumulated evidence from our behavioral studies with LI children suggest that: (1) a common mechanism underlies the discrimination of verbal *and* nonverbal acoustic stimuli characterized by rapid change in the temporal domain; and (2) disruption of this auditory temporal processing ability impairs *both* the ability to discriminate speech sounds and nonverbal stimuli such as tone pairs. Given these results, one can introduce the evolutionary hypothesis that auditory temporal processing represents a "precursor" to speech processing, and further, that left hemisphere specialization for this basic process might be expected in other species. To assess this hypothesis, we designed a series of studies to investigate the potential origins of left hemisphere specialization for speech processing in an animal model.

While other researchers have identified left-hemisphere specialization for the discrimination of species-typical calls in both monkeys and mice (Ehret 1987; Heffner and Heffner 1986; Petersen et al. 1978), these results have typically been interpreted as evidence of left-hemisphere specialization for communicative information processing. Such an interpretation, however, is called into question by findings that monkeys exhibit left-hemisphere specialization for performing complex auditory discriminations of stimuli with no communicative relevance (Dewson 1977; Gaffan and Harrison 1991), and also findings that the key information used by monkeys in discriminating species-typical calls is peak frequency position, a specifically temporal cue (May, Moody, and Stebbins 1989). Thus, we would argue that the preceding results may reflect left-hemisphere specialization for auditory temporal processing in other species, and that this mechanism is critical to the discrimination of both coo calls in monkeys and ultrasonic noise bursts in mice.

To further investigate this hypothesis, Fitch, Brown, and Tallal (1992) trained adult rats in a modified operant conditioning procedure which culminated in a test paradigm similar to a human dichotic listening test. Sequences of two tones separated by an inter-stimulus interval were presented selectively to the right or left ear, while white noise was presented to the contralateral ear. Rats were trained to use a go/no go strategy to identify one "target" sequence out of three other possible negative sequences. Correct responses resulted in water reinforcement. It is important to note that these tone sequences carried no intrinsic communicative relevance for the rat. Results showed that adult male rats were significantly better at discriminating these tone sequences with the right as compared to the left ear, a finding that has been replicated in two additional studies. (Fitch, Brown, and Tallal 1992; see also Fitch et al. 1993).

Interestingly, human dichotic listening tests and tests of language recovery after left-hemisphere damage have shown a gender difference suggesting stronger left-hemisphere specialization of language function in males (e.g., see Kimura and Harshman 1984; McGlone 1980). We were interested in whether this result might reflect stronger lateralization of auditory temporal processing in males and, if so, whether the same effect might be seen in a nonlingual species. Thus adult male and female rats were simultaneously tested in the paradigm just described. Results showed a highly significant interaction between sex and ear advantage across two separate studies; male rats were, in fact, significantly more lateralized to the left hemisphere than females.

These results are of significant interest for two reasons. First, they support the critical importance of a basic, nonlingual process—auditory temporal processing—to the existence of left hemisphere specialization for language processing in humans, by suggesting that critical precursors to this function can be found in other species. Thus, in addition to studies with LI children which argue that basic temporal processing abilities are critical to the development of speech processing, we now argue that this function may underlie the very evolution of speech processing mechanisms as well. Second, the identification of neural mechanisms for this critical function in an animal model provides the opportunity for asking questions that cannot be easily addressed in human subjects. Further studies are currently in progress to: (1) examine the effects of hormonal manipulations and stress on lateralization for auditory temporal processing; (2) examine the effects of specific neuropathologies that mimic those observed in adult dyslexic brains on auditory temporal discrimination in rats; and (3) to assess the relative organization of this function within the CNS.

The long-term goal of our studies is to shed light not only on key issues underlying the mystery of developmental language and reading disorders, but also on fundamental questions pertaining to the neurobiological basis of phonological systems in humans and the origins of hemispheric specialization for language.

REFERENCES

Beitchman, J. H., Nair, R., and Patel, P. G. 1986. Prevalence of speech and language disorders in 5-year-old kindergarten children in the Ottawa-Carlton region. *Journal of Speech and Hearing Disorders* 51:98–110.

Blumenstein, S., and Cooper, W. E. 1974. Hemispheric processing of intonation contours. *Cortex* 10:146–58.

Cutting, J. E. 1974. Two left hemisphere mechanisms in speech perception. *Perception and Psychophysics* 16:601–12.

Dewson, J. H. III. 1977. Preliminary evidence of hemispheric asymmetry of auditory function in monkeys. In *Lateralization in the Nervous System*, eds. S. Harnad, R. W. Doty, L. Goldstein, J. Jaynes, and G. Krauthamer. New York: Academic Press.

Elliot, L. L., Hammer, M. A., and Scholl, M. E. 1989. Fine-grained auditory discrimination in normal children and children with language-learning problems. *Journal of Speech and Hearing Research* 32:112–19.

Ehret, G. 1987. Left hemisphere advantage in the mouse brain for recognizing ultrasonic communication calls. *Nature* 325:249–51.

Fiez, J. A. 1992. Functional anatomy of lexical processing: PET activation and performance studies. Unpublished dissertation, St. Louis, MO: Washington University

Fiez, J. A., Tallal, P., Miezin, F. M., Dobmeyer, S., Raichle, M. E., and Petersen, S. E. 1992. PET studies of auditory processing: Passive presentation and active detection. *Society for Neuroscience Abstracts* 18:932.

Fiez, J. A., Tallal, P., Raichle, M. E., Miezin, F. M., Katz, W. F., and Petersen, S. E. in press. PET studies of auditory and phonological processing: Effects of stimulus characteristics and task demands. *Journal of Cognitive Neuroscience.*

Fitch, R. H., Brown, C., and Tallal, P., 1992. Left hemisphere specialization for auditory discrimination in male and female rats, *Society for Neuroscience Abstracts* 18:1039.

Fitch, R. H., Brown, C. P., and Tallal, P. 1993. Left hemisphere specialization for auditory temporal processing in rats. In Temporal Information Processing in the Nervous System: Special Reference to Dysphasia and Dyslexia, eds. P. Tallal, A. M. Galaburda, R. R. Llinás, and C. von Euler. *Annals of the New York Academy of Sciences* 682:346–47.

Fitch, R. H., Brown, C., O'Connor, K., and Tallal, P. 1993. Functional lateralization for auditory temporal processing in male and female rats. *Behavioral. Neuroscience* 107(5):844–50.

Gaffan, D., and Harrison, S. 1991. Auditory-visual associations, hemispheric specialization and temporal-frontal interaction in the rhesus monkey. *Brain* 114:2133–44.

Galaburda, A. and Livingstone, M. 1993. Evidence for a magnocellular defect in developmental dyslexia. In Temporal Information Processing in the Nervous System: Special Reference to Dysphasia and Dyslexia, eds. P. Tallal, A. M. Galaburda, R. R. Llinás, and C. von Euler. *Annals of the New York Academy of Sciences* 682:70–82.

Gazzaniga, M. S. 1970. *The Bissected Brain.* New York: Appleton-Century-Crofts.

Goswami, U. Phonological skills and learning to read. In Temporal Information Processing in the Nervous System: Special Reference to Dysphasia and Dyslexia, eds. P. Tallal, A. M. Galaburda, R. R. Llinás, and C. von Euler. *Annals of the New York Academy of Sciences* 682:296–311.

Heffner, H. E., and Heffner, R. S. 1986. Effects of unilateral and bilateral auditory cortex lesions on the discrimination of vocalizations by Japanese macaques. *Journal of Neurophysiology* 56:683–701.

Hugdahl, K. (Ed.). 1988. *Handbook of Dichotic Listening: Theory, Methods and Research.* New York: John Wiley & Sons.

Jernigan, T., Hesselink, J., and Tallal, P. 1991. Cerebral structure on magnetic resonance imaging in language-learning impaired children. *Archives of Neurology* 48:539–45.

Johnston, R. B., Stark, R. E., Mellits, E. D., and Tallal, P. 1981. Neurological status of language-impaired and normal children. *Annals of Neurology* 10:159–63.

Katz, W. F., Curtiss, S., and Tallal, P. 1992. Rapid automatized naming and gesture by normal and language-impaired children. *Brain and Language* 43:623–41.

Katz, W. F., Curtiss, S., and Tallal, P. 1993. Naming and gesture by normal and language-impaired children: Evidence from a modified rapid automatized naming test. In Temporal Information Processing in the Nervous System: Special Reference to Dysphasia and Dyslexia, eds. P. Tallal, A. M. Galaburda, R. R. Llinás, and C. von Euler. *Annals of the New York Academy of Sciences* 682:359–62.

Kimura, D. 1961. Cerebral dominance and the perception of verbal stimuli. *Canadian Journal of Psychology* 15:166–71.

Kimura, D., and Archibald, Y. 1974. Motor function of the left hemisphere. *Brain* 97:337–50.

Kimura, D., and Harshman, R. 1984. Sex differences in brain organization for verbal and non-verbal functions. In *Progress in Brain Research*, vol. 61, eds. G. J. DeVries et al. Amsterdam: Elsevier Science Publishers.

Liberman, A. M. 1993. In speech perception, time is not what it seems. In *Temporal Information Processing in the Nervous System: Special Reference to Dysphasia and Dyslexia*, eds. P. Tallal, A. M. Galaburda, R. R. Llinás, and C. von Euler. *Annals of the New York Academy of Sciences* 682:264–71.

Liberman, I. Y., and Shankweiler, D. 1985. Phonology and the problems of learning to read and write. *Remedial and Special Education* 6:8–17.

Llinás, R. 1993. Is dyslexia a dischronia? In Temporal Information Processing in the Nervous System: Special Reference to Dysphasia and Dyslexia, eds. P. Tallal, A. M. Galaburda, R. R. Llinás, and C. von Euler. *Annals of the New York Academy of Sciences* 682:48–56.

Lovegrove, W. 1993. Weakness in the transient visual system: A causal factor in dyslexia? In Temporal Information Processing in the Nervous System: Special Reference to Dysphasia and Dyslexia, eds. P. Tallal, A. M. Galaburda, R. R. Llinás, and C. von Euler. *Annals of the New York Academy of Sciences* 682:57–69.

May, B., Moody, D. B., and Stebbins, W. C. 1989. Categorical perception of conspecific communication sounds by Japanese macaques, *Macaca fuscata*. *Journal of the Acoustical Society of America* 85:837–47.

McGlone, J. 1980. Sex differences in human brain asymmetry: A critical review. *Behavioral and Brain Sciences* 3:215–63.

Merzenich, M. M., Schreiner, C., Jenkins, W., and Wang, X. 1993. Neural mechanisms underlying temporal integration, segmentation, and input sequence representations: Some implications for the origin of learning disabilities. In Temporal Information Processing in the Nervous System: Special Reference to Dysphasia and Dyslexia, eds. P. Tallal, A. M. Galaburda, R. R. Llinás, and C. von Euler. *Annals of the New York Academy of Sciences* 682:1–22.

Milner, B. 1962. Laterality effects in audition. In *Interhemispheric Relations and Cerebral Dominance*, ed. V. Mountcastle. Baltimore: Johns Hopkins University Press.

Ojemann, G. A. 1984. Common cortical and thalamic mechanisms for language and motor function. *American Journal of Physiology* 246:R901–03.

Ojemann, G. A., and Mateer, C. 1979. Human language cortex: Localization of memory, syntax, and sequential motor-phoneme identification systems. *Science* 205:1401–03.

Petersen, M. R., Beecher, M. D., Zoloth, S. R., Moody, D. B., and Stebbins, W. C. 1978. Neural lateralization of species-specific vocalizations by Japanese macaques *(Macaca fuscata)*. *Science* 202:325–27.

Phillips, D. P. 1993. Neural representation of stimulus times in the primary auditory cortex. In Temporal Information Processing in the Nervous System: Special Reference to Dysphasia and Dyslexia, eds. P. Tallal, A. M. Galaburda, R. R. Llinás, and C. von Euler. *Annals of the New York Academy of Sciences* 682:104–18.

Schwartz, J., and Tallal, P. 1980. Rate of acoustic change may underlie hemispheric specialization for speech perception. *Science* 207:1380–81.

Stark, R., and Tallal, P. 1979. Analysis of stop consonant production errors in developmentally dysphasic children. *Journal of the Acoustical Society of America* 66:1703–12.

Stark, R. E., and Tallal, P. 1981. Selection of children with specific language deficits. *Journal of Speech and Hearing Disorders* 46:114–22.

Steffens, M. L., Eilers, R. E., Gross-Glenn, K., and Jallad, B. 1992. Speech perception in adult subjects with familial dyslexia. *Journal of Speech and Hearing Research* 35:192–200.

Tallal, P. 1980. Auditory temporal perception, phonics, and reading disabilities in children. *Brain and Language* 9:182–98.

Tallal, P., Curtiss, S., and Kaplan, R. 1988. The San Diego longitudinal study: Evaluating the outcomes of preschool impairment in language development. In *International Perspectives on Communication Disorders*, eds. S. E. Gerber, and G. T. Mencher. Washington, DC: Gallaudet University Press.

Tallal, P., and Newcombe, F. 1978. Impairment of auditory perception and language comprehension in dysphasia. *Brain and Language* 5:13–24.

Tallal, P., and Piercy, M. 1973a. Defects of non-verbal auditory perception in children with developmental aphasia. *Nature* 241:468–69.

Tallal, P., and Piercy, M. 1973b. Developmental aphasia: Impaired rate of nonverbal processing as a function of sensory modality. *Neuropsychologia* 11:389–98.

Tallal, P., and Piercy, M. 1974. Developmental aphasia: Rate of auditory processing and selective impairment of consonant perception. *Neuropsychologia* 12:83–93.

Tallal, P., and Piercy, M. 1975. Developmental aphasia: The perception of brief vowels and extended stop consonants. *Neuropsychologia* 13:69–74.

Tallal, P., Sainburg, R., and Jernigan, T. 1991. Neuropathology of developmental dysphasia. *Reading and Writing* 4:65–79.

Tallal, P., and Stark, R. E. 1981. Speech acoustic-cue discrimination abilities of normally developing and language-impaired children. *Journal of the Acoustical Society of America* 69:568–74.

Tallal, P., Stark, R., Kallman, C., and Mellits, D. 1981. A reexamination of some nonverbal perceptual abilities of language-impaired and normal children as a function of age and sensory modality. *Journal of Speech and Hearing Research* 24:351–57.

Tallal, P., Stark, R. E., and Curtiss, S. 1976. Relation between speech perception and speech production impairment in children with developmental dysphasia. *Brain and Language* 3:305–17.

Tallal, P., Stark, R. E., and Mellits, D. 1985a. The relationship between auditory temporal analysis and receptive language development: Evidence from studies of developmental language disorder. *Neuropsychologia* 23:527–34.

Tallal, P., Stark, R. E., and Mellits, D. 1985b. Identification of language-impaired children on the basis of rapid perception and production skills. *Brain and Language* 25:314–22.

Tomblin, J. B., Freese, P. R., and Records, N. L. 1992. Diagnosing specific language impairment in adults for the purpose of pedigree analysis. *Journal of Speech and Hearing Research* 35:832–43.

Wolff, P. H. 1993. Impaired temporal resolution in developmental dyslexia. In *Temporal Information Processing in the Nervous System: Special Reference to Dysphasia and Dyslexia*, eds. P. Tallal, A. M. Galaburda, R. R. Llinás, and C. von Euler. *Annals of the New York Academy of Sciences* 682:87–103.

Zatorre, R. J., Evans, A. C., Meyer, E., and Gjedde, A. 1992. Lateralization of phonetic and pitch discrimination in speech processing. *Science* 256:846–49.

Zeigler, M., Tallal, P., and Curtiss, S. 1990. Selecting language impaired children for research studies: Insights from the San Diego Longitudinal Study. *Perceptual and Motor Skills* 71:1079–89.

Chapter • 9

Phonologic Mediation in Skilled and Dyslexic Reading

Guy C. Van Orden
Stephen D. Goldinger

Dyslexic children read poorly compared to non-dyslexic children of the same age, background, intelligence, and instructional level. Dyslexia may last into adulthood and have a pernicious effect on quality of life. Many dyslexics show qualitative differences from non-dyslexics in simple reading and language tasks.[1] Specifically, their performance differs systematically from younger non-dyslexic children who successfully read words at about the same level (i.e., *reading-age* control subjects; see Rack, Snowling, and Olson 1992, for review). These "developmental phonological dyslexics" show specific performance deficits on tasks that require constructive use of phonology (e.g., phonological awareness tasks and pseudoword naming tasks, described shortly). This form of dyslexia is the subject of our chapter, and we will use the term *dyslexia* synonymously with developmental phonological dyslexia. Our goal in this chapter is to provide an account of dyslexia that is integrated with our previous account of phonology's role in skilled reading (Van Orden and Goldinger 1994; Van Orden, Pennington, and Stone 1990). This goal requires that we introduce hypotheses concerning covariant learning and self consistency,

---

[1]Sometimes dyslexic children's poor performance resembles that of younger, reading-age, control subjects who successfully read words at about the same level (Manis et al. in press). These dyslexics appear to be developmentally delayed, but are otherwise not systematically different from non-dyslexic readers.

from which we derive our accounts of both skilled and dyslexic reading. But to begin, we will examine the performance deficits of dyslexics in a little more detail.

Correct performance in phonological awareness tasks depends upon fine-grain, "phoneme-size" knowledge of words' phonology. These tasks typically require subjects to manipulate or judge the phonology of words. In a "pig Latin" task, for example, the first phoneme of a word must be moved to the end and pronounced with /AY/ (e.g., /dog/ becomes /og day/). Dyslexics perform very poorly on this task, relative to reading-age control subjects, even when they need only recognize whether *someone else* has produced correct pig Latin (Pennington et al. 1990). Poor performance on such phonological awareness tasks is a primary symptom of dyslexia (Bradley and Bryant 1978; Liberman et al. 1985; Liberman, and Shankweiler 1979; Olson et al. 1990; Olson et al. 1989; Pratt and Brady 1988; Wagner and Torgesen 1987).

Pseudoword naming requires knowledge of how letter strings translate into phonology. In this task, a subject is presented with a letter string such as BINT that shares spelling structure with actual words (consider MINT, BIN, etc.—pseudowords are pronounced analogous to words by skilled readers [Seidenberg et al. 1994]). Dyslexic readers are much slower at naming pseudowords and produce more "impossible" pronunciations than reading-age controls (Baddeley et al. 1982; Holligan and Johnston 1988; Kochnower, Richardson, and DiBenedetto 1983; Manis et al. 1988; Olson 1985; Olson et al. 1989; Siegel and Ryan 1988; Snowling 1981). As with pig Latin, they also perform poorly when they need only judge whether *someone else* has produced a "possible" pronunciation of a pseudoword (Snowling 1980). Deficits in pseudo-word naming are typically correlated with deficits in phonological awareness, and both deficits appear to be hereditary (e.g., see Olson et al. 1989; Olson and Wise 1986; Pennington et al. 1990; Smith et al. 1986).

All these findings motivate the hypothesis that dyslexia is a deficit in fine-grain knowledge of phonology and its relation to print in alphabetic languages. The importance of phonology in dyslexia agrees with current models of skilled reading in which phonology plays a crucial role. The crux of reading is perception of individual printed words (Perfetti 1985); but the centrality of phonology in word perception has been a long-standing controversy (Crowder 1982; Gibson and Levin 1975; Huey 1908; Rayner and Pollatsek 1989; Smith 1971). Our view of perception as an emergent dynamic between stimulus forms and their functions clarifies phonology's mediating effect on word perception in silent reading (Van Orden and Goldinger 1994).

A resonant dynamic between a word's visual form and its pho-nologic function is the earliest source of constraint in its perception. We call this the *phonologic coherence hypothesis* (Van Orden 1991; Van

Orden, Pennington, and Stone 1990), and we believe it explains why phonology is a *primary* constraint in word perception, not a secondary or occasional constraint, as is usually assumed (Coltheart 1978; Paap et al. 1982; Seidenberg and McClelland 1989). In this chapter, we describe this hypothesis and the broader complex systems metaphor whence it derives, en route to an account of dyslexia. In doing so, we distinguish the phonologic coherence hypothesis from traditional, flow-chart views of phonologic mediation. But more importantly, we use this example to illustrate a deeper *self-consistency principle* that characterizes emergent structure in cognitive systems (see also Stone 1994; Van Orden and Goldinger 1994). Eventually, we explain dyslexia with respect to self-consistency effects.

Next, we outline the theoretical basis of a recurrent "neural" network model, and we clarify the complex systems metaphor that such models embody. Recurrent network models are computationally demanding, in the sense of processing resources required for computer simulations. Once grasped, however, their underlying metaphor is quite simple and elegant. The next sections introduce two key constructs: Resonance and Attractors. Following that, we apply these constructs in the case of printed word perception to explain phonologic mediation. We conclude with an account of dyslexia that entails a failure to develop fine-grain visual-phonologic constraints on perception of printed words.

RESONANCE

Imagine a fictitious neural system that functions in perception of printed words. This system comprises a family of neurons affiliated with vision and a family of neurons affiliated with language (see figure 1). The vision neurons are richly connected to the language neurons and the language neurons are richly connected back to the vision neurons. Now, imagine a specific pattern of activation across the vision neurons, due to the presentation of a printed word. This visual pattern induces a pattern of activation across the linguistic neurons, which, in turn, feed activation back to the vision neurons. If this feed-back pattern confirms the visual pattern that initiated the dynamic, then the visual pattern gains force in re-activating the linguistic pattern that, in turn, re-activates the visual pattern, and so on. Within limits, this *resonance* is self-perpetuating and binds the respective patterns of activation into a coherent whole. The visual pattern initiating such interactive-activation need not be a perfect match to the pattern returned by linguistic feedback; cooperative–competitive dynamics smooth out small mismatches, but large mismatches prohibit resonance (Grossberg 1982; Grossberg and Stone 1986; Stone and Van Orden 1989; Van Orden and Goldinger 1994).

This fictitious neural system is only for exposition; we find it helpful to think of words' features as neurons, and their statistical

Linguistic Neurons

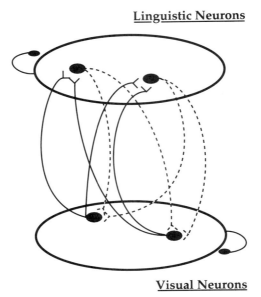

Visual Neurons

Figure 1. A fictitious neural system made up of visual neurons, linguistic neurons, within-level inhibition, and between-level excitatory connections.

interconnections as synapses. However, the analogy between cognitive and neural systems is only slightly stronger than analogies that might be drawn to other complex systems, such as weather or turbulent flow. Coherent, recurrent feedback explains coherent dynamic structure in physical, chemical, biological, cognitive, and social systems (Abraham, Abraham, and Shaw 1991; Grossberg 1982; Nowak, Szamrej, and Latané 1990; Prigogine and Stengers 1984; Smith and Thelen 1993; Stone and Van Orden 1989; Thelen and Smith 1994; Vallacher, and Nowak 1994; Van Orden and Goldinger 1994). These varied systems are not equally reducible to neural accounts. Consequently, word perception is perhaps better described in (admittedly vague) cognitive terms: When a pattern of activation across visual features (however conceived) activates a pattern of linguistic features (however conceived), the linguistic features, in turn, feed activation back to visual features. If the stimulus-driven visual pattern adequately matches the fed-back linguistic pattern, then the visual features and linguistic features coalesce in a coherent dynamic whole—a resonance.

Resonance manifests holism, which greatly adds to its appeal as a theoretical tool. The problems that holistic phenomena have traditionally posed for psychology are well-known (Kohler 1947). Word perception illustrates holism, because printed words are more readily perceived as words than as collections of letters (Reicher 1969; Wheeler 1970). In traditional symbolic theories, representations of wholes are either assumed, a priori, or constructed by juxtaposing representations of parts. In the former case, parts are subordinate to wholes in a hierarchy of representations. A model of word perception might include letter representations B_1 and E_2 that, together, specify a whole-word representation BE. In the latter case, rules are assumed to combine parts, and wholes are created by fiat. A model of word perception might include a rule that joins the parts B_1 and E_2 to form the whole B_1E_2 (cf., Fodor and Pylyshyn 1988).

Neither of the traditional solutions fully confronts the problem of holism. A priori representation of wholes merely acknowledges the problem; it does not solve it (Fodor and Pylyshyn 1988). The rule-solution, on the other hand, solves the problem by decree. A combinatorial rule says B_1 and E_2 are a whole, therefore they are a whole. Wholes created by mere juxtaposition of parts, however, are the literal sum of those parts—the antithesis of holism. This disrespects the maxim: *The whole is greater than the sum of its parts*, which is certainly true when a letter string is perceived as a word.

By contrast, in resonance, parts become an irreducible whole through a form of reciprocity. The dynamic character of each part affects the dynamic character of every other part (Stone 1994). In word perception, for example, a word's "name function" (Berent and Perfetti 1995; Chastain 1981; Lesch and Pollatsek 1993; Perfetti, Bell, and Delaney 1988; Van Orden 1987) and its "meaning function" (Azuma and Van Orden 1996; Balota, Ferraro, and Connor 1991; Strain, Patterson, and Seidenberg 1995) coalesce with its "visual form" in the earliest moments of perception. Consequently, the perceived form of a printed word is bound inextricably to its phonology and meaning. The "parts" or dimensions of these form-function resonances emerge secondarily as a function of development. Following Smith (1989), we suggest that " . . . objects [are] perceived as unitary wholes, and attributes and features [are] secondarily derived from wholes" (p. 148). The eventual contrast between dyslexic and non-dyslexic word perception in this chapter may illustrate the developmental priority of holistic relations, followed by later-emerging dimensional structure. Dyslexia is a failure of perceptual development to derive fine-grain dimensions of word perception that are implicit in holistic visual-phonologic resonances.

ATTRACTORS

Resonance is a construct from dynamical systems theory, which provides additional tools for describing the behavior of complex systems. For example, the behavior of a system may be described in a topology of *attractors* across a *state space* (Abraham, Abraham, and Shaw 1991; Killeen 1989, 1992). A state space comprises all possible states that a system may occupy; the space for printed word naming may be constructed from visual and articulatory features. (This space is clearly incomplete because naming is affected by semantic features as well, Strain, Patterson, and Seidenberg 1995). In this streamlined example, each stimulus (visual) feature and each response (articulatory) feature is a single dimension of a high-dimensional state space. Points in the state space are unique combinations of visual and articulatory features. Performance is correlated with movement between points in the state space (Killeen 1989).

A word naming trial begins with presentation of a printed word, which "activates" visual and articulatory dimensions. The combination of visual and articulatory dimensions entailed in this initial feedforward activation comprises the *initial conditions* of word naming. These include both appropriate and inappropriate feature dimensions. For example, because _INT is pronounced differently in PINT and MINT, an initial encoding of PINT will include some articulatory features of MINT (Kawamoto and Zemblidge 1992; Van Orden, Pennington, and Stone 1990; Van Orden and Goldinger 1994). More generally, the initial state of a cognitive system includes all functional dimensions previously associated to a stimulus form, each activated in proportion to its statistical association with the stimulus form.[2] Following this initial state, cooperative-competitive dynamics begin. Eventually, in typical dynamics, appropriate dimensions are fully activated and inappropriate dimensions are inhibited. Such "clean-up" dynamics move the encoding from its initial point to an *attractor point*[3]—the point in the state space comprising the feature dimensions that eventually come into resonance.

Because the state space of word naming is continuous, it includes all potential feature combinations (potential resonances), which would entail all pronounceable letter strings. However, only a subset of these

---

[2]This is an over-simplification because feedback will also activate initially all dimensions of form previously associated to stimulus functions. This is the basis of the feedback consistency effects (Stone, Vanhoy, and Van Orden in press) discussed later in the chapter.

[3]Alternatively, behavior may be described using cyclic attractors called limit cycles, or even more complex attractors. For example, we could expand our notational scheme for phonology to allow dynamics that unfold over time, more like an actual naming response. Simple dynamic analogies include certain chemical reactions (Prigogine and Stengers 1984) and predator-prey relations (May 1976), but more complex behavioral patterns ("unfoldings") may also be modeled in this framework (e.g., see Abraham and Shaw 1992; Thompson and Stewart 1987). Within the framework of dynamical systems theory, it is even plausible that each time-slice of performance, taken as a whole, is unique. In this extreme possibility, each instance of coordinated activity will be different, if only slightly—even for "identical" tokens of the same stimulus type (cf., Freeman 1991; Freeman and Grajski 1987; Skarda and Freeman 1987).

possible combinations actually occurs in a given language, and is learned. *Attractors* develop as a consequence of this learning. The relations between words' forms and functions vary arbitrarily across languages. Because arbitrary relations must be learned, *developmental history* is a primary determinant of the attractor topology for word perception. However, both skilled reading and dyslexia must also be understood with respect to *evolutionary history*, due to established patterns of heritability. Evolutionary history shapes form-function attractor topologies across the successive lives of many individuals (Killeen 1989, 1992; Kohonen 1988; Rumelhart and McClelland 1986b; Shepard 1989). Functional environmental regularities may be "selected" by evolutionary processes and show themselves behaviorally in form-function attractors that reliably emerge in development. Such regularities may include dimensions of phonology, and a failure of those dimensions to emerge may be the primary basis of the dyslexic profile.[4]

Each attractor in a state space is bounded by a *separatrix*—a high dimensional boundary that circumscribes an attractor basin. Within the attractor basin, dynamics move encodings toward the respective attractor point; beyond the separatrix, encodings fall in the basin of some other attractor (compare Maddox and Ashby's 1993 discussion of decision boundaries in perceptual categorization). Word naming experiments typically collect response time and accuracy data. With regard to dynamics, the distance traveled in an attractor basin between the initial encoding and the attractor point is positively correlated with response time (Kawamoto 1993, 1994; Kawamoto, Farrar, and Kello 1994; Kawamoto and Kitzis 1991; Kawamoto and Zemblidge 1992; Seidenberg and McClelland 1989; Van Orden 1987; Van Orden, Pennington, and Stone 1990), and the attractor point usually comprises visual and articulatory features consonant with a correct naming response. On occasion, however, naming errors occur, as when PINT is mispronounced to rhyme with MINT. Such naming errors result when encodings fall into false–positive attractor basins, typically basins that adjoin the correct attractor basin (Hinton and Shallice 1991; Kawamoto 1993, 1994; Kawamoto and Kitzis 1991; Kawamoto and Zemblidge 1992; Plaut and Shallice 1993; Van Orden, Pennington, and Stone 1990; Van Orden, Pennington, and Stone 1996). Naming errors usually resemble correct responses because adjoining attractor basins share many visual-articulatory dimensions.

---

4 Please note, we do not propose to dissociate evolutionary history and developmental history. "[O]ntogeny is a matter of nested causal systems whose functional order is a result of the running of the system, not of any one set of its constituents . . . " (Oyama 1985, p. 159). All behavior reflects combined, interdependent constraints of nature and nurture (Bronfenbrenner and Ceci 1994).

Relative distances between attractors, and between encodings and attractors, may be estimated on ordinal scales. We are restricted to ordinal scales because independent and dependent variables in psychological experiments lack trustworthy interval properties. For example, when we manipulate the relatedness of meaning between a "prime" and a "target"—as when DOCTOR is chosen as a related prime for NURSE versus an unrelated prime such as CHAIR—we manipulate the relationship "more than," but we do not know "by how much." Likewise, when we observe "structured" errors—as when PINT is mis-pronounced to rhyme with MINT—we only know that the error is more similar to the correct response than if PINT had been mis-pronounced to rhyme with ZUCCHINI. In both cases, only the ordinal properties of these relations are trustworthy (see the discussion of "error scores" in Van Orden, Pennington, and Stone 1990).

Traditional analyses in cognitive psychology trust the interval properties of response time to measure the durations of component functions in complex behavior (Posner 1978; Sternberg 1969). However, this analysis requires that some component functions (structures) are independent of other component functions (structures), so they can make independent contributions to overall response time. The assumption of independent causal structures is the (somewhat circular) basis for mapping independent sources of variance that are discovered in data onto independent representations or processes (cf. Stone and Van Orden's 1993, discussion of *first-order empirical isomorphism*). However, because the present framework embraces recurrent feedback as its primary theoretical tool, it cannot also embrace discrete, independent structures and processes. In recurrent feedback dynamics, there are no independent sources of constraint, nor are there discernible lines between stimulus forms and functions. Consequently, although response times may reveal reliable ordinal relations (i.e., earlier versus later satisfaction of constraints), interval properties of dynamics cannot be derived.

We can illustrate this problem using our model state space of word naming. Naming time may be interpreted as distance traveled between an initial encoding and an attractor point. The attractor point corresponds to the observed pronunciation (e.g., PINT pronounced to rhyme with MINT). Ideally, the interval properties of an observed naming time translate onto intervals along a trajectory in state space. However, to make this translation, we require privileged knowledge of the events leading to resonance. This includes knowledge of the initial conditions, the topology of the attractor basin, and the route traveled through the state space to the attractor point. If empirical studies could reveal exactly which feature values were activated initially, which feature values compose the attractor point, and the precise path traveled in-between, we could dissect dynamics using the interval properties of naming time. Unfortunately, such attempts to track dynamics backwards in time, from the final attractor back to the initial encoding, confront an impenetrable *barrier of uncertainty* (Prigogine and Stengers 1984). The source of this barrier is the information loss inherent in empirical analysis.

For example, suppose we wish to recover the initial conditions preceding an observed naming time to the word PINT (i.e., the time from PINT's appearance until the subject's vocalization triggers a voice key). Assume that we know one millisecond of naming time equals one unit movement in state space (velocity is constant) and that we know dynamics travel in a straight line to the attractor point. Next, we require knowledge of the exact visual and linguistic features that resonate in a pronunciation of PINT, entailing knowledge of the true dimensions of the state space. With this ideal state of knowledge, we could use naming time to measure back from the attractor point to the initial conditions.

In principle, this is impossible. Even if we knew the true dimensions of the state space, the exact visual and linguistic features that resonate in a pronunciation of PINT, that velocity was a constant, and that dynamics always traveled in a straight line, we would not find a single point at the origin of the trajectory. Rather, we would find *spherical surface of points, equidistant from the observed pronunciation,* and *infinite* in number. At this point we have exhausted all our data. The precise character of PINT's observed pronunciation was used to establish the attractor point, and its naming time was used to find the sphere of possible initial conditions. There are no data that can further limit the infinite set of candidate initial conditions, even in these idealized circumstances.

Worse yet, in practice we will never confront such ideal circumstances. Our assumptions of constant velocity and straight trajectories are certainly false; velocity changes as a function of the direction and strength of competing attractors that pull on an encoding. The trajectory between PINT's initial conditions and its attractor is lined with competing pronunciations, which deflect encodings from a straight line through the attractor basin. Vagaries in performance imply countless deviations from a straight trajectory, due to multiple sources of constraint and systemic noise. Consequently, any point on, within, or outside of the previous sphere becomes a candidate for initial conditions. Practical knowledge of all competition would entail knowing the complete history of a system (each subject) to determine its unique attractor landscape. This is all clearly impossible.

Abraham, Abraham, and Shaw (1991) also describe this general barrier of uncertainty that stands between an observer and knowledge of initial conditions:

> [N]ear a point attractor, the flow of trajectories converge. Here earlier distinct points eventually become indistinct experimentally and extrapolation backwards tells us nothing about initial states. Thus, **converging flows** provide **decreasing information** about past initial states. **Information is lost** about the past. (p. II-77, emphasis in original).

From this complex systems' perspective, it appears impossible to deduce a set of internal causal structures that create human behavior; "the behavior of the complex system is not reducible to the events that generated it." (Uttal 1990, p. 192). This limit on mapping out a state space is closely related to limits on prediction. In strongly nonlinear systems, even a minute miscalculation of initial conditions will be amplified by feedback and may result in gross qualitative differences in system performance (see Gleick's 1987 description of the *butterfly effect*). Thus, the limit on specifying initial conditions limits the predictability of system performance. However, we *can* discern the topology of a state space, using the directions and relative magnitudes of reliable effects. Perhaps most importantly, we can track patterns of interaction among variables, strictly limiting the set of possible trajectories through the state space (Stone and Van Orden 1993).

PRINTED WORD PERCEPTION

The previous sections introduced a complex systems framework in which we may formalize the resonance metaphor. In this section, we describe word perception within this framework. We then describe hypotheses concerning two design principles, *covariant learning* and *self consistency*, that together predict empirical findings across a vast literature (see also Van Orden and Goldinger 1994; Van Orden, Pennington, and Stone 1990).

Design principles refer jointly to patterns in data and in models' behavior (Stone and Van Orden 1994; Van Orden, Pennington, and Stone 1990); they are reliable patterns in behavior that can be seen from the perspective of modeling frameworks. When behavior appears to have the same design from the perspective of two or more models, then these models share a design principle (e.g., the various models that all predict frequency effects). Ideally, a design principle can be represented graphically as a trajectory through a state space (cf. Killeen 1989, 1992; Newell 1990). (This ideal is superbly illustrated by van der Maas and Molenaar's [1992] use of trajectories through control planes in their application of catastrophe theory to stagewise cognitive development.) By emphasizing design principles rather than model architectures, we acknowledge that no single mechanism can be proven as a necessary basis of human performance (Dunn and Kirsner 1988, 1989; Uttal 1990; Stone and Van Orden 1993, 1994; Van Orden, Pennington, and Stone 1995). At most, we may identify families of mechanisms that are sufficient to mimic complex patterns of observed behavior (Donahue and Palmer 1989).

Initial Conditions

Assume that presentation of a stimulus word initiates a massive spread of activation from visual features to linguistic features. Imagine this spread of activation in a model that includes visual, phonologic, and semantic subsymbols, and all their interconnections. We could unfold this interconnected network and lay it out as a triangular sheet of nodes (see figure 2), with visual subsymbols in one corner, phonologic subsymbols in a second corner, and (to keep things simple) semantic subsymbols in the third corner. Readers familiar with connectionist models of word identification may notice a resemblance between this interactive–activation triangle and the figures that illustrate those models (e.g., McClelland and Rumelhart 1981; Seidenberg and McClelland 1989). Be careful how you interpret this resemblance, however: The illustrated units are *arbitrary*, as are their segregations. Any notational structures in a subsymbolic model could just as well be derived dynamically using finer-grain notational structures (subsymbols); we return to this point shortly.

Referring to figure 2, stimulus presentation initiates a pocket of activation in the visual corner which spreads simultaneously to the phonologic and semantic corners. (This initial spread of activation is indicated in the figure by bold arrows.) A discrete approximation (simulation) of this spread would be accomplished in one step: A visual vector would be multiplied by a matrix that would transform it into a phonologic/semantic (linguistic) vector. This first time-step would end with diffuse patterns of activation, including all phonologic and semantic subsymbols previously associated to active visual subsymbols. Take careful note of this initial state: The only apparent structure derives from the identities of the subsymbols. But, again, there is no behaviorally meaningful structure in the separate identities of these notations. Subsymbols (nodes) are relatively arbitrary notations chosen at a grain-size of form-function correspondence that is fine enough to predict performance (Van Orden, Pennington, and Stone 1990). This point can be a stickler for cognitive scientists who, like us, were trained to search for structures of mind, but it is clarified by example.

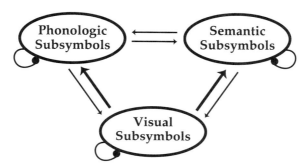

Figure 2.   An interconnected network of subsymbols for modeling printed word perception.

Consider the variation in visual features that make up a letter. In truth, each letter of the alphabet connotes an intricate local topology of feature-sets that share a family resemblance. "Letters" are not canonical entities; they are categories, with full natural variability. Some feature combinations are more typical, as in common typefaces. However, instances of a letter can differ substantially, as the visual characteristics of letters differ across type fonts, when written in script, or when spelled out in the shards of a broken mirror. Categorical entities such as letters or phonemes are not explicit in a cognitive system; they are only explicit in models and illustrations. On this point, it should be clear that the theoretical basis of subsymbolic models departs from more traditional views (Van Orden, Pennington, and Stone 1990). Behaviorally meaningful structure arises via feedback. We cannot discover "atoms" of behavior, nor corresponding atomic mental structures. Observed behavior is emergent in the structural coupling (resonance) of an organism and its environment (Van Orden and Goldinger 1994; Varela, Thompson, and Rosch 1991, and cf. Gibson 1986; Turvey and Carello 1981).

After the initial spread of activation, cooperative–competitive dynamics begin among all subsymbol families. Coherent behavioral structures emerge as relatively stable feedback loops (resonance). Thus, high-level structure, crudely approximated by our notational scheme, would not exist independent of resonance. In particular, "orthographic structure" is a consequence of visual-linguistic dynamics; it does not originate in discrete, a priori, spelling representations, as is typically assumed. A complex systems view emphasizes the emergence of behavior via cooperative–competitive dynamics, and thus must accept a purely narrative function for notations, such as "nodes," in models. A more fantastic notational simplification is entailed in the separation of semantic subsymbols from visual and phonologic subsymbols. Semantic subsymbols stand in for a vast continuous range of sensorimotor ensembles (compare *image schemas*, Gibbs 1994; Gibbs et al. 1994; Johnson 1987; Lakoff 1987). Within this range, the dimensions of a semantic subsymbol may overlap with the dimensions of a visual or phonologic subsymbol. Consider an example from Allport (1983):

> The object-concept of telephone, for example, must involve the convolution not only of many different complex properties of shape, surface texture, size and so forth that are codable in visual and tactile attribute domains, but also properties specific to auditory and to action-coding domains of representation, including manipulation and speech. (p. 52).
>
> The essential idea is that the same neural elements that are involved in coding the sensory attributes of a (possibly unknown) object presented to eye or hand or ear also make up the elements of the . . . activity-patterns that represent familiar object-concepts in 'semantic memory'. This model

is, of course, in radical opposition to the view, apparently held by many psychologists, that 'semantic memory' is represented in some abstract, modality-independent, 'conceptual' domain remote from the mechanisms of perception and of motor organization. (p. 53).

Although Allport's speculation is perhaps too literally neural, this does not detract from his observation that a false dichotomy is typically assumed between concepts and sensorimotor organization (cf. Churchland 1990; Rockwell 1994; Smith and Katz in press). We contend that resonance among many sensory and motor dimensions is a proper analogy for the "glue" that instantiates perceptual and conceptual objects. All behaviors and meaningful experiences have their basis in recurrent feedback between forms and functions.

Consider another example that may be inflammatory to most "word nerds" (scientists like us who obsess over strings of letters and phonemes). The meaningful experience of a pseudoword (e.g., DASK) is due to the coherence of sensorimotor ensembles that typically participate in the dynamics of perceiving actual words. This allows us to judge its "proper" pronunciation, etc. A reliable conventional "meaning" of a pseudoword may even emerge (e.g., PSYCHOLOXY) when dynamics are tightly constrained (cf., Forster 1992; Rueckl and Olds 1993). The scientific convention, however, is to assume that pseudowords lack semantics of any sort. For example, this convention is a bedrock assumption in (otherwise subtle and technically brilliant) work in cognitive neuroscience (e.g., see Petersen et al. 1988), but it has no empirical basis. A current promising approach to semantics grounds meaning in bodily experience (Gibbs 1994; Gibbs et al. 1994; Johnson 1987; Lakoff 1987). With respect to bodily experience, a necessary and sufficient basis for distinguishing semantics and surface form cannot exist. Next, we move past initial conditions and discuss covariant learning and self-consistency.

Covariant Learning

The covariant learning hypothesis concerns the development of word perception, in which visual forms come to shape, and be shaped by, their linguistic functions (Van Orden 1987; Van Orden, Pennington, and Stone 1990). This hypothesis predicts a characteristic profile of development:

1. Forms and functions are associated on a stimulus-specific basis. Thus, early in development, performance is governed by relatively stimulus-specific attractors.
2. Eventually, finer-grain rule-like performance emerges as the attractor topology is shaped by correlations across form-function pairs.

3. Finally, with sufficient experience of individual form-function relations, performance may converge on an asymptote.

Thus, effects of inconsistency may be diminished or eliminated for high frequency form-function relations. The design principle that this hypothesis entails describes verb past-tense acquisition (MacWhinney and Leinbach 1991; Rumelhart and McClelland 1986a; Plunkett and Marchman 1991) and German definite article acquisition (MacWhinney et al. 1989), in addition to the development of printed word perception (Seidenberg and McClelland 1989; Van Orden 1987; Van Orden, Pennington, and Stone 1990).

Consistent *crosstalk* will enhance performance whenever the same visual-linguistic correspondence is shared across a neighborhood of words. Consistent crosstalk extracts positive correlations between forms and functions and across families of form-function pairs. In word naming, consistent crosstalk is the source of many common effects, such as rule-strength effects and word frequency effects. Rule strength is estimated by a count of all words that share a particular grapheme-phoneme correspondence (e.g., K - /k/). Strong-rule words (e.g., DESK) and pseudowords (e.g., DASK) are named faster and more accurately than weak-rule words (e.g., FIZZ) and pseudowords (e.g., NOZZ) (Rosson 1985; Van Orden, Pennington, and Stone 1996; see also Johnson and Venezky 1976; Ryder and Pearson 1980). Also, high frequency words are named faster and more accurately than low frequency words (Forster and Chambers 1973). Figure 3 illustrates how these effects emerge in covariant learning. BE and BY share a relatively strong rule (B - /b/), and BE is the more frequent word (in the figure). One purpose of this illustration is to clarify how covariant learning and self-consistency are confounded in the performance of some models.

In figure 3a, a BE learning trial increases four pairs of connection weights to bring four pairs of subsymbols into collective resonance: $B_1 \leftrightarrow /b/_1$, $B_1 \leftrightarrow /i/_2$, $E_2 \leftrightarrow /b/_1$, and $E_2 \leftrightarrow /i/_2$. At this point in the model's development, the resonance $B_1 E_2 \leftrightarrow /b_1 i_2/$ is a continuous "encapsulated" whole. Although the modeler can see potential subresonances in the a priori relations between letter and phoneme nodes, this substructure is not reflected in the model's behavior. If it were presented again with the letters B and E, the activation values of the same four nodes would grow symmetrically toward resonance. Thus the model's behavior would exhibit only coarse-grain, word-size knowledge. This simple figure illustrates how dimensionally nonspecific (holistic) relations may emerge behaviorally (and experientially) prior to relational rule-like knowledge (Smith 1989; Thelen and Smith 1994). The later emergence of rule-like knowledge is illustrated in panels 3b and 3c.

A subsequent BY trial, shown in 3b, adjusts four pairs of connection weights to bring its four pairs of subsymbols into collective resonance:

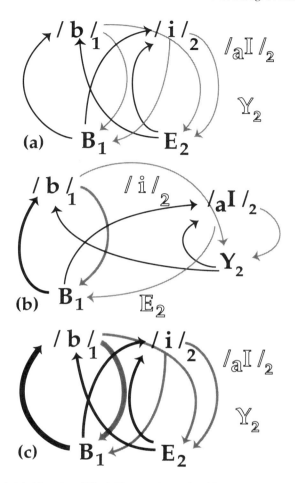

Figure 3.   A highly simplified illustration of self-consistent crosstalk in a recurrent network. a: The consequences for the connections between the visual subsymbols (bottommost in each panel) and phonologic subsymbols (topmost in each panel) of a learning trial for the word BE. b: Likewise for the word BY. c: A second learning trial for the word BE. The presence of a line between two subsymbols indicates an increase in the connection weights between those two subsymbols. The width of the lines ranks the self-consistency of the relations that accumulates across learning trials. Notice across the figures that the self-consistency (width of lines) between B_1 and $/b/_1$ increases faster than the self-consistency of other relations. (Also notice that covariant learning and self-consistency are confounded in this figure.)

$B_1 \leftrightarrow /b/_1$, $B_1 \leftrightarrow /a^I/_2$, $Y_2 \leftrightarrow /b/_1$, and $Y_2 \leftrightarrow /a^I/_2$. Notice at this point that the connections between B_1 and $/b/_1$ have been adjusted more often than any other connections. If, in turn, another BE learning trial occurs (3c), then the four pairs of connection weights: $B_1 \leftrightarrow /b/_1$, $B_1 \leftrightarrow /i/_2$, $E_2 \leftrightarrow /b/_1$,

and $E_2{\leftrightarrow}/i/_2$ are adjusted again to promote the four component resonances. Because B correlates with the same pronunciation in BY and
BE, the configuration of weights promoting the resonance $B_1{\leftrightarrow}/b/_1$ is
tuned toward a single strong attractor more often than configurations
promoting other component resonances. It emerges as a strong rule.

Strong-rule resonances, such as B↔/b/, are examples of local
dynamics exhibiting relatively high *self-consistency*. After learning, the
component resonances of a strong-rule word show themselves behaviorally as they coalesce quickly and facilitate naming. Consequently, even
a relatively unfamiliar word may be named quickly if it is composed of
strong rules (Rosson 1985). Additionally, pseudoword (BINT) naming
is primarily constrained by these fine-grain dynamic structures. This
will prove important in our discussion of dyslexia. We may describe
dyslexia as perceptual development's failure to derive fine-grain
dimensions of word perception. We provide an explicit illustration of
this hypothesis at the end of this chapter, but first we review findings
from skilled reading that typify the self-consistency principle.

Figure 3 illustrates how we may understand performance with
respect to self-consistency, a more inclusive construct than invariant
rules. Self-consistency effects are observed in all network models that
self-organize performance through recurrent feedback (e.g., Grainger
and Jacobs in press; Grossberg 1982; Hinton and Sejnowski 1986; Jacobs
and Grainger 1992; Kawamoto, Farrar, and Kello 1994; Kawamoto and
Zemblidge 1992; McClelland and Rumelhart 1981; Smolensky 1986a,
1986b). In recurrent network models, self-consistency effects are due to
the strength of the feedback received by a set of subsymbols, relative to
competitors who also receive feedback. Put another way, self-consistency estimates subsymbols' capacity to *conserve* their own activation as
dynamics proceed. Subsymbols conserve their activation when they
"send" it to other subsymbols that will "return" that activation in relatively exclusive feedback. Inconsistent crosstalk, in either direction, dissi-
pates activation and increases the competition for resonance. Frequency
of previous occurrence also affects the likelihood of resonance. There is a
large advantage for frequent, self-consistent relations in cooperative-
competitive dynamics. Self-consistent relations such as $B_1{\leftrightarrow}/b/_1$ yield
powerful subword-size attractors that cohere earlier than less self-consistent relations (e.g., C - /s/). Likewise, the form-function relations that
make up a high frequency word (e.g., $B_1E_2{\leftrightarrow}/b_1i_2/$ in figure 3) are
strong word-size attractors that cohere earlier than low frequency words
(all else equal).

Fine-Grain Self-Consistency

As we noted previously, strong-rule words and pseudowords are named
faster and more accurately than weak-rule words and pseudowords

(Rosson 1985; Van Orden, Pennington, and Stone 1995). In fact, low frequency strong-rule words are named almost as fast as high frequency words! Rule-strength effects emerge from fine-grain, visual-phonologic self-consistency. Letters and phonemes co-occur much more frequently than the syllables and words they compose. Moreover, the covariation between many letters and phonemes is relatively consistent ("regular"), which effectively conserves activation. Thus, these fine-grain pockets of self-consistency are typically the strongest local attractors. This means they will cohere first and supply the earliest local constraints in printed word identification. Fine-grain self-consistency is also a primary basis for pseudoword naming, and will provide a basis for our account of dyslexia (as dyslexics perform poorly on pseudoword naming tasks).

Berent and Perfetti (1995) reported a series of experiments that elegantly demonstrate the fine-grain microstructure of self-consistency. Their results track the topology of letter-phoneme relations predicted by self-consistency (although the authors offer an alternative account). Their paradigm involves identification of masked words: Subjects are shown a word (e.g., RAKE) very briefly (for either 15 or 30 msec). This word is then replaced by a pseudoword, which is either a pseudohomophone (RAIK), a foil that shares all of the word's consonants (RIKK, a consonant preserving pseudoword), a foil that shares a consonant and vowel (RAIB, a vowel preserving pseudoword), or a foil that shares no letters with the word (BLIN). The pseudoword is also shown very briefly (30 msec), before it is replaced by a pattern mask. (These authors reported numerous experiments; these timing parameters are only representative.) The subject's task is to identify the flashed word.

With this procedure, Berent and Perfetti (1995) found a combination of predictable and surprising results. On the predictable side, subjects were least accurate in word identification when the word (RAKE) was replaced with a completely dissimilar pseudoword (BLIN) and most accurate when the word (RAKE) was replaced by a homophone (RAIK). In a model, RAKE and RAIK would share identical phonologic subsymbols. Presentation of RAIK should thus benefit resonant dynamics that include RAKE's phonology (e.g., phonologic-semantic dynamics). This translates into a benefit for word identification in these extreme (brief presentation, pattern masking) conditions that may be attributed to the pseudohomophone "mask" (Perfetti, Bell, and Delancy 1988; Perfetti and Bell 1991). On the surprising side, the intermediate conditions also produced reliable differences: When the word (RAKE) was exposed very briefly (15 msec), replacing it with a vowel-preserving pseudoword (RAIB) was less beneficial to identification than replacing it with a consonant-preserving pseudoword (RIKK). However, when the word (RAKE) was exposed for slightly longer (30 or 45 msec), this difference vanished.

In terms of a resonance model, these results may be summarized as follows: Letters corresponding to consonants achieve visual-phonologic coherence (resonance) faster than letters corresponding to vowels. This is evident because benefits to word identification accrue more quickly when the trailing pseudoword preserves the target word's consonants than when it preserves the target word's vowel. From our perspective, the most interesting aspect of this result is its predictability via fine-grained self-consistency. Irregularities and inconsistencies in English words are almost always due to the variable nature of vowel pronunciations. The self-consistency of consonant letters is generally quite high—most consonant letters (e.g., L, M, Z) are pronounced only one way in all their instantiations. Even the less self-consistent consonant letters rarely have more than two pronunciations (e.g., C - /k/ and C - /s/).

Vowel letters, on the other hand, are often extremely ambiguous with respect to phonology. The letter O, for example, occurs in ROD, ROAD, ROOF, ROYAL, COMB, etc. In dynamics, the presence of an O in a letter string will initiate vast competition among visual-phonologic subsymbols; contextual constraints are necessary to achieve a singular resonance. Dynamics involving consonants reach coherence quickly, and then form the contextual basis for disambiguating vowel phonology.

"Regular," fine-grain, visual-phonologic effects were originally interpreted to indicate *grapheme-phoneme correspondence* (*GPC*) *rules* (Coltheart 1978; Coltheart et al. 1993), as symbolic analysis seeks regularities that qualify as invariant rules. In contrast, subsymbolic analysis assumes a more inclusive, statistical form of regularity (Jared, McRae, and Seidenberg 1990; Van Orden, Pennington, and Stone 1990). It is more inclusive because it accommodates previous versions of regularity plus relations that entail weaker correlations. The special case of *invariance* is merely a form-function correlation that approaches unity.

Intermediate-Grain Self-Consistency

Recent work by Kawamoto and Zemblidge (1992) provides direct evidence that fine-grain and intermediate-grain self-consistency are predictably the earliest constraints on naming. They studied cases in which relatively self-consistent, subword, visual-phonologic attractors are at odds with global, whole-word visual-phonologic attractors. Such cases are not common, but they clearly demonstrate the early coherence of fine- and intermediate-grain visual-phonologic dynamics, relative to coarse-grain (whole-word) visual-phonologic dynamics and later semantic dynamics. For example, the word PINT has subword structure like MINT, LINT, HINT, TINT, PIN, SIN, PIT, etc. Consequently, the more frequent (hence, more self-consistent) visual-phonologic relations encourage an erroneous naming response to PINT that rhymes with MINT.

In a naming experiment, PINT was misnamed to rhyme with MINT on about 25% of trials (Kawamoto and Zemblidge 1992). More interesting, the naming times for these "regular" errors to PINT were faster than the naming times for correct "irregular" responses (601 vs. 711 msec). Fast regularization errors indicate the faster coherence of the more self-consistent ("regular") relation.[5] Correct naming of PINT requires that the self-consistency of the "false-positive" visual-phonologic attractor (the rhyme with MINT) is weaker than the self-consistency of the correct visual-phonologic attractor. But, if this were true, correct naming times of PINT would be faster than incorrect naming times. Apparently, the false-positive attractor is more self-consistent. Consequently, correct naming requires that some other constraint (perhaps, a correct phonologic-semantic attractor) counters the false-positive attractor. Because correct naming times are slower than incorrect naming times, correct performance must rely on constraints that emerge *after* visual-phonologic attractors begin to cohere. Consequently, phonologic-semantic dynamics must cohere after visual-phonologic dynamics. Kawamoto and Zemblidge (1992) simulated this performance profile in an attractor network. In their simulation, dynamics traveled initially toward a local "regular" visual-phonologic attractor, but were usually captured by the global (word-size) attractor that maximizes global self-consistency. The global dynamic entails PINT's correct pronunciation, but it takes longer to cohere than its respective local dynamics.

Another recent study demonstrates effects of intermediate-grain self-consistency in a manner that is particularly germane to a complex systems perspective. Recall that behavior in a dynamic system is only realized via recurrent dynamics—feedforward and feedback loops that converge to resonance. As we have noted several times, stimuli with ambiguous form-function relationships (i.e., relatively low self-consistency) take longer to achieve a single, correct resonance. This is demonstrated by *regularity* or *consistency effects* in lexical decision or naming (Glushko 1979; Paap, Noel, and Johansen 1992; see also *neighborhood* effects: Andrews 1989; 1992; Coltheart et al. 1977; Grainger et al. 1989, 1992; Jaredg, McRae, and Siedenberg 1990; Taraban and McClelland 1987). For example, subjects name the word PINT relatively slowly because _INT is phonologically ambiguous. From our perspective, these effects

---

[5]We chose to illustrate the phonologic coherence hypothesis with regularization errors to PINT because, in this example, phonologic coherence works against correct performance. This example illustrates the inevitability of early visual-phonologic coherence because performance is drawn to an error by the strength of local "regular" attractors. However, the primary finding of Kawamoto and Zemblidge (1992) is that lower frequency regular pronunciations of homographs like LIVE are produced as fast or faster than alternative, high frequency, irregular pronunciations. Presumably, the strength of local regular attractors more than compensates for lower word frequency. This result also supports our claim that fine- and intermediate-grain self-consistency of visual-phonologic relations are the earliest source of structure in word perception and naming.

occur because the letter string PINT generates ambiguous feedforward activation of phonology, supporting both correct and incorrect pronunciations; perception must resist false-positive attractors, which adds time to its trajectory.

To this point, researchers have only considered consistency in a *feedforward* direction: Classic experiments on regularity and consistency have only asked the feedforward question, "Does it matter in word perception that a *spelling* may have more than one *pronunciation?*" (e.g., _INT as in MINT or PINT). From a modular information-processing perspective, this is the only sensible question: The letter string is unambiguous to subjects (it is right in front of their eyes); the only potential ambiguity arises with respect to derived (phonologic) representations. Once we consider perception as a product of resonance, however, the concept of perceptual ambiguity must be generalized—we must consider consistency in the *feedback* direction as well. Now we ask the feedback question, "Does it matter in *visual* word perception that a *pronunciation* may have more than one *spelling?*" From the perspective of resonant dynamics, feedback consistency should affect performance as strongly as classic, feedforward consistency.

Stone, Vanhoy, and Van Orden (in press) examined both feedforward and feedback consistency effects in lexical decision. They compared several types of words: In bidirectionally consistent words (e.g., SUCK), the spelling body (_UCK) can only be pronounced one way, and the pronunciation body (/_uk/) is only spelled one way. In feedforward inconsistent words (e.g., MOTH), the spelling body can be pronounced in multiple ways (e.g., BOTH), but the pronunciation body (/_ôth/) is only spelled one way. In feedback inconsistent words (e.g., HURL), the spelling body is pronounced in only one way, but the pronunciation body can be spelled in more than one way (e.g., GIRL). In bidirectionally inconsistent words (e.g., WORM), the spelling body can be pronounced in multiple ways and the pronunciation body can be spelled in multiple ways. Their results provide clear evidence for perception as a "two-way street", correct "word" recognition times were equally (and strongly) slowed by feedforward and feedback inconsistency.

The feedback consistency effect is particularly compelling, for several reasons. First, it underscores the importance of bidirectional dynamics in perception. Second, it demonstrates that stimulus function (in this case, a word's "name function") lends perceptual structure to stimulus form. Note the non-intuitive nature of this phenomenon—the letter string is clearly visible to the subject, and it remains visible until a response is recorded. But if phonologic feedback suggests that some *other* letter-string *could have* been presented, recognition is slower. Third, it is a phenomenon that could only be predicted by a theory emphasizing bidirectional dynamics. One of the criticisms we have frequently heard is that the resonance framework is too powerful and flexible—it explains many phenomena while predicting none. The feedback consistency effect is a clear counterpoint to this critique; it is a non-intuitive effect that we predicted only because the entailments of resonance, attractors, covariant learning, and self-consistency made it inescapable.

Coarse-Grain Self-Consistency

The perceptual and empirical unity of a word's form with its linguistic functions is due to word-size (coarse-grain) self-consistency (cf. Healy 1976). Previously, word-size self-consistency effects have been attributed to *dictionary units* (Triesman 1960), *logogens* (Morton 1969), *lexical entries* (Forster 1979), *direct access* (Coltheart 1978), *addressed phonology* (Patterson 1982), and so forth. These symbolic constructs always entail structural unity, explaining word-size effects via causal properties of discrete representations and their corresponding processes. Consequently, the number of hypothesized representations and processes grows almost as fast as the number of observed effects. The present metaphor is more fluid, allowing a variety of word-size effects to emerge via common dynamic processes (Stone and Van Orden 1989; Van Orden and Goldinger 1994). There is no better example of emergent word-size effects than phonologic mediation.

PHONOLOGIC MEDIATION

The visual-phonologic dynamic of printed word perception coheres before the phonologic-semantic or visual-semantic dynamics. This is not due to a "flow chart" of information processing from shallow to deep levels; it is due to relative self-consistency. The visual-phonologic dynamic is primary because the self-consistency between visual forms and phono-logic functions is generally greater than the self-consistency between either of these surface patterns and meaning. Context-conditioned variation between words and their meanings is much more widespread than the variation between spelling and phonology. Moreover, although frequency greatly benefits a word's visual-phonologic dynamics, frequency and consistency of meaning are not so correlated. The more frequent a word, the greater the variety of meanings it will typically express (Jastrzembski 1981). If a word has one pronunciation, but a variety of meanings, then during covariant learning, its visual-phonologic dynamic must become more self-consistent than the concurrent dynamic structures forming between these surface patterns and meaning. The resonance that emerges between visual and phonologic features becomes a coherent foundation for building "higher-level" resonances. This is the phonologic coherence hypothesis (Van Orden, Pennington, and Stone 1990; Van Orden 1991).

Phonology "mediates" word identification via early coherence. Notice that our use of *mediate* in the phonologic coherence hypothesis is different from the use of *mediate* in flowchart models (e.g., Coltheart 1978). *Mediate* has several definitions as a transitive and intransitive verb from the *American Heritage Dictionary* (Morris 1982):

> —*tr.* **1.** To resolve or settle (differences) by acting as an intermediary agent between two or more conflicting parties. **2.** To bring about (a settlement, for example) by action as an intermediary. **3.** *To convey or transmit as an intermediary agent or mechanism [italics added].*—*intr.* **1.** To intervene between two or more disputing parties in order to effect an agreement, settlement or compromise. **2.** To settle or reconcile differences.

Flowchart models make exclusive use of the transitive verb *mediate*'s meaning number **3** (the emphasized meaning). This is why phonologic mediation appears inefficient and counterintuitive (Paap, Noel, and Johansen 1992; Seidenberg 1992). It requires extra computational steps: Why should information processing traverse the same "psychological distance" in two steps (step one: orthographic representation to phonologic representation; step two: phonologic representation to lexical representation) rather than one step (orthographic representation to lexical representation)? To retain economy of processing, most theories of skilled reading remain "stubbornly nonphonological" (Liberman 1991, p. 242), in whole or in part. These theories cling tenaciously to null phonology effects (Coltheart et al. 1991; Fleming 1993; Jared and Seidenberg 1991; Seidenberg 1992), despite overwhelming positive evidence that phonology constrains word perception (Berent and Perfetti 1995; Carello, Turvey, and Lukatela 1992; Perfetti, Zhang, and Berent 1992).

The phonologic coherence hypothesis provides an economical interpretation of phonology's mediating effect on word perception. Coincidentally, its dynamic metaphor invokes the remaining definitions of *mediate* listed above—the meanings left unused by flowchart models. Highly self-consistent feedback from phonology rapidly organizes the system, mediating local competitions that would "structure" the visual stimulus. Subsequently, a coherent visual-phonologic dynamic *mediates* competitions between alternative global interpretations—their chances for survival are enhanced if they are maximally consistent with extant, coherent, visual-phonologic dynamics. In this system, phonologic *mediation* is not merely efficient but inescapable, due to the dense, powerfully self-consistent, visual-phonologic attractor topology. The psycholinguist Jakobson observed that, "we speak in order to be heard, in order to be understood" (Jakobson, Fant, and Halle 1963, p. 13). The phonologic mediation hypothesis suggests that, "we read in order to 'hear,' in order to understand." The phonologic coherence hypothesis explains this resemblance in the time course of resonant dynamics.

Phonologic mediation is demonstrated empirically when effects due to properties of a word (e.g., ROSE) are *mediated* by presentation of its homophone (ROWS) or pseudohomophone (ROZE). For example, subjects' familiarity with ROSE, estimated by word frequency, predicts the likelihood that ROWS will be falsely categorized as A FLOWER (Jared and Seidenberg 1991; Van Orden 1987; Van Orden, Johnston, and Hale 1988; Wydell, Patterson and Humphreys 1993). Likewise, the frequency of ROSE predicts the likelihood of lexical decision, categorization and proofreading errors to ROZE (Van Orden 1991; Van Orden, Johnston, and Hale 1988; Van Orden et al. 1992) but ROSE never appears in these experiments. Performance expected from the familiarity of ROSE is *mediated* by the phonology of ROWS or ROZE. Because this phenomenon is observed across a variety of simple reading tasks, despite explicit warnings to accept only correctly spelled targets (cf., Coltheart et al. 1991), it conclusively demonstrates phonologic mediation.

ROSE's semantic priming potential is also brought about by presentation of ROWS or ROZE. In a naming task, when ROSE precedes FLOWER, naming of FLOWER is facilitated, relative to a baseline condition. However, ROZE also facilitates naming of FLOWER, and the magnitude of ROZE's "pseudopriming effect" is equal to that of ROSE (Lukatela and Turvey 1991). Prior presentation of ROWS also facilitates naming of FLOWER, although ROWS's effect is sensitive to the time course of prime and target presentation. The pseudopriming effect of ROWS is as large as the priming effect of ROSE when ROWS is presented for only 40 msec and only 100 msec passes from its onset until presentation of FLOWER (facilitation due to ROWS = 20-35 msec in Lukatela, Lukatela and Turvey; 1993, facilitation due to ROSE = 32 msec in Fleming 1993). Likewise, ROWS and ROSE produce equal but smaller effects when these primes are replaced by a pattern mask after 50 msec (Lesch and Pollatsek 1993). However, only a small and nonsignificant priming effect is observed when 200 msec passes before the primes are replaced by the pattern mask (Lesch and Pollatsek 1993), or when 250 msec passes from the onset of ROWS to the onset of FLOWER (Fleming 1993).

The overall pattern of these pseudopriming effects agrees with the account that we prefer. The visual features of ROWS activate all associated linguistic features. The self-consistent relation between visual and phonologic features insures that dynamics favor semantic subsymbols of both ROSE and ROWS, at least initially. In time, however, dynamics are drawn into a correct interpretation of ROWS. As ROWS's correct visual-semantic resonance coheres, it naturally reduces ROWS's capacity to produce a pseudopriming effect for FLOWER. ROZE has no pre-existing visual-semantic attractor, so its priming effect is robust over time. Notice that this empirical pattern—dynamics traveling toward a strong false-positive attractor, to be corrected by later emerging constraints—parallels the pattern of fast regularization errors to PINT

(Kawamoto and Zemblidge 1992). The same design principle is observed at different grain-sizes.

The most direct evidence of phonologic mediation comes from experiments in which homophones such as ROWS or ROZE are misidentified as their homophonic mate. For example, subjects in a categorization task typically make many false-positive errors to homophone foils (e.g., ROWS or ROZE misidentified as A FLOWER), in comparison to control foils, even when subjects get a good look at the homophone foils (Banks, Oka and Shugarman 1981; Bosman 1994; Bosman and de Groot, in press; Coltheart et al. 1991; Jared and Seidenberg 1991; Llewellen et al. 1993; Meyer and Gutschera 1975; Nielson 1991; Nielson and Van Orden 1992; Van Orden 1987; Van Orden, Johnston, and Hale 1988; Van Orden et al. 1992). Wydell, Patterson, and Humphreys (1993) recently reported a dramatic demonstration of this phenomenon. They observed inflated categorization error-rates to Japanese Kanji homophones. Kanji characters lack the alphabetic properties thought to promote phonologic mediation. Consequently, from a traditional perspective, Wydell, Patterson, and Humphreys' study provides a most unexpected demonstration of phonologic mediation. From our perspective, visual-phonologic resonances should precede semantic resonances for any language in which the relation between spelling and sound is more self-consistent than the relation between surface forms and meaning.

Our final example clarifies the biasing effect of the category name (A FLOWER) on whether ROWS will be misidentified as ROSE. When A FLOWER precedes presentation of ROWS, the semantic subsymbols common to FLOWER and ROSE are active prior to presentation of ROWS (Stone and Van Orden 1989; Van Orden, Pennington, and Stone 1990). Preactivated subsymbols bias dynamics toward resonances that include those subsymbols. As a consequence, phonologic-semantic dynamics that agree with context better conserve their activation and better compete with alternative dynamics.

Context's biasing effect is evident in categorization of high-frequency target homophones that have low-frequency homophone mates. If ROWS was a high-frequency word and ROSE was a low-frequency word, then ROWS's correct phonologic-semantic attractor(s) would be strong, relative to ROSE's phonologic-semantic attractor(s), all else equal. Consequently, "high-frequency" ROWS should be correctly interpreted, irrespective of phonologic mediation. However, in typical categorization experiments, ROWS's frequency has no discernible effect (Jared and Seidenberg 1991; Van Orden 1987; Van Orden, Johnston, and Hale 1988; Wydell, Patterson, and Humphreys 1993). But, when the context is weakened—as when the category A LIVING THING precedes ROWS—high-frequency homophones are correctly interpreted (Jared and Seidenberg 1991). Presumably, the category designation A

LIVING THING activates fewer semantic subsymbols unique to ROSE than does A FLOWER, and the biasing effect of context is reduced.

DYSLEXIA

Accepting that phonologic mediation is fundamental to skilled reading, then developmental dyslexia might be explained by an absence of phonologic mediation. Lacking coherent phonology, dyslexics must rely on less stable dynamic relations. It turns out, however, that "absent phonology" is far too strong a hypothesis (Bruck 1988; Olson et al. 1985). For example, developmental dyslexics' performance to homophone foils in a categorization task clearly indicates phonologic mediation (see table 1).

The categorization results summarized in table 1 come from an unpublished study of adult dyslexics (Van Orden, Pennington, and Green 1996). In this experiment, every dyslexic subject, except one, makes many more categorization errors to homophones (ROWS categorized as A FLOWER) than to control items, and the single subject who failed to produce this pattern was at ceiling. Dyslexic subjects' data resemble the data from (reading-age) control subjects in the overall percentage of errors to homophones (53.3%, SE=4.8, versus 55.9%, SE=4.0, respectively) and control items (15%, SE=3.5, versus 12.5%, SE=3.4, respectively) although the data are not identical—especially the pattern of means to control items. These dyslexic subjects came from families in which linkage studies have established genetic correlates to their dyslexic profile. Moreover, they all exhibited deficits in phonological awareness as indicated by extremely poor performance on "pig Latin" tasks (the subjects were the 15 familial dyslexics described by Pennington et al. 1990).

Table 1   Percentage of trials in which a homophone (Hom) such as ROWS or control (Con) such as ROBS was incorrectly categorized as an exemplar of a preceding category such as A FLOWER. The top scores, subjects D1 - D15, are adult dyslexics and the bottom scores, subjects R1 - R15, come from yoked, reading-age, control subjects.

							Percent Categorization Errors								

Adult Developmental Dyslexics

	D1	D2	D3	D4	D5	D6	D7	D8	D9	D10	D11	D12	D13	D14	D15
Hom	50	30	20	85	80	70	60	0	65	75	45	75	45	45	55
Con	0	0	5	50	50	30	5	0	10	30	10	25	5	0	5

Reading-Age Control Subjects

	R1	R2	R3	R4	R5	R6	R7	R8	R9	R10	R11	R12	R13	R14	R15
Hom	40	25	50	85	60	60	30	85	65	70	70	35	40	65	58.9
Con	10	0	15	20	5	15	10	0	10	20	0	5	5	0	72.2

The paradox for the "absent phonology" hypothesis is that these same dyslexic subjects show both positive and negative phonology effects. A strong positive phonology effect was found in their categorization data, and a strong negative phonology effect was found in their phonological awareness data. Such demonstrations of negative phonology effects are the basis of the absent phonology hypothesis (Bruck 1988). A key difference between these tasks may be the added constraints in the categorization task supplied by the category name. As we noted in the previous section, these constraints are enough to bias skilled readers toward misinterpreting even high-frequency homophone words. This source of constraint may be sufficiently potent to make dyslexics' performance appear similar to reading-age controls' (cf., Stanovich, Nathan, and Vala-Rossi 1986). It must do so, however, by enhancing ("cleaning up") available phonologic constraints, as indicated by the very high error rate to homophone foils (see table 1). Thus, our ability to observe phonology effects in the performance of dyslexics is partly a function of the task in which such effects are assessed (cf., Johnston, Rugg, and Scott 1987, 1988). We propose next that different tasks may emphasize different grain-sizes of phonology, and these different grain-sizes of phonology are entailed in the respective positive and negative effects. (Although our account is not a symbolic account, it shares several key behavioral predictions with previous symbolic accounts, see, e.g., Frith 1985; Manis et al. in press; Olson et al. 1985; Perfetti, Zhang, and Berent 1992; Rack, Snowling, and Olson 1992).

Haphazard Connections

Earlier in this chapter, we used a simple neural analogy as a metaphorical basis for the term *resonance*. We do the same in this section to introduce our account of dyslexia. Postmortem studies have found anatomical anomalies in the brains of dyslexics (Drake 1968; Galaburda and Kemper 1979; Galaburda et al. 1985; Humphreys, Kaufmann, and Galaburda 1990). These anomalies may be due to subtle anomalies in neuronal migration. Locally small anomalies in neural positioning may cause large changes in the pattern of interconnectivity between neurons in different regions of the brain. These anatomical findings inspired our "haphazard connections" hypothesis concerning the phonologic deficits of dyslexics (Van Orden, Pennington, and Green 1996). (Please do not interpret this rough analogy as a claim to anatomical plausibility. We merely wish to acknowledge the inspiration for our hypothesis.)

Figure 4 illustrates a haphazard pattern of connectivity between visual and phonologic subsymbols. You should compare this figure to figure 3, in which all connections are symmetrical. We can easily track the outcome for covariant learning and self-consistency, given this haphazard connectivity. Once again, consistent crosstalk extracts positive correlations between forms and functions and across families of form-function pairs. However, although BE and BY share a relatively strong rule (B - /b/), the rule does not emerge as a self-consistent subdynamic in the behavior of our model system. This is the key to our account. The illustration in figure 3 confounded covariant learning and self-consistency. They are disconfounded in figure 4, as we explain next.

In figure 4a, a BE learning trial increases six connection weights to bring four subsymbols into collective resonance: $B_1 \rightarrow /b/_1$, $B_1 \leftrightarrow /i/_2$, $E_2 \leftarrow /b/_1$, and $E_2 \leftrightarrow /i/_2$. As in figure 3a, at this point in the model's development, the resonance $B_1E_2 \leftrightarrow /b_1i_2/$ is a continuous whole. The model would produce correctly the whole-word phonology of BE, but its behavior is opaque to substructure such as $B_1 \leftrightarrow /b/_1$. A subsequent BY trial, shown in 4b, adjusts five connection weights to bring four pairs of subsymbols into collective resonance: $B_1 \rightarrow /b/_1$, $B_1 \leftarrow /a^I/_2$, $Y_2 \leftrightarrow /b/_1$, and $Y_2 \rightarrow /a^I/_2$. Notice the difference at this point between panel b in figure 3 and the corresponding panel in figure 4. The feedforward connection weight $B_1 \rightarrow /b/_1$ grows faster than other connections in the resonance $B_1E_2 \leftrightarrow /b_1i_2/$, due to covariant learning. However, the subword relation $B_1 \leftrightarrow /b/_1$ does not grow in self-consistency. The haphazard connectivity between B_1 and $/b/_1$ in figure 4b does not allow the emergence of the subword attractor $B_1 \leftrightarrow /b/_1$, and this state of affairs is not changed by adding another BE trial (4c).

Despite the a priori correlation between B and /b/, the subword attractor $B_1 \leftrightarrow /b/_1$ does not emerge as a relatively independent dynamic structure. Consider the dynamics for the word BE following the learning trials depicted in figure 4. The advantage due to covariant learning between B_1 and $/b/_1$ may still affect performance. The relatively stronger connection $B_1 \rightarrow /b/_1$ would promote a faster overall time to resonance for the word BE. The node $/b/_1$ is strongly activated by B_1, and $/b/_1$ conserves this strong activation for the whole-word resonance when it feeds activation back to E_2. In turn, E_2 feeds this activation forward to $/i/_2$, $/i/_2$ feeds it back to B_1 and E_2, and the strong activation has been conserved in a *word-size feedback loop*. At no time, however, did a *subresonance* $B_1 \leftrightarrow /b/_1$ emerge in the behavior of the model.

We noted previously that pseudoword (BINT) naming is primarily dependent upon fine-grain dynamic structures such as $B_1 \leftrightarrow /b/_1$. These powerful structures are necessary to insure the integrity of pseudoword pronunciation. However, these fine-grain attractors do not emerge reliably in a model with haphazard connectivity. The failure to develop such fine-grain attractors translates behaviorally into a deficit in pseudoword naming. Skilled pseudoword naming is a fairly pre-dictable function of the statistical relation between words' spellings and pronunciations (Seidenberg et al. 1994). With haphazard connec-tivity, pseudowords are robbed of their strongest source of information about how words' spellings relate to phonology. A model

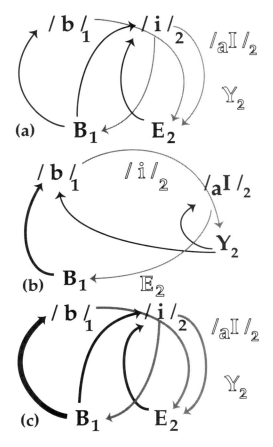

Figure 4.   A highly simplified illustration of the failure of development to derive fine-grain self-consistent structures in word perception. a: The consequences for the connections between the visual subsymbols (bottommost in each panel) and phonologic subsymbols (topmost in each panel) of a learning trial for the word BE when visual and phonologic subsymbols are haphazardly connected. b: Likewise for the word BY. c: A second learning trial for the word BE. The presence of a line between two subsymbols indicates an increase in the connection weights between those two subsymbols. The width of the lines ranks the effects of covariant learning, but only symmetric bi-directional changes would affect self-consistency. Notice across the figures that the self-consistency between B_1 and $/b/_1$ does not change even though covariant learning strengthens the relation $B_1 \rightarrow /b/_1$. The emergence of fine-grain, self-consistent relations such as $B_1 \leftrightarrow /b/_1$ requires dense symmetrical connectivity between subsymbols.

analogous to our simple illustration would fail to derive a full complement of fine-grain attractors necessary to mimic skilled pseudoword naming. Thus, dyslexia is a failure of perceptual development to derive fine-grain self-consistent dimensions of word perception.

While it is not explicit in figure 4, intermediate-grain attractors would be less affected by fine-grain haphazard connectivity than fine-grain attractors. The extent of this effect—from no effect to a large effect—depends on the grain-size of connectivity and the distribution of asymmetric connections. Intermediate-grain attractors could emerge to the same degree as in a symmetrical model, and they would typically emerge more robustly than fine-grain attractors. This may explain why developmental dyslexics produce regularity effects of the same magnitude as reading-age control subjects, despite significant pseudoword reading deficits (Olson et al. 1985; Rack, Snowling, and Olson 1992). As we noted previously, the most reliable demonstrations of regularity effects entail manipulations of intermediate-grain self-consistency (Jared, McRae, and Seidenberg 1990; Stone, Vanhoy, and Van Orden 1995). Additionally, the effect of covariant learning in figure 4—i.e., faster global word-size resonance $B_1E_2 \leftrightarrow /b_1i_2/$ due to the strong local connection $B_1 \rightarrow /b/_1$—would contribute to regularity effects.

The essential point for implementing our scheme is that haphazard connectivity blocks the emergence of fine-grain dynamic structures (attractors) that may act relatively independently of the coarse-grain structures from which they derive. These fine-grain structures are necessary to mimic the full range of performance to printed language. We could even expand our simple notations for phonology and propose haphazard connectivity between acoustic and articulatory subsymbols, thus precluding the development of proper "phoneme," radial-category structures (Lakoff 1987). In this way, we might extend our explanation to poor performance on phonological awareness tasks. The crux of our account is merely its capacity to mimic performance profiles of dyslexic subjects: Positive phonologic mediation effects accompanied by poor performance in pseudoword naming and phonological awareness tasks. We propose that this profile is reasonably described as a relative failure of perceptual development to derive fine-grain self-consistency between words' visual forms and phonologic functions.

SUMMARY

Phonologic mediation is explained by the phonologic coherence hypothesis. The phonologic coherence hypothesis derives from covariant learning and self-consistency—behavioral principles that are also seen in the behavior of recurrent neural network models. Highly self-consistent relations correspond to resonances that are strongly self-perpetuating. They are more likely to survive competitive dynamics than less self-consistent relations, and they strongly constrain global dynamics toward a state consonant with their survival. Covariant learning tracks the self-consistency of form-function relations, including the relations between words' visual forms, pronunciations, and meanings.

In such models, dynamics are drawn over time toward successive local attractors reflecting "expected values" from previous experience, and eventually, to the global attractor that strikes the best balance among local attractors (i.e., the global attractor that best mediates lasting dispositions and contextual eccentricities). A gradient of self-consistency is correlated with the grain-size of form-function relations, and is the basis of hierarchically structured behavior (cf., Simon 1973). The initial powerful attraction to reliable local states is revealed in fast regularization errors (Kawamoto and Zemblidge 1992) and early consonant effects in backward masking paradigms (Berent and Perfetti 1995); the eventual weaker attraction to global states is revealed in the time course of pseudopriming effects (Fleming 1993; Lesch and Pollatsek 1993; Lukatela, Lukatela, and Turvey 1993) and in fluid context effects (Jared and Seidenberg 1991). The developmental priority of global states is revealed in the developmental trend toward finer-grain effects in performance (Van Orden, Pennington, and Stone 1990), and the failure of perceptual development to derive fine-grain phonologic structures in dyslexia.

Our hypotheses do not concern cognition's architecture, they concern behavior's design. With respect to behavior's design, phonologic mediation appears fundamental to reading, and the phonologic coherence hypothesis explains why this is so. This account, based primarily on two simple design principles, provides a coherent explanation of word perception. Interdependence of form and function explains phonologic mediation in skilled and dyslexic reading.

ACKNOWLEDGEMENTS

Preparation of this chapter was funded by a National Institute of Health FIRST award (CMS 5 R29 NS26247-05) to Guy Van Orden. We thank Roger Schvaneveldt and Mark Seidenberg for conversations that helped delimit the content of this chapter, and we thank Ray Gibbs, Marian Jansen op de Haar, Heather Kleider, Ken Paap, Bruce Pennington, and Greg Stone for comments on previous versions. The hypothesis proposed here concerning developmental dyslexia originated in our ongoing collaboration with Bruce Pennington.

REFERENCES

Abraham, F. D., Abraham, R. H., and Shaw, C. D. 1991. *A Visual Introduction to Dynamical Systems Theory for Psychology*. Santa Cruz, CA: Aerial Press.

Abraham, R. H., and Shaw, C. D. 1992. *Dynamics: The Geometry of Behavior*. Redwood City, CA: Addison-Wesley.

Allport, D. A. 1983. Distributed memory, modular subsystems and dysphasia. In *Current Perspectives in Dysphasia*, eds. S. Newman and R. Epstein. London: Churchill Livingstone.

Andrews, S. 1989. Frequency and neighborhood size effects on lexical access: Activation or search? *Journal of Experimental Psychology: Learning, Memory and Cognition* 15:802–14.

Andrews, S. 1992. Frequency and neighbourhood effects on lexical access: Lexical similarity or orthographic redundancy? *Journal of Experimental Psychology: Learning, Memory and Cognition* 18:234–54.

Azuma, T., and Van Orden, G. C. 1996. *Why SAFE is better than FAST: The relatedness between a word's meanings affects lexical decision performance.* (Manuscript submitted for publication.)

Baddeley, A. D., Ellis, N. C., Miles, T. R., and Lewis, V. J. 1982. Developmental and acquired dyslexia: A comparison. *Cognition* 11:185–95.

Balota, D. A., Ferraro, F. R., and Connor, L. T. 1991. On the early influence of meaning in word recognition: A review of the literature. In *The Psychology of Word Meanings,* ed. P. J. Schwanenflugel. Hillsdale, NJ: Lawrence Erlbaum Associates.

Banks, W. P., Oka, E., and Shugarman, S. 1981. Recoding of printed words to internal speech: Does recoding come before lexical access? In *Perception of Print,* eds. O. J. L. Tzeng and H. Singer. Hillsdale, NJ: Lawrence Erlbaum Associates.

Berent, I., and Perfetti, C. A. 1995. A rose is a REEZ: The two cycles model of phonology assembly in English visual word recognition. *Psychological Review* 102:146–84.

Bosman, A. M. T. 1994. Reading and spelling in children and adults: Evidence for a single-route model. Doctoral dissertation, University of Amsterdam, Dissertatie reeks 1994–2, Faculteit Psychologie.

Bosman, A. M. T., and de Groot, A. M. B. in press. Phonologic mediation is fundamental to reading: Evidence from beginning readers. *The Quarterly Journal of Experimental Psychology.*

Bradley, L., and Bryant, P. 1978. Difficulties in auditory organization as a possible cause of reading backwardness. *Nature* 271:746–47.

Bronfenbrenner, U., and Ceci, S. J. 1994. Nature-nurture reconceptualized in developmental perspective: A Bioecological model. *Psychological Review* 101:568–86.

Bruck, M. 1988. The word recognition and spelling of dyslexic children. *Reading Research Quarterly* 23:51–69.

Carello, C., Turvey, M. T., and Lukatela, G. 1992. Can theories of word recognition remain stubbornly nonphonological? In *Orthography, Phonology, Morphology, and Meaning,* eds. R. Frost and L. Katz. Amsterdam: North-Holland.

Chastain, G. 1981. Phonological and orthographic factors in the word-superiority effect. *Memory and Cognition* 9:389–97.

Churchland, P. M. 1990. A deeper unity: Some Feyerabendian themes in neurocomputational form. *Minnesota Studies in the Philosophy of Science, Vol. 15.* Minneapolis: University of Minnesota Press.

Coltheart, M. 1978. Lexical access in simple reading tasks. In *Strategies in Information Processing,* ed. G. Underwood. London: Academic Press.

Coltheart, M., Curtis, B., Atkins, P., and Haller, M. 1993. Models of reading aloud: Dual-route and parallel distributed processing approaches. *Psychological Review* 100:589–608.

Coltheart, M., Davelaar, E., Jonasson, J. T., and Besner, D. 1977. Access to the internal lexicon. In *Attention and Performance VI*, ed. S. Dornic. Hillsdale, NJ: Lawrence Erlbaum Associates.

Coltheart, V., Avons, S. E., Masterson, J., and Laxon, V. 1991. The role of assembled phonology in reading comprehension. *Memory and Cognition* 19:387–400.

Crowder, R. G. 1982. *The Psychology of Reading: An Introduction*. New York: Oxford University Press.

Donahue, J. W., and Palmer, D. C. 1989. The interpretation of complex human behavior: Some reactions to Parallel Distributed Processing, eds. J. L. McClelland, D. E. Rumelhart, and the PDP Research Group [Book Review]. *Journal of the Experimental Analysis of Behavior* 51:399–416.

Drake, W. E. 1968. Clinical and pathological findings in a child with a developmental learning disability. *Journal of Learning Disabilities* 1:9–25.

Dunn, J. C., and Kirsner, K. 1988. Discovering functionally independent mental processes: The principle of reversed association. *Psychological Review* 95:91–101.

Dunn, J. C., and Kirsner, K. 1989. Implicit memory: Task or process? In *Implicit Memory: Theoretical Issues*, eds. S. Lewandowsky, J. C. Dunn, and K. Kirsner. Hillsdale, NJ: Lawrence Erlbaum Associates.

Easton, T. A. 1972. On the normal use of reflexes. *American Scientist* 60:591–99.

Fleming, K. K., 1993. Phonologically mediated priming in spoken and printed word recognition. *Journal of Experimental Psychology: Learning, Memory, and Cognition* 19:272–84.

Fodor, J. A., and Pylyshyn, Z. W. 1988. Connectionism and cognitive architecture: A critical analysis. *Cognition* 28:3–71.

Forster, K. I. 1979. Levels of processing and the structure of the language processor. In *Sentence Processing: Psycholinguistic Studies Presented to Merrill Garrett*, eds. W. E. Cooper and E. C. T. Walker. Hillsdale, NJ: Lawrence Erlbaum Associates.

Forster, K. I. 1992. Memory-addressing mechanisms and lexical access. In *Orthography, Phonology, Morphology, and Meaning*, eds. R. Frost and L. Katz. Amsterdam: North- Holland.

Forster, K. I., and Chambers, S. M. 1973. Lexical access and naming time. *Journal of Verbal Learning and Verbal Behavior* 12:627–35.

Freeman, W. J. 1991. What are the state variables for modeling brain dynamics with neural networks? In *Nonlinear Dynamics and Neuronal Networks*, ed. H. G. Schuster. New York: VCH Publishers.

Freeman, W. J., and Grajski, K. A. 1987. Relation of olfactory EEG to behavior: Factor analysis. *Behavioral Neuroscience* 101:766–77.

Frith, U. 1985. Beneath the surface of developmental dyslexia. In *Surface Dyslexia*, eds. K. E. Patterson, J. C. Marshall, and M. Coltheart. London: Routledge and Kegan Paul.

Galaburda, A. M., and Kemper, T. L. 1979. Cytoarchitectonic abnormalities in developmental dyslexia: A case study. *Annals of Neurology* 6:94–100.

Galaburda, A. M., Sherman, G. F., Rosen, G. D., Aboitiz, F., and Geschwind, N. 1985. Developmental dyslexia: Four consecutive cases with cortical anomalies. *Annals of Neurology* 18:222–33.

Gibbs, R. W. 1994. *The Poetics of Mind: Figurative Thought, Language, and Understanding*. New York: Cambridge University Press.

Gibbs, R. W., Beitel, D. A., Harrington, M., and Sanders, P. E. 1994. Taking a stand on the meanings of *Stand*: Bodily experience as motivation for polysemy. *Journal of Semantics* 11:231–51.

Gibson, E. J., and Levin, H. 1975. *The Psychology of Reading*. Cambridge, MA: MIT Press.

Gibson, J. J. 1986. *An Ecological Approach to Visual Perception*. Hillsdale, NJ: Lawrence Erlbaum Associates. (Original work published 1979).

Gleick, J. 1987. *Chaos: Making a New Science*. New York: Viking Press.

Glushko, R. 1979. The organization and activation of orthographic knowledge in reading aloud. *Journal of Experimental Psychology: Human Perception and Performance* 5:674–91.

Grainger, J., and Jacobs, A. M. in press. A three-process model of lexical decision and word recognition. *Psychological Review*.

Grainger, J., O'Regan, J. K., Jacobs, A. M., and Segui, J. 1989. On the role of competing word units in visual word recognition: The neighborhood frequency effect. *Perception and Psychophysics* 45:189–95.

Grainger, J., O'Regan, J. K., Jacobs, A. M., and Segui, J. 1992. Neighborhood frequency effects and letter visibility in visual word recognition. *Perception and Psychophysics* 51:49–56.

Grossberg, S. 1982. *Studies of Mind and Brain*. Dordrecht, The Netherlands: D. Reidel.

Grossberg, S., and Stone, G. O. 1986. Neural dynamics of word recognition and recall: Priming, learning, and resonance. *Psychological Review* 93:46–74.

Healy, A. F. 1976. Detection errors on the word *the*: Evidence for reading units larger than letters. *Journal of Experimental Psychology: Human Perception and Performance* 2:235–42.

Hinton, G. E., and Sejnowski, T. J. 1986. Learning and relearning in Boltzmann machines. In *Parallel Distributed Processing: Explorations in the Microstructure of Cognition. Vol. 1: Foundations*, eds. D. E. Rumelhart and J. L. McClelland. Cambridge, MA: MIT Press.

Hinton, G. E., and Shallice, T. 1991. Lesioning an attractor network: Investigations of acquired dyslexia. *Psychological Review* 98:74–95.

Holligan, C., and Johnston, R. 1988. The use of phonological information by good and poor readers in memory and reading tasks. *Memory and Cognition* 16:522–32.

Huey, E. B. 1908. *The Psychology and Pedagogy of Reading*. New York: Macmillan. (Republished: Cambridge, MA: MIT Press, 1968.)

Humphreys, P., Kaufmann, W. E., and Galaburda, A. M. 1990. Developmental dyslexia in women: Neuropathological findings in three cases. *Annals of Neurology* 28:727–38.

Jacobs, A. M., and Grainger, J. 1992. Testing a semistochastic variant of the interactive activation model in different word recognition experiments. *Journal of Experimental Psychology: Human Perception and Performance* 18:1174–88.

Jakobson, R., Fant, G., and Halle, M. 1963. *Preliminaries to Speech Analysis*. Cambridge, MA: MIT Press.

Jared, D., McRae, K., and Seidenberg 1990. The basis of consistency effects in word naming. *Journal of Memory and Language* 29:687–715.

Jared, D., and Seidenberg, M. S. 1991. Does word identification in reading proceed from spelling to sound to meaning? *Journal of Experimental Psychology: General* 120:358–94.

Jastrzembski, J. 1981. Multiple meanings, number of related meanings, frequency of occurrence, and the lexicon. *Cognitive Psychology* 13:278–305.

Johnson, M. 1987. *The Body in the Mind: The Bodily Basis of Meaning, Imagination, and Reason.* Chicago: University of Chicago Press.

Johnson, D. D., and Venezky, R. L. 1976. Models for predicting how adults pronounce vowel digraph spellings in unfamiliar words. *Visible Language* 10:257–68.

Johnston, R. S., Rugg, M. D., and Scott, T. 1987. The influence of phonology on good and poor readers when reading for meaning. *Journal of Memory and Language* 26:57–68.

Johnston, R. S., Rugg, M. D., and Scott, T. 1988. Pseudohomophone effects in 8 and 11 year old good and poor readers. *Journal of Research in Reading* 11:110–32.

Kawamoto, A. H. 1993. Non-linear dynamics in the resolution of lexical ambiguity: A parallel distributed processing account. *Journal of Memory and Language* 32:474–516.

Kawamoto, A. H. 1994. One system or two to handle regulars and exceptions: How time-course of processing can inform this debate. In *The Reality of Linguistic Rules*, eds. S. D. Lima, R. L. Corrigan, and G. K. Iverson. Philadelphia, PA: John Benjamin.

Kawamoto, A. H., Farrar, W. T., and Kello, C. T. 1994. When two meanings are better than one: Modeling the ambiguity advantage using a recurrent distributed network. *Journal of Experimental Psychology: Human Perception and Performance* 20:1233–47.

Kawamoto, A. H., and Kitzis, S. N. 1991. Time course of regular and irregular pronunciations. *Connection Science* 3:207–17.

Kawamoto, A. H., and Zemblidge, J. 1992. Pronunciation of homographs. *Journal of Memory and Language* 31:349–74.

Killeen, P. 1989. Behavior as a trajectory through a field of attractors. In *The Computer and the Brain: Perspectives on Human and Artificial Intelligence*, eds. J. R. Brink and C. R. Haden. Amsterdam: Elsevier.

Killeen, P. 1992. Mechanics of the animate. *Journal of the Experimental Analysis of Behavior* 57:429–63.

Kochnower, J., Richardson, E., and DiBenedetto, B. 1983. A comparison of the phonic decoding ability of normal and learning disabled children. *Journal of Learning Disabilities* 16:348–51.

Kohler, W. 1947. *Gestalt Psychology.* New York: Liveright Publishing Co.

Kohonen, T. 1988. *Self-organization and Associative Memory.* Berlin, Federal Republic of Germany: Springer-Verlag.

Lakoff, G. 1987. *Women, Fire, and Dangerous Things: What Categories Reveal About the Mind.* Chicago: University of Chicago Press.

Lesch, M. F., and Pollatsek, A. 1993. Automatic access of semantic information by phonological codes in visual word recognition. *Journal of Experimental Psychology: Learning, Memory, and Cognition* 19:285–94.

Liberman, A. M. 1991. Observations from the sidelines. *Reading and Writing: An Interdisciplinary Journal* 3:429–33.

Liberman, A. M., and Shankweiler, D. P. 1979. Speech, the alphabet and teaching to read. In *Theory and Practice of Early Reading*, eds. L. Resnick and P. Weaver. Hillsdale, NJ: Lawrence Erlbaum Associates.

Liberman, I. Y., Rubin, H., Duques, S., and Carlise, J. 1985. Linguistic abilities and spelling proficiency in kindergartners and adult poor spellers. In *Biobehavioral*

Measures of Dyslexia, eds. D. Gray and J. Kavanaugh. Parkton, MD: York Press.

Llewellen, M. J., Goldinger, S. D., Pisoni, D. B., and Greene, B. G. 1993. Lexical familiarity and processing efficiency: Individual differences in naming, lexical decision, and semantic categorization. *Journal of Experimental Psychology: General* 122:316–30.

Lukatela, G., Lukatela, K., and Turvey, M. T. 1993. Further evidence for phonological constraints on visual lexical access: TOWED primes FROG. *Perception and Psychophysics* 53:461–66.

Lukatela, G., and Turvey, M. T. 1991. Phonological access of the lexicon: Evidence from associative priming with pseudohomophones. *Journal of Experimental Psychology: Human Perception and Performance* 17:951–66.

MacWhinney, B., and Leinback, J. 1991. Implementations are not conceptualizations: Revising the verb learning model. *Cognition* 40:121–57.

MacWhinney, B., Leinback, J., Taraban, R., and McDonald, J. 1989. Language learning: Cues or rules? *Journal of Memory and Language* 28:255–77.

Maddox, W. T., and Ashby, F. G. 1993. Comparing decision bound and exemplar models of categorization. *Perception and Psychophysics* 53:49–70.

Manis, F. R., Seidenberg, M. S., Doi, L. M., McBride-Chang, C., and Peterson, A. in press. On the bases of two subtypes of developmental dyslexia. *Cognition.*

Manis, F. R., Szeszulski, P. A., Holt, I. K., and Graves, K. 1988. A developmental perspective on dyslexic subtypes. *Annals of Dyslexia* 38:139–53.

May, R. 1976. Simple mathematical models with very complicated dynamics. *Nature* 261:459–67.

McClelland, J. L., and Rumelhart, D. E. 1981. An interactive activation model of context effects in letter perception: Part 1. An account of basic findings. *Psychological Review* 88:375–407.

Meyer, D., and Gutschera, K. D. 1975, November. Orthographic versus phonemic processing of printed words. Paper presented at the meeting of the Psychonomic Society, Denver, CO.

Morris, I. ed., 1982. *American Heritage Dictionary* (Second college edition). Boston, MA: Houghton Mifflin.

Morton, J. 1969. Interaction of information in word recognition. *Psychological Review* 76:165–78.

Newell, A. 1990. *Unified Theories of Cognition*. Cambridge, MA: Harvard Press.

Nielson, C. S. 1991. Phonology affects identification of high frequency printed words. Unpublished honors thesis. Honors College, Arizona State University, Tempe, AZ.

Nielson, C. S., and Van Orden, G. C. 1992, April. Phonology affects identification of high frequency printed words. Presented at the meeting of the Western Psychological Association, Portland, OR.

Nowak, A., Szamrej, J., and Latané, B. 1990. From private attitude to public opinion: A dynamic theory of social impact. *Psychological Review* 97:362–76.

Olson, R. K. 1985. Disabled reading processes and cognitive profiles. In *Biobehavioral Measures of Dyslexia*, eds. D. Gray and J. Kavanagh. Parkton MD: York Press.

Olson, R. K., Kliegel, R., Davidson, B. J., and Foltz, G. 1985. Individual and developmental differences in reading disability. In *Reading Research: Advances in Theory and Practice (Vol. 4)*, eds. G. E. MacKinnon and T. G. Waller. New York: Academic Press.

Olson, R. K., and Wise, B. 1986, November. Heritability of phonetic and orthographic word decoding skills in dyslexia. Paper presented at the meetings
of the Psychonomic Society, New Orleans.

Olson, R. K., Wise, B., Conners, F. A., and Rack, J. P. 1990. Organization, heritability, and remediation of component word recognition and language
skills in disabled readers. In *Reading and its Development: Component Skills
Approaches*, eds. T. H. Carr and B. A. Levy. New York: Academic Press.

Olson, R. K., Wise, B., Conners, F. A., Rack, J. P., and Fulker, D. 1989. Specific
deficits in component reading and language skills: Genetic and environmental
influences. *Journal of Learning Disabilities* 22:339–48.

Oyama, S. 1985. *The Ontogeny of Information: Developmental Systems and
Evolution*. New York: Cambridge University Press.

Paap, K. R., Newsome, S. L., McDonald, J. E., and Schvaneveldt, R. W. 1982. An
activation-verification model for letter and word recognition: The word-
superiority effect. *Psychological Review* 89:573–94.

Paap, K. R., Noel, R. W., and Johansen, L. S. 1992. Dual-route models of print to
sound: Red herrings and real horses. In *Orthography, Phonology, Morphology,
and Meaning*, eds. R. Frost and L. Katz. Amsterdam: North-Holland.

Patterson, K. E. 1982. The relation between reading and phonological coding:
Further neuropsychological observations. In *Normality and Pathology in
Cognitive Functions*, ed. A. W. Ellis. London: Academic Press.

Pennington, B. F., Van Orden, G. C., Smith, S. D., Green, P., and Haith, M. M.
1990. Phonological processing skills and deficits in adult dyslexics. *Child
Development* 61:1753–78.

Perfetti, C. A. 1985. *Reading Ability*. New York: Oxford University Press.

Perfetti, C. A., and Bell, L. C. 1991. Phonemic activation during the first 40
ms of word identification: Evidence from backward masking and masked
priming. *Journal of Memory and Language* 30:473–85.

Perfetti, C. A., Bell, L. C., and Delaney, S. 1988. Automatic (prelexical) phonetic
activation in silent word reading: Evidence from backward masking.
Journal of Memory and Language 27:59–70.

Perfetti, C. A., Zhang, S., and Berent, I. 1992. Reading in English and Chinese:
Evidence for a "universal" phonological principle. In *Orthography,
Phonology, Morphology, and Meaning*, eds. R. Frost and L. Katz. Amsterdam:
North-Holland.

Petersen, S. E., Fox, P. T., Posner, M. I., Mintun, M., and Raichle, M. E. 1988.
Positron emission tomographic studies of the cortical anatomy of single-
word processing. *Nature* 333:585–89.

Plaut, D. C., and Shallice, T. 1993. Deep dyslexia: A case study of connectionist
neuropsychology. *Cognitive Neuropsychology* 10:377–500.

Plunkett, K., and Marchman, V. 1991. U-shaped learning and frequency effects
in a multilayered perceptron: Implications for child language acquisition.
Cognition 38:43–102.

Posner, M. I. 1978. *Chronometric Explorations of Mind*. Hillsdale, NJ: Lawrence
Erlbaum Associates.

Pratt, A. C., and Brady, S. 1988. Relation of phonological awareness to reading
disability in children and adults. *Journal of Educational Psychology* 80:319–23.

Prigogine, I., and Stengers, I. 1984. *Order Out of Chaos: Man's New Dialogue
with Nature*. New York: Bantam Books.

Rack, J. P., Snowling, M. J., and Olson, R. K. 1992. The nonword reading deficit in developmental dyslexia: A review. *Reading Research Quarterly* 27:29–53.

Rayner, K., and Pollatsek, A. 1989. *The Psychology of Reading.* Englewood Cliffs, NJ: Prentice-Hall.

Reicher, G. M. 1969. Perceptual recognition as a function of meaningfulness of stimulus material. *Journal of Experimental Psychology* 81:275–80.

Rockwell, W. T. 1994. On what the mind is identical with. *Philosophical Psychology* 7:307–23.

Rosson, M. B. 1985. The interaction of pronunciation rules and lexical representations in reading aloud. *Memory and Cognition* 13:90–99.

Rueckl, J. G., and Olds, E. M. 1993. When pseudowords acquire meaning: Effect of semantic associations on pseudoword repetition priming. *Journal of Experimental Psychology: Learning, Memory, and Cognition* 19:515–27.

Rumelhart, D. E., and McClelland, J. L. 1986a. On learning the past tense of English verbs. In *Parallel Distributed Processing: Explorations in the Microstructures of Cognition, Vol. 2: Psychological and Biological Models*, eds. J. L. McClelland and D. E. Rumelhart. Cambridge, MA: MIT Press.

Rumelhart, D. E., and McClelland, J. L. 1986b. PDP models and general issues in cognitive science. In *Parallel Distributed Processing: Explorations in the Microstructures of Cognition, Vol. 1: Foundations*, eds. D. E. Rumelhart and J. L. McClelland. Cambridge, MA: MIT Press.

Ryder, R. J., and Pearson, D. D. 1980. Influence of type-to-token frequencies and final consonants on adults' internalization of vowel digraphs. *Journal of Educational Psychology* 72:618–24.

Seidenberg, M. S. 1992. Beyond orthographic depth in reading: Equitable division of labor. In *Orthography, Phonology, Morphology, and Meaning*, eds. R. Frost and L. Katz. Amsterdam: North-Holland.

Seidenberg, M. S., and McClelland, J. L. 1989. A distributed, developmental model of word recognition and naming. *Psychological Review* 96:523–68.

Seidenberg, M. S., Plaut, D. C., Petersen, A. S., McClelland, J. L., and McRae, K. 1994. Nonword pronunciation and models of word recognition. *Journal of Experimental Psychology: Human Perception and Performance* 20:1177–96.

Siegal, L. S., and Ryan, E. B. 1988. Development of grammatical sensitivity, phonological, and short-term memory skills in normally achieving and learning disabled children. *Developmental Psychology* 24:28–37.

Shepard, R. N. 1989. Internal representation of universal regularities: A challenge for connectionism. In *Neural Connections, Mental Computation*, eds. L. Nadel, L. A. Cooper, P. Culicover, and R. M. Harnish. Cambridge, MA: MIT Press.

Simon, H. 1973. The organization of complex systems. In *Hierarchy Theory: The Challenge of Complex Systems*, ed. H. H. Pattee. NY: Braziller.

Skarda, C. A., and Freeman, W. J. 1987. How brains make chaos in order to make sense of the world. *Behavioral and Brain Sciences* 10:161–95.

Smith, F. 1971. *Understanding Reading: A Psycholinguistic Analysis of Reading and Learning to Read.* New York: Holt, Rinehart and Winston.

Smith, L. B. 1989. From global similarities to kinds of similarities: The construction of dimensions in development. In *Similarity and Analogical Reasoning*, eds., S. Vosniadou and A. Ortony. New York: Cambridge Univeristy Press.

Smith, L. B., and Katz, D. B. in press. Activity-dependent processes in perceptual and cognitive development. To appear in *Handbook of Perception and*

Cognition, Vol. 13, eds. R. Gelman and T. Au.

Smith, L. B., and Thelen, E. 1993. *A Dynamic Systems Approach to Development: Applications*. Cambridge, MA: MIT Press.

Smith, S. D., Pennington, B. F., Kimberling, W. J., Fain, P. R., Ing, P. F., and Lubs, H. A. 1986. Genetic heterogeneity in specific reading disability. *American Journal of Human Genetics* 39:A:169.

Smolensky, P. 1986a. Formal modeling of subsymbolic processes: An introduction to harmony theory. In *Advances in Cognitive Science 1*, ed. N. E. Sharkey. New York: Wiley.

Smolensky, P. 1986b. Information processing in dynamical systems: Foundations of harmony theory. In *Parallel Distributed Processing: Explorations in the Microstructures of Cognition: Vol. 1. Foundations*, eds. D. E. Rumelhart, J. L. McClelland, and the PDP Research Group. Cambridge, MA: MIT Press.

Snowling, M. J. 1980. The development of grapheme-phoneme correspondence in normal and dyslexic readers. *Journal of Experimental Child Psychology* 29:294–305.

Snowling, M. 1981. Phonemic deficits in developmental dyslexia. *Psychological Research* 43:219–34.

Stanovich, K. E., Nathan, R. G., and Vala-Rossi, M. 1986. Developmental changes in the cognitive coordinates of reading ability and the developmental lag hypothesis. *Reading Research Quarterly* 21:199–202.

Sternberg, S. 1969. The discovery of processing stages: Extensions of Donders' method. *Acta Psychologica* 30:276–315.

Stone, G. O. 1994. Combining connectionist and symbolic properties in a single process. In *The Reality of Linguistic Rules*, eds. S. Lima, R. Corrigan, and G. Iverson. Philadelphia, PA: John Benjamins.

Stone, G. O., Vanhoy, M., and Van Orden, G. C. in press. Perception is a two-way street: Feedforward and feedback phonology in visual word recognition. *Journal of Memory and Language*.

Stone, G. O., and Van Orden, G. C. 1989. Are words represented by nodes? *Memory and Cognition* 17:511–24.

Stone, G. O., and Van Orden, G. C. 1993. Strategic processes in printed word recognition. *Journal of Experimental Psychology: Human Perception and Performance* 19:744–74.

Stone, G. O., and Van Orden, G. C. 1994. Building a resonance framework for word recognition using design and systems principles. *Journal of Experimental Psychology: Human Perception and Performance* 20:1248–68.

Strain, E., Patterson, K., and Seidenberg, M. S. 1995. Semantic effects in single-word naming. *Journal of Experimental Psychology: Learning, Memory and Cognition* 21:1140–54.

Taraban, R., and McClelland, J. L. 1987. Conspiracy effects in word pronunciation. *Journal of Memory and Language* 26:608–31.

Thelen, E., and Smith, L. B. 1994. *A Dynamic Systems Approach to the Development of Cognition and Action*. Cambridge, MA: MIT Press.

Thompson, J. M. P., and Stewart, H. B. 1987. *Nonlinear Dynamics and Chaos*. New York: Wiley.

Triesman, A. M. 1960. Contextual cues in selective listening. *Quarterly Journal of Experimental Psychology* 12:242–48.

Turvey, M. T. 1977. Preliminaries to a theory of action with reference to vision.

In *Perceiving, Acting, and Knowing,* eds. R. Shaw and J. Bransford. Hillsdale, NJ: Lawrence Erlbaum Associates.

Turvey, M. T., and Carello, C. 1981. Cognition: The view from ecological realism. *Cognition* 10:313–21.

Uttal, W. R. 1990. On some two-way barriers between models and mechanisms. *Perception and Psychophysics* 48:188–203.

Vallacher, R. R., and Nowak, A. 1994. *Dynamical Systems in Social Psychology.* San Diego, CA: Academic Press.

van der Maas, H. L. J., and Molenaar, P. C. M. 1992. Stagewise cognitive development: An application of catastrophe theory. *Psychological Review* 99:395–417.

Van Orden, G. C. 1987. A ROWS is a ROSE: Spelling, sound, and reading. *Memory and Cognition* 15:181–98.

Van Orden, G. C. 1991. Phonologic mediation is fundamental to reading. In *Basic Processes in Reading: Visual Word Recognition,* eds. D. Besner, and G. Humphreys. Hillsdale, NJ: Lawrence Erlbaum Associates.

Van Orden, G. C., and Goldinger, S. D. 1994. Interdependence of form and function in cognitive systems explains perception of printed words. *Journal of Experimental Psychology: Human Perception and Performance* 20:1269–91.

Van Orden, G. C., Johnston, J. C., and Hale, B. L. 1988. Word identification in reading proceeds from spelling to sound to meaning. *Journal of Experimental Psychology: Learning, Memory, and Cognition* 14:371–85.

Van Orden, G. C., Pennington, B. F., and Green, P. 1995. Phonologic mediation and developmental dyslexia. (Unpublished manuscript.)

Van Orden, G. C., Pennington, B. F., and Stone, G. O. 1990. Word identification in reading and the promise of subsymbolic psycholinguistics. *Psychological Review* 97:488–522.

Van Orden, G. C., Pennington, B. F., and Stone, G. O. 1996. What do double dissociations prove? Inductive methods and theory in psychology. (Manuscript submitted for publication).

Van Orden, G. C., Stone, G. O., Garlington, K. L., Markson, L. R., Pinnt, G. S., Simonfy, C. M., and Brichetto, T. 1992. "Assembled" phonology and reading: A case study in how theoretical perspective shapes empirical investigation. In *Orthography, Phonology, Morphology, and Meaning,* eds. R. Frost, and L. Katz. Amsterdam: North-Holland.

Varela, F. J., Thompson, E., and Rosch, E. 1991. *The Embodied Mind: Cognitive Science and Human Experience.* Cambridge, MA: MIT Press.

Wagner, R. K., and Torgesen, J. K. 1987. The nature of phonological processing and its causal role in the acquisition of reading skills. *Psychological Bulletin* 101:192–212.

Wheeler, R. M. 1970. Processes in word recognition. *Cognitive Psychology* 1:59–85.

Wydell, T. N., Patterson, K. E., and Humphreys, G. W. 1993. Phonologically mediated access to meaning for Kanji: Is a *Rows* still a *Rose* in Japanese Kanji? *Journal of Experimental Psychology: Learning, Memory, and Cognition* 19:491–514.

Part • V

Functional Neural Imaging

When Franz Joseph Gall was a schoolboy around the turn of the 19th century, he noted that those of his classmates who excelled in mathematics appeared to have protruding eyeballs. He reasoned that this peculiar trait was the result of an expansion of the brain regions located behind the eyes thereby forcing them out, and that this focal enlargement of brain mass in mathematically gifted individuals indicated that that region of the brain was specialized for this function. Thus was the field of phrenology created.

Phrenology is based on three tenets: (1) Behavioral traits ("faculties") are located in specific regions of the brain; (2) one's ability in a particular faculty leads to either an increase or decrease in brain size in the area subsuming that faculty; and (3) that this enlargement or decrease of focal brain regions is reflected as either bumps or depressions on the overlying skull. Thus, by knowing what regions of the brains subsumed what functions, Gall could determine individuals' behavioral traits by palpating the bulges or dents of their crania. The scientific underpinnings of phrenology were, at best, suspect, and Gall didn't particularly help himself when he performed a phrenologic analysis of Descartes' skull. After finding the area of the skull purportedly overlying the higher reasoning center of the brain to be remarkably small, Gall remarked that perhaps the French philosopher was not such a great thinker after all.

We now know, of course, that phrenology is hogwash. Yet the importance of Gall's contribution to modern cognitive neuroscience should not be overlooked. Until phrenology was espoused, the brain's role in the control of behavior was considered, when it was considered at all, to be "holistic" in the sense that each part of the brain was thought to operate the same as any other. With the introduction of phrenology, scientists began to consider the possibility that there were regions of specialized functions within the human brain. Broca's and Wernicke's descriptions in the mid 1800s of language localization to specific regions of left hemisphere were undoubtedly informed by the ongoing localizationist debates spurred by phrenology.

In the period after Broca and Wernicke, however, the pendulum of neurological thought began to swing away from localization of function. With a few notable exceptions (Dejerine, for example), most workers, while acknowledging lateralization of the brain for language, thought that most other higher cognitive functions were likely not to be localized. It was not until the mid portion of this century that an increasingly large number of neurologists and neuroscientists began to consider once again that individual regions of the brain could underlie specific functions. The work that fueled this renaissance of localizationist thinking was based on the careful study of the behavioral deficits associated with specific focal brain injury, as well as investigations of animal models.

But there are always questions raised concerning this type of research. In the case of the human "natural experiments," one could control neither the location nor the extent of lesion. In the case of animal experimentation, the ability to generalize to the case of the human had to be considered. And for both types of experiments, the notion that simply because there was a correlation between the loss of a specific brain region and some alteration in behavior did not necessarily indicate that that portion of the brain alone was responsible for that function. What was clearly needed to further the arguments was a way of visualizing the brain in action. This is where the advent of functional imaging came to the fore.

Some of the most exciting advances in our understanding of the role of brain and behavior have been fueled by the introduction of functional imaging techniques. These techniques, including functional MRI, positron emission tomography (PET), and magnetoencephalography (MEG) allow us to peek at the brain while it processes information. Schwartz and Gallen, for example, present evidence indicating the advantages of MEG for determining electrical function of the brain in terms of spatial and temporal resolution. The chapter of Fiez, Petersen, and Raichle details how two different pathways of the brain are activated when performing tasks requiring word generation based on visually or auditorally presented input. Their emphasis on pathways of information processing illustrates quite well how this type of work has enabled cognitive neuroscience to move beyond the simple notions of phrenology and more toward a view of the brain as a complex processor of information. The promise of these techniques for the study of dyslexia lies not only in the basic understanding of normal language processing, but in future research on how dyslexics process linguistic information.

Chapter • **10**

Identification of Two Pathways Used for Verbal Response Selection

Julie A. Fiez
Steven E. Petersen
Marcus E. Raichle

The design and interpretation of experiments conducted by our research group are based on the idea that performance of a task requires specific types of information processing. No one area of the brain is devoted to a very complex function such as "syntax" or "semantics." Rather, any task or "function" utilizes a set of brain areas that form an interconnected, parallel, and distributed hierarchy. Each area within the hierarchy makes a specific contribution to the performance of the task (Posner et al. 1988).

The value of PET activation studies is that they can help identify the types of information processing performed by specific brain regions, as well as how different regions may interact with each other. The basic rationale underlying PET activation studies is that performance of any task leads to changes in neural activity in various functional areas of the brain. Changes in neuronal activity produce changes in local blood flow that can be measured with PET (Raichle 1989). Because of this relationship, we will refer to local blood flow increases as functional activations.

The use of PET activation studies based on a subtraction method and image averaging to identify functional activations is a fairly recent development: the first PET study of language processing using the methodological advances described below was published only seven years ago (Petersen et al. 1988; Petersen et al. 1989). This report was designed to examine, at several levels, the processing of single words. The study looked at three levels of change: passive presentation of nouns (compared to simple fixation), repetition aloud of the nouns (compared to passive presentation), and generation aloud of a verb appropriate to the presented nouns (compared to repetition). Each of these levels was assessed in one set of scans with visual input, and in another set of scans with auditory input. The logic of the subtraction analysis was that the passive presentation-fixation subtraction would isolate areas involved in passive sensory processing, the repetition-passive presentation subtraction would isolate areas involved in articulatory output and motor programming, and the verb generation-repetition would isolate areas involved in high-level processes such as semantic and syntactic analysis.

In its most simple form, the type of hierarchical subtraction method used for the design and analysis of this survey study involves accepting the premise that processing done by previously added areas does not change with the addition or deletion of new areas, i.e., each area is functionally isolated. Also assumed in this approach is that the subject does not change strategies with the addition of another task, and that the task combinations do not interact with each other (Donders 1969; Kulpe 1909; Sternberg 1969).

The limitations of the "additive" method were first discussed in terms of reaction time studies of human performance. For PET studies, some empirical testing of the assumptions involved in the subtraction method is possible: the locations of areas added at different stages in a task hierarchy can be identified, and the magnitude of their activity at each level in the scan sequence can be monitored. If a brain area is not functionally isolated, then the magnitude of its activity will be modulated by the addition of new tasks.

While, theoretically, changes in the activity of a region across different levels of a hierarchy can be detected, a number of issues complicate selecting an appropriate statistical measure to detect such changes in PET subtraction images. First, PET is a noisy technique, and data must be combined in some manner across individual subtraction images. Second, the locations of significant change may not be known or hypothesized a priori; this presents a difficult statistical problem, because each image is composed of a large number of spatial locations (over 300,000 pixels), with a small number of observations (usually 8-12 subjects perform each active and control task).

One approach has been to use thresholding techniques in order to define statistically significant responses without a priori regions of interest (e.g., see Ford et al. 1991; Fox and Mintun 1989; Fox et al. 1988; Friston et al. 1991; Worsley et al. 1992). In the analysis used previously by Petersen et al. (1988, 1989), one such thresholding technique was used to identify regions of change for each of the comparisons in the task hierarchy. The greatest limitation of thresholding techniques is that it is difficult to select a threshold that minimizes false positives, while including most reliable regions of change (Hunton et al. 1994). Typically, fairly conservative thresholds have been used. Thus, while the identified responses are likely to reflect real biological changes, many other real regions of change may be overlooked.

Detection of small changes, which may not exceed threshold values for significance, is particularly critical in order to test the assumptions of the additive approach. For this reason, in further evaluating the data from the Petersen et al. (1988, 1989) study, we began with a less conservative approach for describing magnitude changes across levels of the task hierarchy. The reanalysis revealed three regions that appeared unlikely to be functionally isolated. The pattern of activation across tasks in these three regions was then investigated more rigorously in a second group of subjects.

GENERAL PET METHODS

A brief description of PET activation methods follows. For more comprehensive reviews, see (Haxby et al. 1991; Raichle 1989; Stytz and Frieder 1990). For specific details regarding the data analyzed below, see (Petersen et al. 1988; Petersen et al. 1989; Raichle et al. 1994).

A PET scanner is a doughnut-shaped machine consisting of a circular array of radiation detectors. The scanner is used to generate images of the distribution of previously administered radiation within cross-sectional slices of the human body. For images of brain blood flow, the subject's head is inserted into the scanner aperture, and images are made from computer-generated slices cut transaxially through the head. Most activation studies in normal subjects currently measure blood flow using a radioactive form of oxygen ([15]-O) as a tracer, which is incorporated into a saline solution as [15]-O-labeled water and then injected into the blood stream. Following the tracer injection, the scanner is turned on, and the distribution of radioactivity emitted from the head is measured for about a minute. Because [15]-O decays rapidly, and the data acquisition time is so short (usually 60 sec or less), multiple (usually 5-10) scans can be performed in a single session.

To place the images into a standard format that allows comparisons to be made across subjects, two steps are performed. First, the number of counts measured in each image is normalized to 1000. This linear normalization negates the effect of global fluctuations in activity and variations in amount of isotope injected (Fox et al. 1987). Therefore, magnitude data is given in terms of normalized counts (e.g., a peak in a subtraction image with a magnitude of +100 counts represents roughly a 10% increase in tissue radioactivity—a measure that is linearly related to blood flow—[Fox, Perlmutter, and Raichle 1985; Herscovitch, Markham, and Raichle 1983]).

Second, the image is transformed into a standard anatomical space (based upon skull dimensions and section placement information obtained from a lateral skull x-ray) (Fox, Perlmutter, and Raichle 1985; Talairach and Tournoux 1988), and a 49-slice linearly interpolated image is created from the seven slices of each reconstructed image (Fox et al. 1988).

Since multiple scans can be made in a scan session, different tasks can be performed in each subject. The basis of all data analysis in our laboratory is a comparison of neuronal activity (indirectly imaged with the scanner) under two conditions. To isolate areas of activity change between task conditions, an image generated during performance of one task is subtracted, on a pixel by pixel basis, from the image generated during performance of another task. The resultant images will be referred to as *individual difference images*.

Because the images are cast into the space of the Talairach and Tournoux stereotactic atlas (Talairach and Tournoux 1988), each focus of activity change can be reported in terms of x, y, and z coordinates. The x-coordinate is the distance in mm to the right (+) or left (–) of midline, the y-coordinate is the distance in mm anterior (+) or posterior (–) to a vertical plane through the anterior commissure, and the z-coordinate is the distance in mm above (+) or below (–) a horizontal plane that cuts through the anterior-posterior commissures. Coronal and transverse sections will be presented with the left hemisphere to the left of midline.

REANALYSIS OF LANGUAGE DATA (ACTIVATION ACROSS LEVELS OF TASK HIERARCHY)

In this section, data from Petersen et al. (1988, 1989) are reanalyzed, in order to test the assumptions of the additive method used in the design of the study. For this reanalysis, we used a regions-of-interest approach to examine the magnitude changes across the stages of the language task hierarchy used by Petersen and collaborators.

Methods

Data used for analysis. Data was collected by Petersen and collaborators as part of a survey study of language processing. The paradigm and methods for data collection and original analysis are described fully by the original investigators (Petersen et al. 1988; Petersen et al. 1989). Only a very brief description follows.

Words were presented at a rate of one per second, and subjects performed one of three tasks: passively look at or listen to presented nouns (passive task), say aloud the presented nouns (noun repetition task), or think of and say aloud an appropriate use (verb) for the presented nouns (verb generation task). Most subjects performed each task once with visually presented words, and once with auditorily presented nouns.

Six different subtraction conditions formed the basis of the original data analysis used by Petersen et al. (1988, 1989) (see table 1). At the lowest level in the subtraction hierarchy were the auditory and visual passive-noun repetition difference images. At the second level in the subtraction hierarchy were the auditory and visual noun repetition-passive difference images. At the third, and highest level in the subtraction hierarchy were the auditory and visual verb generation-noun repetition difference images.

In the reanalysis, the same six subtraction conditions used by Petersen et al. (1988, 1989) were examined. The subject composition of the images varied somewhat, however. Developments in assessing artifacts caused by subject movement between scans suggested some subjects included in the original analysis did not meet current criteria for movement (an average of one subject per image, range of 0-3), while a few others that had been excluded fell within the limits (an average of two subjects per image, range of 1-4). In addition, due to improvements in the automatization and standardization of skull x-ray information, there were some differences in the factors used for stereotactic normalization of each subject (see General PET Methods). These changes resulted in fairly minor differences between the two sets of images.

Regions of interest definition.   The purpose of the reanalysis was to investigate the activity of areas identified at one stage in the task subtraction hierarchy across the other two levels. The areas of interest were based upon those identified by Petersen and collaborators (1988, 1989), who used a thresholding approach to analyze the average difference images for the six subtraction conditions. The areas of change they isolated across the subtraction conditions are displayed in figure 1, and briefly described below.

Passive presentation of words appeared to activate modality-specific primary and extraprimary sensory-processing areas. When words are presented visually (without any task demands), several areas of extrastriate visual cortex are activated. These include areas in both hemispheres. The presentation of auditory words activated

Table I.   Subtraction Hierarchy

Control State	Stimulated State	Task Differences
visual fixation point only	passive words (vis. or aud. presentation)	passive sensory processing word-level coding
passive words (vis. or aud. presentation)	repeat words (vis. or aud. presentation)	articulatory coding motor programming & output
repeat words (vis. or aud. presentation)	generate verbs (vis. or aud. presentation)	semantic association selection for action

Table showing the three hierarchical subtractions used in the study by Petersen et al. (1988, 1989). Some hypothesized cognitive operations isolated by each comparison are represented in the third column.

REGIONS OF INTEREST ACROSS CONDITIONS
AUDITORY PRESENTATION   VISUAL PRESENTATION

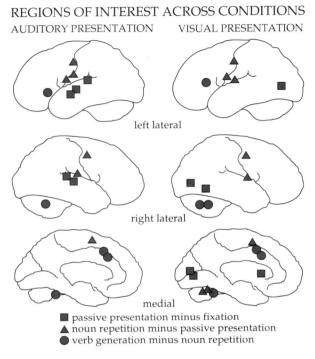

left lateral

right lateral

medial

■ passive presentation minus fixation
▲ noun repetition minus passive presentation
● verb generation minus noun repetition

Figure 1:   Regions of interest across conditions in language hierarchy. Regions of interest were selected based upon an outlier analysis that identified significant foci of change across three subtraction conditions in two modalities. Squares indicate foci identified from the auditory and visual passive word presentation-fixation average difference images. Triangles indicate foci identified from the auditory and visual noun repetition-passive presentation average difference images. Circles indicate foci identified from the auditory and visual verb genera-tion-noun repetition average difference images. The activation for each of these regions across levels of the hierarchy is shown in figures 2a-f.

areas bilaterally along the superior temporal gyrus, as well as a left-lateralized area in the temporoparietal cortex.

When the repetition tasks were compared to the passive tasks, similar areas of activation for auditory and visual presentations were found. For both auditory and visual cues, speech output produced activation in areas that have been implicated in some aspect of motor coding or programming, including primary sensorimotor mouth cortex, the supplementary motor area (SMA), and regions of the cerebellum. Several areas that might be considered lateral premotor regions in Sylvian-insular cortex and a left-lateralized region on the lateral surface of the frontal cortex at or near inferior area 6 were also activated.

The generate verb task made additional processing demands. Here the subtraction condition was the repetition condition, so the sensory input was identical in the active and control condition, and the motor output was very similar. For the generate subtraction, two foci in anterior cingulate cortex were activated, several regions of the left anterior inferior prefrontal cortex, as well as the right inferior lateral cerebellum.

The areas of change identified by Petersen et al. (1988, 1989) defined the regions of interest for the reanalysis (see figure 1); each region of interest consisted of a spherical volume with a 7 mm radius centered at a given focus of change.

Assessment of regional magnitudes across subtraction conditions. Once the set of regions had been defined, regional magnitudes were then computed for each of the six conditions in the subtraction hierarchy. For example, one region was a primary motor cortex region defined on the basis of a focus identified in the noun repetition (visual presentation)—passive visual presentation average difference image. The average regional magnitude was computed for the individual difference images comprising the six average difference images: (1) passive auditory presentation–fixation, (2) passive visual presentation–fixation, (3) auditory noun repetition–passive auditory presentation, (4) visual noun repetition–passive visual presentation, (5) verb generation for auditory nouns–auditory noun repetition, and (6) verb generation for visual nouns– visual noun repetition.

In addition to computing a mean regional magnitude value for each condition, one sample t-tests were also used to determine whether the magnitude changes were significantly different from zero. These values should be considered to be primarily descriptive in nature, given the large number of comparisons that were performed, and the relatively small number of subjects (ranging from 8 for the three auditory conditions to 14 for the visual noun repetition–passive visual presentation condition).

The logic of the analysis was that if an area identified at one level of the hierarchy is affected by the addition of the next task in the hierarchy, then the change should be detected in another subtraction image. For instance, primary motor cortex may not be active when subjects passively look at visually presented nouns. When subjects have to repeat the noun, however, the area may become active. If this occurs, a positive change in regional activation should be detected in the repetition-passive image, while the change in regional activation should be near zero in the passive-fixation image.

At the highest task level, when subjects are required to say aloud verbs for the presented nouns, the motor cortex might remain active at the same level as in the noun repetition task, since for both tasks a motor output is required. If this is so, then regional activation in the verb generation-noun repetition image should also be near zero. Alternatively, the activity of the motor cortex might be changed. For instance, because subjects did not always produce a verb for each noun, fewer words were spoken during the verb generation task; one might hypothesize that activity in the primary motor cortex should decrease, and therefore the regional activity in the verb generation-noun repetition image might be negative.

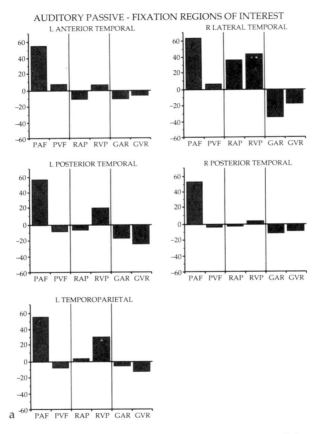

Figures 2 a-f: Regional magnitudes across subtraction conditions: auditory and visual passive, repetition, and generation regions. Each of the foci shown in figure 1 defined the center of a regular spherical region. They are divided into groups on the basis of the condition in which the foci were identified as significant outliers. Each graph represents the magnitudes for a single region. The light gray bars indicate the magnitude in the auditory and visual passive presentation-fixation conditions (PAF and PVF, respectively). The dark gray bars indicate the magnitude in the auditory and visual noun repetition-passive presentation conditions (RAP and RVP, respectively). The black bars indicate the magnitudes in the auditory and visual generation-repetition conditions (GAR and GVR, respectively). Magnitude changes that differ significantly from zero are marked with asterisks (*p<.05; **p<.01; one-sample two-tailed t-test). Magnitude changes in the condition that gave rise to the region of interest are marked with a pound (#) sign. All graphs are scaled from −60 to +65 counts.

Results

The results of the regional analysis are graphically presented in figures 2a-f. The hypothesis was that each area should be functionally isolated. That is, it should only become active when its particular type of processing is required to perform a task, and as long as the same processing is required it should remain active. Thus, the strong prediction would be that across the subtraction conditions the regional activation of each area should only change once, given the hierarchical design of the subtraction conditions.

The data do not support such a prediction. Few areas appear to be changed only in one condition. A variety of explanations may account for the observed changes. Some (perhaps many) of these changes are just noise; many of the changes are slight in comparison to the magnitude of responses that are typically found to be significant using an thresholding approach to examine data. Other changes might be real. For instance, they might reflect enhancements in certain areas related to differences in task difficulty and/or attentional state. The changes might also reflect spread

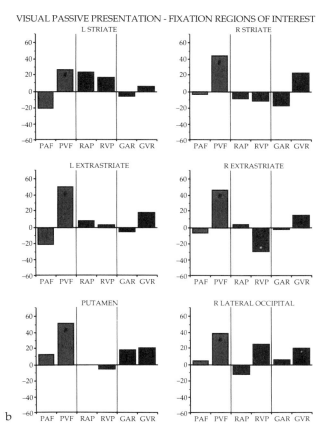

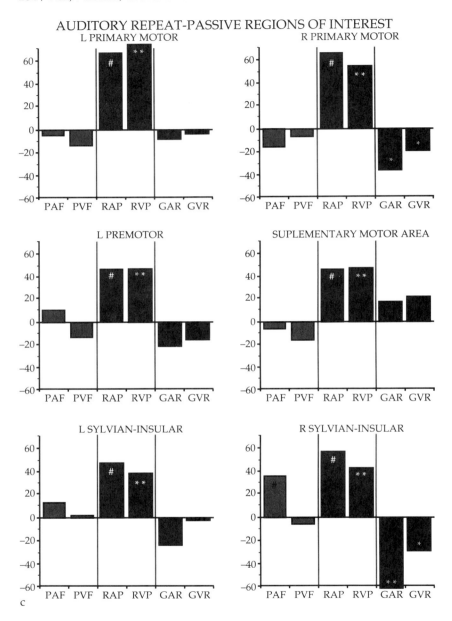

AUDITORY REPEAT-PASSIVE REGIONS OF INTEREST

c

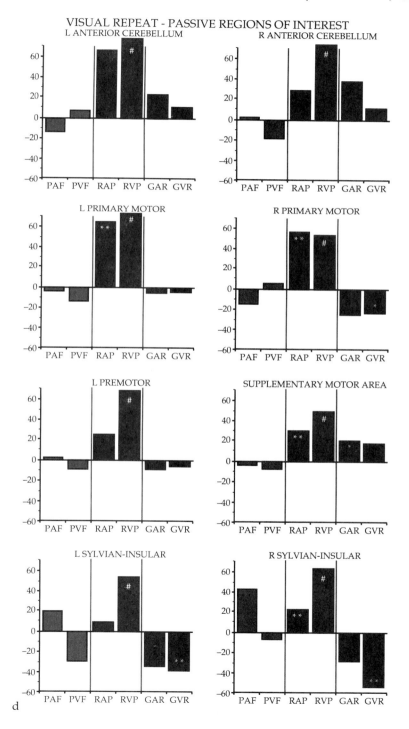

VISUAL REPEAT - PASSIVE REGIONS OF INTEREST

d

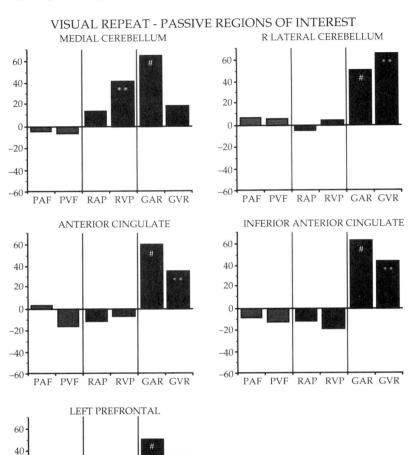

VISUAL REPEAT - PASSIVE REGIONS OF INTEREST

VISUAL GENERATE - REPEAT REGIONS OF INTEREST

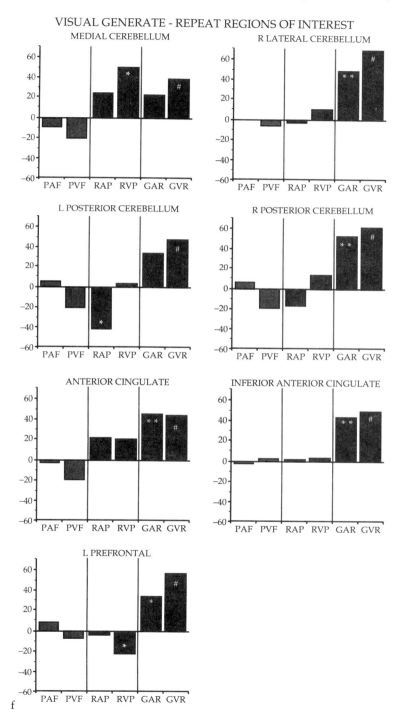

f

of activation from a distant, but strongly activated area; the regional analysis does not provide information about where the center-of-mass of a regional activation is located. Some of the changes might reflect a shift in the strategy used to perform a task. This should produce a change in the types of required processing, and an area active for a task at one stage in the hierarchy might not be active at the next stage. This is theoretically the most interesting type of change. (See figure 3 for an illustration of how these changes could be seen across subtraction conditions.)

In viewing the results, three areas were found with a pattern of activation most consistent with a shift in subject strategy: the left and right Sylvian-insular regions, and the left prefrontal cortex. The regional activation in the Sylvian-insular regions was positive in the noun repetition-passive presentation conditions (for both auditory and visual nouns), but negative in the verb generation-noun repetition conditions (for both auditory and visual nouns). In other words, Sylvian-insular regions are less active during performance of the verb generation task than during

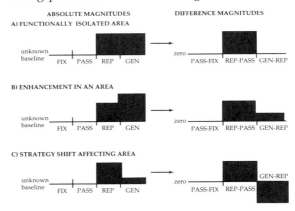

Figure 3: Correlation between changes in activation and changes seen in difference images. The activation observed in a hypothetical brain area is diagrammed under three conditions. In the left column, the absolute magnitude of radioactive counts within the area is given for four different tasks. The differences in absolute magnitudes in the different conditions gives rise to the observed changes shown in the right column. For a functionally isolated area, a change should be observed in only one task condition, representing the first time that area is recruited to perform a particular task. For instance, this area might represent primary motor cortex, which presumably should be active in both the repetition and verb generation tasks, since articulation is required in both instances. For an area that shows some enhancement in activity, a large change might be seen in one subtraction condition, and another, smaller, change might also be seen in another subtraction condition. For an area that is differentially used across different tasks, positive and negative changes should be seen in different subtraction conditions. Illustrated is a positive change representing the initial recruitment of the area in the repeat task. When a task that no longer uses the area (such as the verb generation task) is compared to the repeat task, a negative change is now seen in the subtraction images.

the noun repetition task, and so when the noun repetition task is subtracted from the verb generation task a negative regional activation is
detected (see figures 4 and 5).

A converse pattern of results is seen in a left frontal region. The
left frontal regions (auditory and visual) were originally identified
from positive foci of change in the verb generation-noun repetition
images, and thus a positive regional activation in the verb generation-
noun repetition conditions is found. In contrast, in the noun repetition-
passive presentation conditions (both visual and auditory) a negative
left frontal regional activation was found; this result suggests frontal
regions might be inhibited relative to the passive control and or fixation
during the noun repetition task (see figure 6).

The left frontal and bilateral Sylvian-insular areas were selected for
further investigation. The selection was made on the basis of the regional
magnitude data presented in this section. Particular emphasis was placed
on identifying regions for which: (1) similar patterns observed across the
visual and auditory presentation conditions, (2) the t-tests suggested that

LEFT SYLVIAN-INSULAR REGION

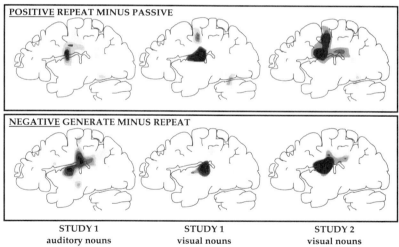

| POSITIVE REPEAT MINUS PASSIVE |
| NEGATIVE GENERATE MINUS REPEAT |

| STUDY 1 | STUDY 1 | STUDY 2 |
| auditory nouns | visual nouns | visual nouns |

Figure 4:   Left Sylvian-insular activation across conditions and studies.
Shown are sagittal sections 39 mm to the left of the midline, for both the noun
repetition-passive presentation and verb generation-noun repetition conditions.
The color bar has been set to display the absolute value of the activation, from
white (0 counts) to black (± 60 counts). In the noun repetition-passive condition (top row), *positive changes* in activation can be seen, with both auditory
stimulus presentation (left-most column), and visual stimulus presentation
(middle column). These positive changes were replicated in a second group
of subjects with visual stimulus presentation (right-most column). In the verb
generation-noun repetition condition (bottom row), *negative changes* in activation can be seen.

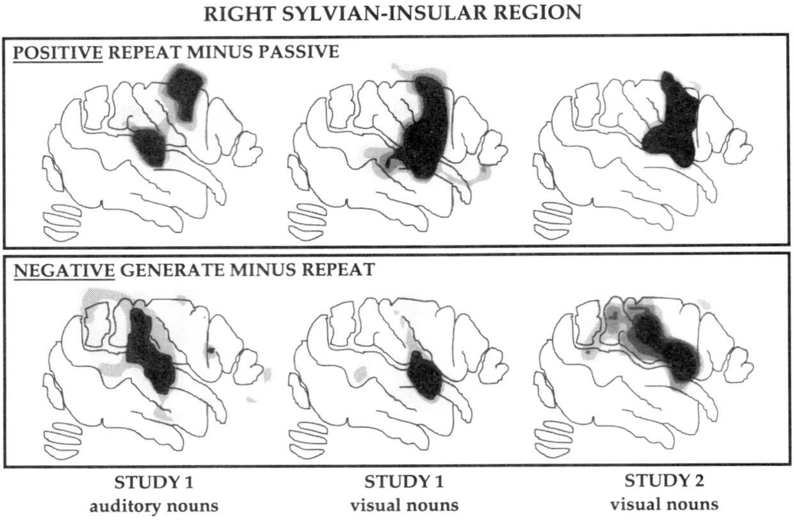

RIGHT SYLVIAN-INSULAR REGION

STUDY 1
auditory nouns

STUDY 1
visual nouns

STUDY 2
visual nouns

Figure 5: Right Sylvian-insular activation across conditions and studies. Shown are sagittal sections 55 mm to the right of the midline, for both the noun repetition-passive presentation and verb generation-noun repetition conditions. The color bar has been set to display the absolute value of the activation, from white (0 counts) to black (columns 1 and 2: ± 50 counts, column 3: ± 75 counts). In the noun repetition-passive condition (top row), *positive changes* in activation can be seen, with both auditory stimulus presentation (left-most column), and visual stimulus presentation (middle column). These positive changes were replicated in a second group of subjects with visual stimulus presentation (right-most column). In the verb generation-noun repetition condition (bottom row), *negative changes* in activation can be seen.

the changes were reliable across the subjects in the original study, and (3) the foci of positive and negative changes were similarly located and not due to large changes in fairly distant areas. None of the other areas met these selection criteria, though they may represent interesting areas for future investigations.

REPLICATION OF SYLVIAN-INSULAR AND LEFT FRONTAL TASK-DEPENDENT ACTIVATION

Activation in bilateral Sylvian-insular and the left frontal cortex during noun repetition and verb generation was measured in a second group of twelve subjects. The paradigm used for the second study is described fully in Raichle et al. (1994). Only data from the first three scans was used for this analysis. In the first scan, subjects passively looked at visually presented nouns. In the second scan, subjects repeated aloud the visually presented nouns, and in the third scan subjects generated appropriate verbs for the visually presented nouns.

LEFT FRONTAL REGION

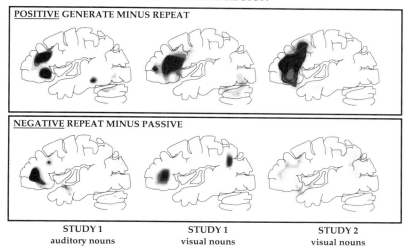

POSITIVE GENERATE MINUS REPEAT

NEGATIVE REPEAT MINUS PASSIVE

| STUDY 1 | STUDY 1 | STUDY 2 |
| auditory nouns | visual nouns | visual nouns |

Figure 6: Left frontal activation across conditions and studies. Shown are sagittal sections 45 mm to the left of the midline, for both the noun repetition-passive presentation and verb generation-noun repetition conditions. The color bar has been set to display the absolute value of the activation, from white (0 counts) to black (columns 1 and 2: ± 60 counts, column 3: ± 80 counts). In the noun repetition-passive condition (top row), *negative changes* in activation can be seen, with both auditory stimulus presentation (left-most column), and visual stimulus presentation (middle column). These negative changes did not replicate in a second group of subjects with visual stimulus presentation (right-most column). In the verb generation-noun repetition condition (bottom row), *positive changes* in activation can be seen, which do replicate in the second group of subjects.

The presentation rate for this second study was slower (one noun every 1.5 seconds) than in the original study (one noun every one second), because behavioral studies demonstrated that at the slower rate subjects were able to respond with a verb to nearly every presented noun. The set of presented nouns was also modified slightly from the original study to avoid presentation of nouns with similar verb associates (e.g., the verb "cut" is appropriate for both the nouns "razor" and "knife").

Methods

Three regular regions were defined. A left Sylvian-insular region was centered at x=–37, y=–16, z= 15 and a right Sylvian-insular region was centered at x=55, y=–7, z=11; these correspond to foci identified in the noun repetition-passive presentation average difference images from the first study. A left frontal region was centered at x=–37, y=31, z=11;

this corresponds to a focus identified in the verb generation for visually presented nouns-visual noun repetition condition.

For each region, individual regional magnitudes were computed for both the noun repetition-passive presentation and verb generation-noun repetition individual difference images across the 12 subjects. For each region, a one sample t-test was used to test whether the regional activation in either condition was significantly different from zero. The resulting p-values were Bonferroni corrected for 6 comparisons (3 regions x 2 conditions).

Results

The results are summarized in figures 4 to 6. In the right Sylvian-insular region significant positive regional activation was once again found in the noun repetition-passive presentation condition (mean=54 counts, t=6.16, df=11, p=.0006, Bonferroni corrected for 6 comparisons) and significant negative regional activation was found in the verb generation-noun repetition condition (mean=–38; t=–3.37, df=11, p=.037, Bonferroni corrected for 6 comparisons). In the left Sylvian-insular region positive regional activation was nearly significant following correction for multiple comparisons (mean=30 counts, t=3.06, df=11, p=.065 Bonferroni corrected for 6 comparisons), and significant negative regional activation was found in the verb generation-noun repetition condition (mean=–49; t=–3.99, df=11, p=.013, Bonferroni corrected for 6 comparisons). In the left frontal region, significant positive activation in the verb generation-noun repetition condition was replicated (mean= 57; t=7.45, df=11, p=.0006, Bonferroni corrected for 6 comparisons), but not the negative activation in the noun repetition-passive presentation condition (mean=–15; t=–2.19, df=11, p=.31, Bonferroni corrected for 6 comparisons).

The lack of left frontal negative activation may reflect paradigm differences between the original and second study. The most likely factors are: (1) the change in presentation rate (from one per second to one per 1.5 seconds), (2) scan order (in the original study the task order varied across subjects, while in the second study noun repetition always followed the passive presentation task), (3) task repetition (some of the data analyzed from the first study came from the second repetition of the task, though in a different modality, while all of the data analyzed from the second study came from the first performance of the task). Most important, though, is the observation that the left frontal regional activation is not positive during the noun repetition condition. The left frontal, anterior cingulate, and right lateral cerebellar regions thus all appear to be significantly changed only in the verb generation-noun repetition condition. This suggests these areas are recruited during performance of the verb generation task, but not during noun repetition.

DISCUSSION

The results suggest that when subjects either repeat a presented noun or produce appropriate verbs for the presented nouns, similar sensory input and motor output regions (such as extrastriate cortex and primary motor cortex) are active. However, the areas used to select an appropriate response differ between the two tasks. When subjects are asked to repeat a word they also activate Sylvian-insular areas. When required to generate an appropriate verb for a presented noun they activate left frontal, anterior cingulate, and cerebellar areas, but not Sylvian-insular areas.

The following discussion will first explore converging evidence from behavioral investigations in normals and in patients which supports a distinction between word repetition and other language tasks. Then, evidence will be presented from converging PET studies that suggests a more general distinction between the role of the frontal and anterior cingulate, and the Sylvian-insular regions. Next, it will be shown that these distinctions map onto information processing models developed in cognitive psychology, and they are consistent with other data about the functions of each area.

The role of the cerebellum is discussed in other publications (Fiez and Petersen 1993; Fiez et al. 1992). This area, while important, is not always activated in conjunction with frontal and anterior cingulate regions. For this reason it is not considered an integral part of the two selection pathways discussed below.

Converging Evidence for Two Speech Production Routes

Normal performance. Evidence from performance studies in normals suggests there may be a fundamental difference between merely repeating a word and requiring subjects to generate a response based upon a stimulus input. Slamecka and Graf (1978) compared recall of the second item of a word pair following performance of one of the following tasks: (1) read aloud both words in the pair, and (2) read aloud the first word in each pair, and think of and say aloud a synonym for the first word, given the initial letter of the target word (e.g., in response to the display "rapid f-", say "rapid" and "fast"). Recall of the items that were generated was found to be significantly better than recall of the items that were simply read aloud, regardless of whether or not subjects were informed that a memory test would follow performance of the generation and repetition tasks. Subsequent investigations have confirmed and extended the initial finding to a number of different generation rules and paradigm manipulations (e.g., Greenwald and Johnson 1989; Johns and Swanson 1988; McElroy 1987; Payne, Neely, and Burns 1986).

Patient performance. Behavioral investigations in patients have also demonstrated that performance on word and sentence repetition tasks can be dissociated from performance on other types of production and/or comprehension tasks. The syndrome of conduction aphasia is characterized by an impaired ability to perform auditory repetition tasks in conjunction with relatively intact spontaneous speech and comprehension. In some, but not all cases, patients may also show relatively spared comprehension of written material, while being unable to read aloud written words (Benson et al. 1973; Damasio 1992; Goodglass and Kaplan 1983). Some investigators, based on extensive evaluation of single patients, have suggested that the repetition impairments they show reflect an inability to access automatically motor representations for visually and auditorily presented words (Friedrich, Glenn, and Marin 1984; Strub and Gardner 1974). Other interpretations have been made, however, such as an underlying short-term memory impairment (e.g., Caramazza et al. 1981; Warrington and Shallice 1969), and a disconnection between sensory and motor speech areas (e.g., Geschwind 1965; Kinsbourne 1972).

The converse dissociation—a preserved ability to repeat words despite significant impairments in speech production and/or comprehension—has also been described (though less frequently). Patients with this pattern of abilities are classified as sensory, motor, or mixed transcortical aphasics. In its most extreme form, patients with mixed transcortical aphasia may spontaneously repeat words and sentences (echolalia), but be unable to comprehend their meaning or produce them spontaneously. Similarly, their ability to read aloud may be intact, though comprehension of written material is severely impaired (Benson 1979; Damasio 1992; Goldstein 1948). These patients provide compelling evidence that word repetition is a task that can be retained despite nearly total loss of other linguistic functions.

Based on such divergent patterns of dissociations, Lichtheim (1885) proposed a 2-route model of speech production, such that repetition could be impaired by damage to a route between sensory images of words and motor images of words, although spontaneous speech could still be mediated via a route between "concept centers" and motor images of words. As a test of this model, McCarthy and Warrington (1984) tested two patients with conduction aphasia and one patient with transcortical motor aphasia on a variety of tasks. They showed, in support of the Lichtheim model, that repetition tasks that required semantic processing were performed better by the conduction aphasics than the transcortical motor aphasic, while the converse was true for repetition tasks in which the semantic components were minimized.

Not only do the patterns of deficits shown by conduction and transcortical aphasic patients support a distinction between word repetition and other language tasks, the loci of anatomical damage associated with each of these syndromes is consistent with the PET data suggesting noun repetition activates Sylvian-insular regions, while verb generation activates frontal and cingulate areas. Patients with conduction aphasia (impaired repetition with preservation of other language functions) commonly (but not always) have damage extending into the left insula (Benson 1979; Damasio and Damasio 1980), while the left Sylvian-insular cortex usually remains undamaged in patients with even the most severe forms of transcortical aphasia (intact repetition with loss of speech production and comprehension) (Benson 1979; Bogousslavsky, Regli, and Assal 1988; Geschwind, Quadfasel, and Segarra 1968).

Converging Results From Other PET Studies

Behavioral studies of both normal and patient performance provide converging evidence to support the PET data that suggests noun repetition and verb generation activate anatomically distinct pathways. Evidence from several other PET studies suggests the dichotomy between Sylvian-insular versus prefrontal and anterior cingulate activation may extend beyond the domain of language.

Lateral Sylvian activation similar to that produced during noun repetition was also found in a study of selective and divided attention to visual features of color, speed and shape (Corbetta et al. 1991). In the selective conditions, a subject made judgments about changes in one, and only one, of the attributes during the scan, while in the divided condition the subjects monitored for changes in all of the attributes simultaneously. For each of the selective conditions, a lateral Sylvian activation was found, but none was seen in the divided condition.

In contrast, both anterior cingulate and lateral prefrontal activation has been seen in several other conditions: in the conflict condition of the Stroop color naming task (where subjects name the color of ink in which a word is printed rather than to say aloud the word itself, e.g., to say "green" when the word RED is presented in green ink) (Pardo et al. 1990); in a divided attention condition where subjects were asked to simultaneously monitor visual arrays for changes in the color, shape, or speed of a visual stimulus (Corbetta et al. 1991); and in a condition in which subjects were asked to pick an arbitrary direction for movement when given a signal to move (Frith et al. 1991).

Although the pattern of frontal and cingulate activation tends to occur in more difficult conditions, such as generating a word versus noun repetition, the results reported by Corbetta et al. (1991) discussed above provide evidence against a general task difficulty interpretation of cingulate and prefrontal activation. As measured by d', a psychophysical measure of discriminability (Green and Swets 1966), the selective color discrimination was nearly as difficult as the discrimination required in the divided condition; in contrast to the similarity in performance, there was no evidence of cingulate activation in the selective color condition, but clear activation in the divided condition.

These findings would be consistent with the idea that across a range of cognitive domains, responses can be produced through two different processes. If there is a strong association between a stimulus and response, subjects use a Sylvian-insular pathway; when this condition is not met, further analysis occurs using frontal and anterior cingulate regions.

For instance, in the selective visual attention conditions described above, enhanced processing of particular stimulus attributes, such as color, may serve to increase the saliency of the stimulus attribute necessary for making a correct decision. In the divided attention condition, however, no single type of attribute can be selected, and thus further processing has to be done using frontal and cingulate regions.

Similarly, for the noun repetition condition the relationship between a visual or auditory word, and articulation of that word, is an overlearned association that might be mediated by left medial extrastriate cortex (for visual words) and temporoparietal cortex (for auditory words) in conjunction with premotor Sylvian and insular activation. For the verb generation task, however, strong associates of the presented nouns are not necessarily correct verb responses. For instance, "cat" is more strongly associated with the word "dog" than possible verb answers such as "bark," and so responses may be selected following further analysis involving frontal and cingulate regions.

As a test of this hypothesis, PET and performance studies examined the functional and behavioral effects of practice on the verb generation task (Raichle et al. 1994). Subjects performed the verb generation task (say aloud an appropriate verb for each presented noun) in three different states of practice: (1) naive: initial (unpracticed) performance of the verb generation task, (2) practiced: following 9 blocks of practice with the same set of nouns, and (3) novel: following practice with the task, but with a novel set of nouns as stimuli. As a control state, subjects were asked to merely read aloud the nouns.

Regions most active during naive performance (left prefrontal, right cerebellum, anterior cingulate) were all significantly less active during practiced performance. Conversely, activity in the Sylvian-insular cortex bilaterally increased following practice, to nearly the same level as found in the noun repetition condition. Behavioral evidence demonstrates that practice results in more automatic performance: subjects not only become faster to respond, but they also repeatedly produce many of the same responses. Most of these functional and behavioral effects of practice appear to be item-specific, since introduction of a novel list of nouns produces similar results to those observed during the first performance of the task (naive condition) (Raichle et al. 1994).

Thus, following a brief period of practice (less than 15 minutes), the cortical circuitry used to perform the verb generation task became almost indistinguishable from that used for reading single words. These results provide converging evidence for the existence of two pathways available for the selection of a verbal response, and support the hypothesis that the use of these pathways is strongly affected by the degree to which a particular response is learned, or automatic.

Cognitive Models

The notion that there are at least two different mechanisms available for the selection and production of responses has a long history in the psychological literature. William James (1890) distinguished between "ideo-motor" acts, "wherever movement follows unhesitatingly and immediately the notion of it in the mind," and "willed" acts, where "an additional conscious element in the shape of a fiat, mandate, or expressed consent" is necessary. Nearly a century later, the psychologists Reason and Mycielska (1982) stated a similar concept: "we have two modes of directing our actions, rather like that in a modern aircraft. That is, we can either operate directly (analogous to having our hands on the controls), or we can switch in the automatic pilot."

Reason's investigations of "action slips"—the performance of an unintended action—suggest normal behavior is a finely tuned balance between the two types of control systems. Analysis of subject diaries confirmed what one might intuitively suspect. Many of these slips can be classified as "slips of habit"—the execution of a habitual response in inappropriate circumstances.

Several different models have been developed that capture this sort of balance (e.g., Miller, Galanter, and Pribram 1960; Norman and Shallice 1985; Reason and Mycielska 1982). Though they differ in specifics, all of these models postulate the existence of one system that operates in a relatively open-loop configuration, with a stimulus or goal leading to a cascade of events which operate in a feed-forward manner to produce a response or sequence of action ("automatic system"). The other system operates in a closed-loop manner, utilizing feedback and controlled processing to direct the production of responses ("controlled system").

Converging Evidence From Other Disciplines

As discussed above, the PET evidence suggesting two different mechanisms may exist for response selection is consistent with a number of psychological models of human information processing and response control. The PET data suggests that the "controlled" system involves prefrontal and anterior cingulate regions, while the "automatic" system involves Sylvian-insular regions. The following sections will evaluate the extent to which this processing distinction between frontal, anterior cingulate, Sylvian, and insular regions is consistent with previous observations about each of these areas. Discussions of cortical connections and cytoarchitecture will be based primarily upon studies in non-human primates. Though species differences exist, similar cortical architecture is likely to exist in humans.

Sylvian and insular cortex. The cortical architecture of the insula is heterogeneous, and follows a general ventral to dorsal progression of increasing complexity (Mesulam and Mufson 1985; Sanides 1968). Ventral regions of the insula have strong, reciprocal connections with olfactory, limbic, and paralimbic areas, such as the amygdala and entorhinal cortex. The dorsal insula receives input from a number of sensory areas, such as the somatosensory area SII (Friedman et al. 1986), posterior auditory area Pa (Pandya 1969), and temporal visual area TEm (Mesulam and Mufson 1985). The dorsal insula also has reciprocal connections with a number of motor areas, including regions in the frontal operculum, and the ventral portion of premotor area 6 (Barbas and Pandya 1987; Friedman et al. 1986; Kurata 1991; Matelli et al. 1986). For a comprehensive review of insular cytoarchitecture and cortical connections, see Mesulam and Mufson 1985.

The opercular cortex is situated anterior to the insula, posterior to the prefrontal cortex, and ventral to the inferior portion of premotor area 6. It also is composed of a ventral-dorsal gradient in complexity (Mesulam and Mufson 1985). The dorsal operculum is interconnected with the insula, as mentioned above, and also with the ventral portion of premotor area 6, and prefrontal area 45 (Broca's area) (Barbas and Pandya 1987; Friedman et al. 1986; Kurata 1991; Matelli et al. 1986).

Area 6 is a premotor area that lies between prefrontal and primary motor cortex. For several reasons, including patterns of anatomical connections and histochemical staining properties, area 6 has been divided into dorsal and ventral regions. Ventral area 6 is bordered ventrally by the frontal operculum and insula. It has reciprocal connections to a number of areas, including area 45 (Broca's area), anterior cingulate cortex, the dorsal insula, supplementary motor cortex, and frontal opercular regions, as well as the primary motor cortex (Arikuni, Watanabe, and Kubota 1988; Barbas and Pandya 1987; Kurata 1991; Matelli et al. 1986).

Taken as a whole, the pattern of interconnections between dorsal insular, opercular, and ventral area 6 cortical areas provide an architectural substrate for high-level integration of sensory and motor information. The available physiological data also supports such a role. Based in part upon data from single-unit recording studies, it has been suggested that premotor area 6 is involved in the production of movements guided or triggered by sensory signals (Evarts and Wise 1984; Passingham 1985; Rizzolatti, Matelli, and Pavesi 1983). For example, neurons in area 6 have been reported to respond more strongly to movements that are initiated by a visual trigger, rather than being self-paced, or internally determined (Mushiake, Inase, and Tanji 1991; Okano and Tanji 1987). Premotor neurons also appear to be very sensitive to changes in the relationship between presented cues and expected responses (Mauritz and Wise 1986).

Interestingly, Mitz and collaborators (1991) found a significant number of premotor neurons changed activity in association with learning (the majority of neurons showed increased activity, though some decreased). The changes in activity typically occurred only after a visuomotor association had been learned, leading the authors to suggest different cortical regions may be functioning during distinct periods of the learning process. Using a variety of paradigms to manipulate stimulus-response associations, other investigators have also reported experience-dependent changes in premotor neuronal activity (Mauritz and Wise 1986; Mushiake, Inase, and Tanji 1991; Sasaki and Gemba 1982).

Unfortunately, only a few single-unit recording and stimulation studies have been reported for insular and opercular regions, largely because of their buried location within the Sylvian fissure. Neurons responsive to auditory and somasthetic stimulation have been reported in the posterior portions of the insula (Robinson and Burton 1980a; Robinson and Burton 1980b; Sudakov 1971), and electrical stimulation has been reported to produce skeletal movements (Hoffman and Rasmussen 1953; Showers and Lauer 1961).

Anterior cingulate.   The functions of the anterior cingulate have not been well studied, but the available information is consistent with the possibility that it may play an important role in selecting responses based on complex associations to a presented stimulus. Recent single-unit recording work in monkeys has shown greater activation for many anterior cingulate neurons when the animals are performing relatively complex sensory-motor tasks, compared to more simple conditions (Shima et al. 1991). Anatomical tract-tracing studies provide evidence that it has strong, reciprocal connections to a number of other cortical areas, including prefrontal and motor cortex, and the striatum (Goldman-Rakic 1987; Vogt and Pandya 1987).

Patients with large midline lesions including the SMA and anterior cingulate often develop akinetic mutism, a syndrome in which spontaneous speech is extremely rare (Barris and Schuman 1953; Masdeu, Schoene, and Funkenstein 1978; Nielsen and Jacobs 1951). Extensive evaluation of patient groups with more focal, psychosurgical anterior cingulate lesions have failed to detect any impairments across a range of motor and cognitive tasks, however (Ballantine et al. 1975; Corkin, Twitchell, and Sullivan 1979), though a recent single-case study suggested some subtle impairments can be detected (Janer 1991).

Prefrontal cortex. Goldman-Rakic (1988) has outlined an interpretation of prefrontal cortical function consistent with the PET evidence suggesting it is not active when responses can be based upon strong associations with the presented stimuli. She states, "It is my thesis that it is only when internalized or inner models of reality are used to govern behavior that prefrontal cortex is preeminently engaged." Similar interpretations have been made by others (e.g., Duncan 1992; Passingham 1985).

Goldman-Rakic draws on both her own single-unit recording work in macaques, as well as a body of behavioral investigations in both humans and primates with prefrontal lesions, to support her thesis. For instance, she points toward investigations in both patients and primates which demonstrate that damage to prefrontal areas produces impairments in the ability to hold a stimulus in memory (e.g., Chorover 1966; Jacobsen 1935; Mishkin and Manning 1978) or to perform complex stimulus transformations (Luria and Tsvetkova 1964; Shallice 1982).

Analysis of the types of errors made in the absence of normal prefrontal control provides additional, though indirect, information about the operation of a second system of response control. The PET evidence suggests that when activation is not observed in prefrontal regions, the produced responses are strongly associated with the presented stimuli. Abnormal prefrontal function might thus be predicted to result in more "habitual," and stimulus-driven behavior.

Analysis of both primates and humans with prefrontal lesions confirms this prediction. For instance, frontal patients are impaired at performing the Wisconsin card sorting task, in which subjects are required to form a sorting principle that is dependent on analysis of the color, number, or shape of items presented on each card. The sorting criteria is covertly changed periodically throughout the test, and subjects must attempt to discern the new principle, through trial and error. Frontal patients tend to repeatedly apply a previously correct sorting principle despite feedback that the principle is no longer correct (Milner 1963; Robinson et al. 1980). Similarly, monkeys performing a visual discrimination task have difficulty overcoming their preestablished preferences for a particular response (Brush, Mishkin, and Rosvold 1961; Meyer et al. 1964).

Another prediction would be that both patients and monkeys with prefrontal lesions should be able to perform well in routine, largely stimulus-driven situations. One of the clearest demonstrations of this preserved ability was reported by Luria and Tsvetkova (1964). They investigated the performance of a patient with an extensive right frontal lesion on a pattern construction task, in which the subject was given a geometrical pattern that had to be reproduced from a set of blocks. While the patient successfully performed constructions in which the actions could be determined by the perceived patterns, he failed when the perceived pattern had to be "decoded" into elements forming the basis of the reconstruction. This failure could be overcome, however, by providing a set of simple steps for "decoding" the pattern. Though not systematically investigated, several other investigators have commented on the preserved abilities of patients and monkeys to perform routine, well-learned tasks (e.g., Jacobsen 1935; Penfield and Evans 1935).

SUMMARY

Data from a survey study of language processing was analyzed using a new approach. Results from this reanalysis suggest the existence of two mutually inhibitory routes through which a word representation can be converted to a motor output representation: a Sylvian-insular and a frontal/cingulate pathway. When subjects are asked to repeat a word they use the Sylvian-insular pathway, and when they are required to generate an appropriate verb for a visually or auditorily presented noun they use the frontal/cingulate pathway. Sensory input and motor output areas appear to be used similarly for both verb generation and noun repetition.

A straightforward interpretation of these results is the following: when a response to a stimulus is overlearned (e.g., the naming of a presented word) the Sylvian-insular pathway is used; when this condition is not met further frontal analysis of the stimuli (through the frontal/cingulate pathway) occurs before a response is made.

This interpretation is consistent with previous suggestions that actions can be either controlled or automatic. It is also supported by data, from both PET and other disciplines, that the prefrontal cortex plays a central role in generating novel, unlearned, and non-associated responses to presented stimuli, while Sylvian-insular areas appear to be involved in high-level integration of sensory-motor processing and the guidance of movement on the basis of sensory cues.

ACKNOWLEDGEMENTS

This work was supported by NIH grants NS06833, EY08775, HL13851, the Charles A. Dana Foundation, and the McDonnell Center for the Study of Higher Brain Function. J. A. Fiez received additional support from the National Science Foundation and the Mr. and Mrs. Spencer T. Olin Program for Women.

REFERENCES

Arikuni, T., Watanabe, K., and Kubota, K. 1988. Connections of area 8 with area 6 in the brain of the macaque monkey. *Journal of Comparative Neurology* 227:21–40.

Ballantine, H. T., Levy, B. S., Dagi, T. F., and Giriunas, I. B. 1975. Cingulotomy for psychiatric illness: Report of 13 years' experience. In *Neurosurgical Treatment in Psychiatry, Pain, and Epilepsy*, ed. W. H. Sweet. Baltimore: University Park Press.

Barbas, H., and Pandya, D. N. 1987. Architecture and frontal cortical connections of the premotor cortex (area 6) in the rhesus monkey. *Journal of Comparative Neurology* 256:211–28.

Barris, R. W., and Schuman, H. R. 1953. Bilateral anterior cingulate gyrus lesions. *Neurology* 3:44–52.

Benson, D. F. 1979. *Aphasia, Alexia, and Agraphia.* New York: Churchill Livingstone.

Benson, D. F., Sheremata, W. A., Bouchard, R., Segarra, J. M., Price, D., and Geschwind, N. 1973. Conduction aphasia: A clinicopathological study. *Archives of Neurology* 28:339–46.

Bogousslavsky, J., Regli, F., and Assal, G. 1988. Acute transcortical mixed aphasia: A corotid occlusion syndrome with pial and watershed infarcts. *Brain* 111:631–41.

Brush, E. S., Mishkin, M., and Rosvold, H. E. 1961. Effects of object preferences and aversions on discrimination learning in monkeys with frontal lesions. *Journal of Comparative and Physiological Psychology* 54:319–25.

Caramazza, A., Basile, A. G., Koller, J. J., and Berndt, R. S. 1981. An investigation of repetition and language processing in a case of conduction aphasia. *Brain and Language* 14:235–71.

Chorover, S. L. 1966. Delayed alternation performance in patients with cerebral lesions. *Neuropsychologia* 4:1–7.

Corbetta, M., Miezin, F. M., Dobmeyer, S., Shulman, G. L., and Petersen, S. E. 1991. Selective and divided attention during visual discrimination of shape, color, and speed: Functional anatomy by positron emission tomography. *The Journal of Neuroscience* 11:2383–402.

Corkin, S., Twitchell, T. E., and Sullivan, E. V. 1979. Safety and efficacy of cingulotomy for pain and psychiatric disorder. In *Modern Concepts in Psychiatric Surgery*, eds. E. R. Hitchcock, H. T. Ballantine Jr., and B. A. Meyerson. New York: Elsevier/North Holland Biomedical Press.

Damasio, A. R. 1992. Aphasia. *New England Journal of Medicine* 326:531–39.

Damasio, H., and Damasio, A. R. 1980. The anatomical basis of conduction aphasia. *Brain* 103:337–50.

Donders, F. C. 1969. On the speed of mental processes. *Acta Psychologica* 30:412–31.

Duncan, J. 1992. Selection of input and goal in the control behaviour. In *Attention: Selection, Awareness, and Control: A Tribute to Donald Broadbent*, eds. A. Baddeley and L. Weiskrantz. Oxford: Oxford University Press.

Evarts, E. V., and Wise, S. P. 1984. Basal ganglia outputs and motor control. In *Functions of the Basal Ganglia Outputs. CIBA Foundation Symposium 107*, eds. D. Evered and M. O'Connor. London: Pitman.

Fiez, J. A., and Petersen, S. E. 1993. PET as part of an interdisciplinary approach to understanding processes involved in reading. *Psychological Science* 4:287–93.

Fiez, J. A., Petersen, S. E., Cheney, M. K., and Raichle, M. E. 1992. Impaired Non-motor Learning and Error Detection Associated with Cerebellar Damage: A Single-Case Study. *Brain* 115:155–78.

Ford, I., McColl, J. H., McCormack, A. G., and McCrory, S. J. 1991. Statistical issues in the analysis of neuroimages. *Journal of Cerebral Blood Flow and Metabolism* 11:A89–A95.

Fox, P. T., Miezin, F. M., Allman, J. M., Van Essen, D. C., and Raichle, M. E. 1987. Retinotopic organization of human visual cortex mapped with positron emission tomography. *Journal of Neuroscience* 7:913–22.

Fox, P. T., and Mintun, M. A. 1989. Noninvasive functional brain mapping by change-distribution analysis of averaged PET images of $H_2^{15}O$. *Journal of Nuclear Medicine* 30:141–49.

Fox, P. T., Mintun, M. A., Reiman, E. M., and Raichle, M. E. 1988. Enhanced detection of focal brain responses using intersubject averaging and change-distribution analysis of subtracted PET images. *Journal of Cerebral Blood Flow and Metabolism* 8:642–53.

Fox, P. T., Perlmutter, J. S., and Raichle, M. E. 1985. A stereotactic method of anatomical localization for positron emission tomography. *Journal of Computer Assisted Tomography* 9:141–53.

Friedman, D. P., Murray, E. A., O'Neill, J. B., and Mishkin, M. 1986. Cortical connections of the somatosensory fields of the lateral sulcus of macaques: Evidence for a corticolimbic pathway for touch. *Journal of Comparative Neurology* 252:323–47.

Friedrich, F. J., Glenn, C. G., and Marin, O. S. M. 1984. Interruption of phonological coding in conduction aphasia. *Brain and Language* 22:266–91.

Friston, K. J., Frith, C. D., Liddle, P. F., and Frackowiak, R. S. J. 1991. Comparing functional (PET) images: The assessment of significant change. *Journal of Cerebral Blood Flow and Metabolism* 11:690–99.

Frith, C. D., Friston, K., Liddle, P. F., and Frackowiak, R. S. J. 1991. Willed action and the prefrontal cortex in man: A study with PET. *Proceedings of the Royal Society of London, Series B-Biological Science* 244:241–46.

Geschwind, N. 1965. Disconnexion syndromes in animals and man, Part 1. *Brain* 88:237–94.

Geschwind, N., Quadfasel, F. A., and Segarra, J. M. 1968. Isolation of the speech area. *Neuropsychologia* 6:327–40.

Goldman-Rakic, P. S. 1987. Circuitry of primate prefrontal cortex and regulation of behavior by representational memory. In *The Handbook of Physiology. Section 1: The Nervous System, Volume V. Higher Functions of The Brain. Part 1*, eds. F. Plum and V. Mountcastle. Bethesda, MD: American Physiological Society.

Goldman-Rakic, P. S. 1988. Topography of cognition: Parallel distributed networks in primate association cortex. *Annual Review of Neuroscience* 11:137–56.

Goldstein, K. 1948. *Language and Language Disturbances: Aphasic Symptom Complexes and Their Significance for Medicine and Theory of Language*. New York: Grune and Stratton.

Goodglass, H., and Kaplan, E. 1983. *The Assessment of Aphasia and Related Disorders* (2nd edition). Philadelphia: Lea and Febiger.

Green, D. M., and Swets, J. A. 1966. *Signal Detection Theory and Psychophysics*. New York: Wiley.

Greenwald, A. G., and Johnson, M. M. S. 1989. The generation effect extended: Memory enhancement for generation cues. *Memory and Cognition* 17:673–81.

Haxby, J. V., Grady, C. L., Ungerleider, L. G., and Horwitz, B. 1991. Mapping the functional neuroanatomy of the intact human brain with brain work imaging. *Neuropsychologia* 29:539–55.

Herscovitch, P., Markham, J., and Raichle, M. E. 1983. Brain blood flow measured with intravenous $H_2^{15}O$. I. Theory and error analysis. *Journal of Nuclear Medicine* 24:782–89.

Hoffman, B. L., and Rasmussen, T. 1953. Stimulation studies of insular cortex of the *macaca mulatta*. *Journal of Neurophysiology* 16:343–51.

Hunton, D. L., Miezin, F. M., Buckner, R. L., Raichle, M. E., and Petersen, S. E. 1994. An assessment of replicability and anatomical variability in functional neuroimaging studies. *Society for Neuroscience Abstracts* 20:354.

Jacobsen, C. F. 1935. Functions of frontal association area in primates. *Archives of Neurology and Psychiatry* 33:558–69.

James, W. 1890. *Principles of Psychology, Vol. 2.* New York: Henry-Holt and Co.

Janer, K. W. 1991. Deficits in selective attention following bilateral anterior cingulotomy. *Journal of Cognitive Neuroscience* 3:231–41.

Johns, E. E., and Swanson, L. G. 1988. The generation effect with nonwords. *Journal of Experimental Psychology: Learning, Memory, and Cognition* 14:180–90.

Kinsbourne, M. 1972. Behavioral analysis of the repetition deficit in conduction aphasia. *Neurology* 22:1126–32.

Kulpe, O. 1909. The Analysis of Compound Reactions. In *Outlines of Psychology*, ed. E. Bradford-Tichener. New York: MacMillan Co.

Kurata, K. 1991. Corticocortical inputs to the dorsal and ventral aspects of the premotor cortex of macaque monkeys. *Neuroscience Research* 12:263–80.

Lichtheim, L. 1885. On aphasia. *Brain* 7:433–84.

Luria, A. R., and Tsvetkova, L. S. 1964. The programming of constructive activity in local brain injuries. *Neuropsychologia* 2:95–107.

Masdeu, J. C., Schoene, W. C., and Funkenstein, H. 1978. Aphasia following infarction of the left supplementary motor area. *Neurology* 28:1220–23.

Matelli, M., Camarda, R., Glickstein, M., and Rizzolatti, G. 1986. Afferent and efferent projections of the inferior area 6 in the macaque monkey. *Journal of Comparative Neurology* 251:281–98.

Mauritz, K.-H., and Wise, S. P. 1986. Premotor cortex of the rhesus monkey: Neuronal activity in anticipation of predictable environmental events. *Experimental Brain Research* 61:229–44.

McCarthy, R., and Warrington, E. K. (1984). A two-route model of speech production: Evidence from aphasia. *Brain* 107:463–85.

McElroy, L. A. 1987. The generation effect with homographs: Evidence for postgeneration processing. *Memory and Cognition* 15:148–53.

Mesulam, M.-M., and Mufson, E. J. 1985. The Insula of Reil in man and monkey: Architectonics, connectivity, and function. In *Cerebral Cortex*, eds. A. Peters and E. G. Jones. New York: Plenum Press.

Meyer, D. R., Treichler, F. R., Yutzey, D. A., and Meyer, P. M. 1964. Precedence effects in discrimination learning by normal and frontal monkeys. *Journal of Comparative and Physiological Psychology* 58:472–74.

Miller, G. A., Galanter, E., and Pribram, K. H. 1960. *Plans and the Structure of Behavior*. New York: Henry Holt and Company.

Milner, B. 1963. Effects of different brain lesions on card sorting. *Archives of Neurology* 9:100–10.

Mishkin, M., and Manning, F. J. 1978. Non-spatial memory after selective prefrontal lesions in monkeys. *Brain Research* 143:313–23.

Mitz, A. R., Godschalk, M., and Wise, S. P. 1991. Learning-dependent neuronal activity in the premotor cortex: activity during the acquisition of conditional motor associations. *Journal of Neuroscience* 11:1855–72.

Mushiake, H., Inase, M., and Tanji, J. 1991. Neuronal activity in the primate pre-motor, supplementary and precentral motor cortex during visually guided and internally determined sequential movements. *Journal of Neurophysiology* 66:705–18.

Nielsen, J. M., and Jacobs, L. L. 1951. Bilateral lesions of the anterior cingulate gyri. *Bulletin of the Los Angeles Neurological Society* 16:231–34.

Norman, D. A., and Shallice, T. 1985. Attention to action: Willed and automatic control of behavior. In *Consciousness and Self-regulation*. New York: Plenum Press.

Okano, K., and Tanji, J. 1987. Neuronal activities in the primate motor fields of the agranular frontal cortex preceding visually triggered and self-paced movement. *Experimental Brain Research* 66:155–66.

Pandya, D. M. 1969. Intra- and interhemispheric connections of the neocortical auditory system in the rhesus monkey. *Brain Research* 14:49–65.

Pardo, J. V., Pardo, P. J., Janer, K. W., and Raichle, M. E. 1990. The anterior cin-gulate cortex mediates processing selection in the Stroop attentional conflict paradigm. *Proceedings of the National Academy of Science USA* 87:256–59.

Passingham, R. E. 1985. Cortical mechanisms and cues for action. *Philosophical Transactions of the Royal Society of London B*, 308:101–11.

Payne, D. G., Neely, J. H., and Burns, D. J. 1986. The generation effect: Further tests of the lexical activation hypothesis. *Memory and Cognition* 14:246–52.

Penfield, W., and Evans, J. 1935. The frontal lobe in man: A clinical study of maximum removals. *Brain* 58:115–33.

Petersen, S. E., Fox, P. T., Posner, M. I., Mintun, M., and Raichle, M. E. 1988. Positron emission tomographic studies of the cortical anatomy of single-word processing. *Nature* 331:585–89.

Petersen, S. E., Fox, P. T., Posner, M. I., Mintun, M., and Raichle, M. E. 1989. Positron emission tomographic studies of the processing of single words. *Journal of Cognitive Neuroscience* 1:153–70.

Posner, M. I., Petersen, S. E., Fox, P. T., and Raichle, M. E. 1988. Localization of cognitive functions in the human brain. *Science* 240:1627–31.

Raichle, M. E. 1989. Developing a functional anatomy of the human brain with positron emission tomography. *Current Neurology* 9:161–78.

Raichle, M. E., Fiez, J. A., Videen, T. O., MacLeod, A. K., Pardo, J. V., Fox, P. T., and Petersen, S. E. 1994. Practice-related changes in human brain functional anatomy during non-motor learning. *Cerebral Cortex* 4:8–26.

Reason, J., and Mycielska, K. 1982. *Absent-minded? The Psychology of Mental Lapses and Everyday Errors*. Englewood Cliffs, NJ: Prentice-Hall, Inc.

Rizzolatti, G., Matelli, M., and Pavesi, G. 1983. Deficits in attention and move-ment following the removal of postarcuate (area 6) and prearcuate (area 8) cortex in macaque monkeys. *Brain* 106:655–73.

Robinson, A. L., Heaton, R. K., Lehman, R. A. W., and Stilson, D. W. 1980). The utility of the Wisconsin Card Sorting Test in detecting and localizing frontal lobe lesions. *Journal of Consulting and Clinical Psychology* 48:605–14.

Robinson, C. J., and Burton, H. 1980a. Organization of somatosensory receptive fields in cortical areas 7b, retroinsula, postauditory, and Granular Insula of M. fascicularis. *Journal of Comparative Neurology* 192:69–92.

Robinson, C. J., and Burton, H. 1980b. Somatic submodality distribution within the second somatosensory (s11), 7b, retroinsular, postauditory, and Granular

Insular cortical areas of M. fascicularis. *Journal of Comparative Neurology* 192:93–108.

Sanides, F. 1968. The architecture of the cortical taste nerve areas in squirrel monkey (Saimiri Sciureus) and their reslationships to insular, sensorimotor, and prefrontal regions. *Brain Research* 8:97–124.

Sasaki, K., and Gemba, H. 1982. Development and change of cortical field potentials during learning processes of visually initiated hand movements in the monkey. *Experimental Brain Research* 48:429–37.

Shallice, T. 1982. Specific impairments of planning. *Philosophical Transactions of the Royal Society of London. B.* 298:199–209.

Shima, K., Aya, K., Mushiake, H., Inase, M., Aizawa, H., and Tanji, J. 1991. Two movement-related foci in the primate cingulate cortex observed in signal-triggered and self-paced forelimb movements. *Journal of Neurophysiology* 65:188–202.

Showers, M. J. C., and Lauer, E. W. 1961. Somatovisceral motor patterns in the insula. *Journal of Comparative Neurology* 117:107–15.

Slamecka, N. J., and Graf, P. 1978. The generation effect: Delineation of a phenomenon. *Journal of Experimental Psychology: Human Learning and Memory* 4:592–604.

Sternberg, S. 1969. The discovery of processing stages: Extensions of Donders' method. *Acta Psychologia* 30:276–315.

Strub, R. L., and Gardner, H. 1974. The repetition defect in conduction aphasia: Mnestic or linguistic? *Brain and Language* 1:241–55.

Stytz, M. R., and Frieder, O. 1990. Three-dimensional medical imaging modalities: An overview. *Critical Reviews in Biomedical Engineering* 18:1–25.

Sudakov, K. 1971. Unit study of exteroceptive inputs to claustrocortex in awake, sitting squirrel monkey. *Brain Research* 28:19–34.

Talairach, J., and Tournoux, P. 1988. *Co-Planar Stereotaxic Atlas of the Human Brain* (Rayport, Mark, Trans.). New York: Thieme Medical Publishers, Inc.

Vogt, B. A., and Pandya, D. N. 1987. Cingulate cortex of the rhesus monkey: II. Cortical afferents. *Journal of Comparative Neurology* 262:271–89.

Warrington, E. K., and Shallice, T. 1969. The selective impairment of auditory verbal short-term memory. *Brain* 92:885–96.

Worsley, K. J., Evans, A. C., Marrett, S., and Neelin, P. 1992. A three dimensional statistical analysis for CBF activation studies in human brain. *Journal of Cerebral Blood Flow and Metabolism* 12:900–18.

Chapter • 11

Neuromagnetic Assessment of Human Cortical Function

Barry Schwartz
Christopher C. Gallen

FUNCTIONAL IMAGING FOR COGNITIVE DEFICITS

For many common disorders of brain function, the diagnosis, determination of mechanism, and assessment of treatment response are based quite often on indirect complex behavioral observations, that are often complicated by ambiguities introduced by subjective and motivational factors. The diagnosis and understanding of such neurological and psychological disorders has awaited the development of tools to map areas of neural function and dysfunction. These disorders include epilepsy, the dementias, head injury, transient ischemic attacks, early stroke, the major psychotic disorders, and the learning and attention disorders.

Cognitive deficits such as dyslexia may well have a variety of genetic, developmental or environmental causes, including, for example, cases involving neuronal migration disorder (Tallal 1991; Galaburda and Kemper 1979). A delay of maturation of some functional neural circuitry may not appear as an imageable structural abnormality on MRI scans, but may well leave clues in the form of sensory and perceptual deficits correlative of aphasia (Geschwind and Behan 1982; Tallal, Stark, and Mellits 1985). Psychophysical deficits that are indicators of dyslexia may well represent tens of milliseconds of activity moving among localized functional centers each occupying only a few cubic millimeters of cortex.

Diagnostic instruments capable of direct, objective assessment and localization and sequencing of functional flows of neural activity would be a boon to studying the mechanisms of dyslexia, as well as to neuro-psychology at large. Such technologies would permit more rigorous testing of models of brain function, more discrete differential diagnostic assessment of functional disorders, more targeted guidance of treatment, and direct assessment of pharmacological response. Clinically relevant brain information processing activities can involve fluctuations of brain activity over a millisecond of time. Distinct brain functional regions can be separated by distances as small as several millimeters. Different functional processing centers may be activated sequentially or with temporal overlap. Some of the clinical disorders producing cognitive dysfunction such as stroke, cerebral lupus, and atherosclerotic processes, can alter blood supply in regions other than those responsible for the clinical symptoms observed. Other diseases of brain dysfunction can involve treatment with pharmacological agents that alter metabolism and/or blood flow more widely than in the dysfunctional area alone.

DIRECT, ELECTROCLINICAL MEASUREMENT OF NEURAL ACTIVITY

Central nervous system activity is predicated on the electrical transmission of signals down nerve membranes to synaptic connections for subsequent chemical transmission. Changes in membrane permeability produce graded alterations of the resting potential, post-synaptic potentials (PSPs) generating a directional electrical vector in the elongated pyramidal cells. The relatively prolonged duration of PSPs in the long, closely packed palisades of cortical pyramidal cells produce multiple parallel and synchronous electrical vectors. When viewed from the distance of subdural or extracranial detectors, these minute vectors summate in time and space to produce a larger net vector generating an electrical field detectable outside the head. These field fluctuations are recorded and used clinically in direct records through leptomeningeal structures (electrocorticography, ECoG), indirectly through placement of electrodes on the scalp (electroencephalography, EEG) or through recordings of the extracranial magnetic field. Fluctuations of this field reflect brain functional activity changes over the timeframe of milliseconds.

Localization of electrical sources using ECoG measurements has been particularly useful clinically since direct recordings provide accurate localization information at least for superficial sources, but are restricted severely in application because of the invasiveness of this procedure. EEG has been widely applied to the task of characterization of brain functional activity, but the localization of sources is complex. The electrical field of the brain is highly distorted and spatially filtered in passing through conductively inhomogeneous layers including cerebrospinal fluid, skull, and scalp. Effective source localization requires complex computations to correct for this distortion and even then the

models used are imperfect, failing to account for significant local variations in skull thickness and conductive breeches resulting from suture
lines or skull orifices. Moreover, the resistance of the skull is about 80-
fold greater than the impedance of the other conductive layers, a ratio
similar to the ratio of skull thickness to head circumference with the
result that an electrode pair placed at any location on the head picks up
the field from all the sources in the head, greatly increasing the number
of possible source regions any localization model must account for.

Magnetoencephalography (MEG) is well suited to detect the rapidly fluctuating, graded changes occurring in long, closely packed palisades of cortical pyramidal cells that produce post-synaptic potentials
(PSP) lasting 10–250 msec. With signal averaging, evoked fields can be
detected outside the head and, in several important clinical applications,
can be modeled as single dipole sources reflecting the intracellular current flow associated with specific sensory events (Williamson and
Kaufman 1987). Precision is aided by the fact that the neuromagnetic
signal passes through brain, cerebrospinal fluid, skull, and scalp undistorted and unattenuated. Since the magnetic field is perpendicular to the
direction of current flow, MEG preferentially detects sources oriented
tangential to the skull surface. Thus far, measurements have been de-
vised to detect a source localizable as a single equivalent current dipole,
although this constraint is surely a temporary one, given the ongoing
development of methods to model multiple dipoles and sources due to
extended areas of cortex (Ioannides et al. 1994).

MEG METHODS FOR MEASURING HUMAN
CORTICAL ACTIVITY

Localization of neuromagnetic sources is an easier task than localization
of electrical signals in several important respects. The MEG signal is
less distorted and simpler to analyze than the EEG signal, facilitating
noninvasive source localization. The brain, cerebrospinal fluid, skull,
and scalp all have nearly the same relative magnetic permeabilities (of
unity) and consequently the neuromagnetic signal passes through these
layers relatively undistorted and unattenuated. Moreover, since magnetic field strength falls off with the inverse square of distance, the
effects of neighboring sources on the activity detected at a particular
locale is diminished. Since the magnetic field is perpendicular to the
direction of current flow, extracranial detectors preferentially detect
sources to the extent that they are oriented on a tangent to a line radiat-
ing from the center of the skull (essentially preferentially seeing sources
oriented parallel to the skull surface). This combination of lack of field
distortion in passage, the attenuation of complicating fields from more
distant sources, the simplified array of sources viewed (by preferentially seeing tangential sources), and the fact that magnetic measure-

ments are not dependent on external referents, all facilitate the use of neuromagnetic fields for source localization. The electromagnetic theory underlying magnetic measurements, shielding, and calculations has been reviewed elsewhere (Okada 1986; Kaufman and Williamson 1986). One important practical problem arises from the fact that the human cerebral magnetic field is exceedingly small, on the order of 50–250 femoTesla (fT, 10^{-15} Tesla). Recordings of this field must occur in the context of substantial noise including the earth (70×10^9 fT), the surrounding laboratory and urban environment (10^{14} fT) and nearby MRI scanners (1.5×10^{15} fT). The small signal and huge noise currently requires very sensitive superconducting quantum interference device based detectors (SQUID) and an extensive magnetically shielded room (MSR) contributing greatly to the price of this technology.

The neuromagnetic field pattern used in the studies described below used a Magnes® Biomagnetometer (Biomagnetic Technologies, Inc.). The 37 detector channels are arrayed in a series of three concentric circles around a central detector. The array diameter is 144 mm. Intrinsic noise in each channel is <10fT/√Hz. The probe is typically placed over a location assessed as relevant to the signal of interest, and may be moved after initial recordings to the most optimal location. The more recent development of dual detector 74 channel arrays allowing bilateral recording of brain magnetic activity allows characterization of brain activities involving bilateral cortical activation. A radio frequency locator system was used to measure the position of the biomagnetometer relative to the patient's head, referring to standard fiduciary points on the skin (left and right preauricular points and nasion). MEG functional localizations are calculated in a three dimensional coordinate system based on extracranial fiducial markers. The combination of MRI anatomical information with magnetoencephalographic (MEG) functional information in a single image is referred to as Magnetic Source Imaging (MSI). MRI scans were obtained in the axial, sagittal, and coronal planes using a GE 1.5T Signa® scanner, with markers to show the auricular points and nasion included on the scans to provide a common frame of reference to MEG. In some cases, three dimensional MRI acquisitions can be combined with three dimensional magnetic resonance angiograms to allow creation of a three dimensional image of the head and blood vessels on to which the functional localizations can be projected. Such three dimensional images are particularly relevant to the problem of relating functional brain maps to the brain surface as visualized in the operating room.

SOMATOSENSORY EVOKED FIELD MEASUREMENTS: MEASURING CORTICAL PLASTICITY

The concept of functional plasticity is likely to be germane to the development of models of compensatory processing related to developmental lags such as those associated with dyslexia.

The concept of neuromagnetic mapping of functional brain areas was demonstrated in careful and laborious studies using an earlier generation of biomagnetometers (Sutherling et al. 1988). Modern instruments with large detector arrays markedly reduce the time of data acquisition and minimize errors in the relative localization of detectors. A clinical somatosensory MSI protocol has been developed and used to aid in planning surgeries for tumors, AVMs, and epilepsy (figures 1–3). The precise mapping of functional areas of somatosensory and motor cortex has aided neurosurgeons in localizing functional areas independent of distortions due to mass effects of tumors or edema prior to surgery (Sobal et al. 1993; Gallen et al. 1993; Gallen et al. in press).

Somatosensory evoked fields were obtained by averaging a series of 256 to 1024 repetitions at a 2/sec rate. A pneumatically driven tactile stimulator applied a brief (30 msec) pulse of pressure to the thumb and to the index finger on the hand contralateral to the measured hemi-

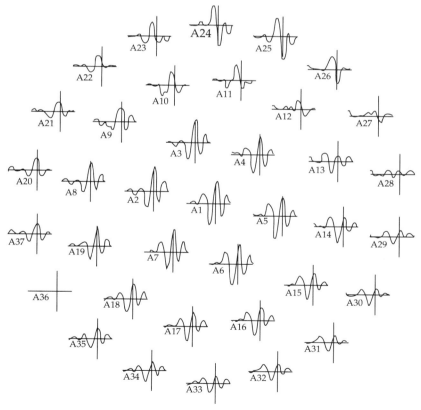

Figure 1. Waveforms for one somatosensory evoked field displayed on an array depicting the sensor coil geometry. Each waveform spans 200 msec. The vertical axis indicates magnetic field strength expressed in femtoteslas (fT).

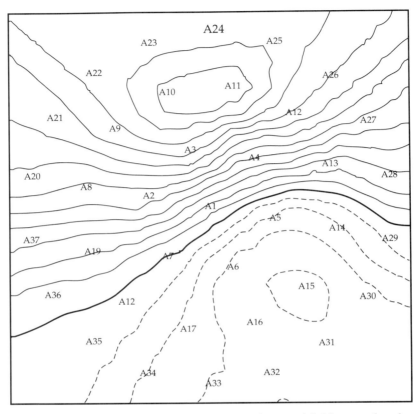

Figure 2. Isocontour plot representing interpolation of field strength values over the 37 detectors at the 68 msec latency following the pneumatic stimulus on the subject's hand. The pattern is consistent with a source midway between the minimum and maximum, at some depth below the detector proportional to the distance between the minimum and maximum.

sphere, or to the lower lip (Schwartz et al 1992). The somatosensory component peaking in the 45–75 msec latency range was identified by reversals of polarity in subsets of the 37 channels. This component has been localized to somatosensory cortex in prior studies comparing electrical and mechanical stimulation (Starr 1981). The 45–75 msec somatosensory ECD observed in these MSI studies has been reported previously, and is known to correspond to primary sensory cortex (S1) and to overlap the source of the N19/P21 electrical evoked response (Hari and Kaukoranta 1985; Hari et al. 1984). The precision of these somatosensory source localizations was assessed with a set of 80 repeated somatosensory measures taken for a single stimulus site on one volunteer subject. Localizations were found to have a point-to-point standard deviation of 5.8 mm, with all localizations falling in the S1 area, posterior to the central sulcus (Gallen et al. 1994). High resolu-

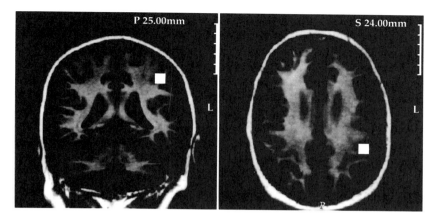

Figure 3. MSI (Magnetic source image): equivalent current dipole solution overlaid on MR slices. The somatosensory source is indicated as a white square. The location of the central sulcus can be seen anterior to the somatosensory source symbol.

tion spatial maps of the homunculus of normal subjects were made with numerous bilateral tactile stimulation sites, demonstrating the ability of MSI to map distinct separations of somatosensory sources from sites on the face, arm, and hand (Yang et al. 1993). The spatial precision of the MSI somatosensory localizations allowed the first observation of cortical plasticity due to deafferentiation in human patients, corresponding to prior research conducted on animals. An experiment was conducted with four patients who had suffered accidental amputation of one arm showing, for the first time in humans a large expansion of the regions associated with shoulder and face into the area abandoned by the missing hand. Comparisons of the abnormal hemisphere with the normal hemisphere showed displacements of up to 35 mm. These displacements were correlated with the psychophysical phenomena of a phantom limb mapped out on the areas of the face and the upper arm or shoulder whose cortical representations were adjacent to that of the hand and lower arm that had been lost (Yang et al. 1994; Ramachandran 1993; Yang et al. 1994b). The possibility can be raised that, with reversible deafferentiation and hyperstimulation, cortical plasticity in normal subjects can be assayed for the primary somatosensory regions, and perhaps the motor regions as well.

AUDITORY EVOKED FIELD MEASUREMENTS: SPATIAL AND TEMPORAL RESOLUTION

Experiments with the perception of simple tones have been employed in the development of MSI as an assay of auditory cortical function.

Pioneering experiments with single channel biomagnetometers showed that a tonotopic map could be made for humans (Romani, Williamson, and Kaufman 1982; Pantev et al. 1988). A study with a large array biomagnetometer localized the evoked auditory responses to primary auditory cortex in the transverse temporal gyrus of Heschl. With 30 repeated measures on the same subject, two separate "components" were found at 93 and 172 msec, the so-called M100 and M200 responses, which were reproducible with standard deviations in each axis of 2 mm and 3 mm respectively. The two components localized to sites separated by 8 mm within the primary auditory cortex in Heschl's gyrus (Pantev et al. 1991).

MEG MAPPING OF SOURCES OF RHYTHMIC ACTIVITY

The clinical use of MSI to detect spontaneous events has focused on abnormal events, such as focal slowing associated with mass lesions (Vieth et al. 1990; Gallen et al. 1993) and inter-ictal spikes associated with epilepsy (Eisenberg et al. 1991; Sutherling et al. 1987; Paetau et al. 1994). Measurements of normal rhythmic cortical activity promise to supply new tools for the analysis of functional cortical events associated with cognitive processes and cognitive deficits.

The presence of a 40 Hz response following sensory stimulation has been hypothesized to mediate the coordination of spatially separated sensory activity centers in the brain (Singer et al. 1990). Studies of evoked responses with auditory tones were extended in a series of experiments that also found a 40 Hz response superimposed on the auditory components during the interval from 20 msec to 130 msec (Ribary 1991). The sequential peaks of the 40 Hz oscillation were localized on a trajectory of sites spanning the 93 msec and 172 msec locations, i.e., within primary auditory cortex (Pantev et al. 1991). The spatial and temporal precision attainable with MSI makes it possible to look selectively at different frequency ranges and thereby identify and localize such relatively low amplitude signals associated with cognitive processing.

In studies of auditory selective attention, it was found that responses to tones in the attended ear evoked larger magnetic responses than did unattended tones in the 50 msec and 100 msec latency ranges. An attentional "difference wave" formed by subtracting the unattended from the attended responses could be fit with a single dipole model and overlaid on MRI to within a few millimeters of the primary auditory locations, suggesting that the activity of primary auditory cortex can be modulated by effects of attention (Woldorff et al. 1993; Hari and Mäkelä 1987).

These and similar results exploiting the spatial and temporal resolution of MSI point the way to experiments on cognitive processes that may distinguish between normals and subjects with developmental lags in sensory processing, or deficits in attention or memory due to disease processes or injury.

Stimulus related changes in rhythmic activity can be observed with changes of attention triggered by light or sound. A marked decrease in amplitude of alpha band (8–13 Hz) activity has long been noted in attention and sensory processing as measured with EEG (Niedermeyer 1993). Occurrence of spindles of alpha activity are reduced markedly and suddenly with visual stimulation. Neuromagnetic mapping of this visual alpha reactivity (VAR) revealed the strongest changes in occipital and parietal areas, consistent with the suppression of multiple, non-synchronous local generators (Gallen et al. 1989; Chapman et al. 1984; Salmelin and Hari 1994).

Alpha reactivity was mapped with MEG in a visual matching task that required the observer to hold in memory a set of shapes against which a target would be judged (Kaufman et al. 1990). Identical stimulus sequences were used with two tasks: a simple reaction time task and a task requiring the subject to identify whether a target stimulus matched one or three recently presented irregular polygon figures. In reaction to the stimulus without the memory task involved, alpha activity decreased markedly within 150 msec and returned quickly (within 500 msec). But in the memory task with the same stimuli, alpha remained suppressed for an average of 1.5 seconds, equal in time to the subjects' latency to press a button to indicate whether the target had matched one of the to-be-remembered sets. The result suggests that visual alpha reactivity indexes a cognitive process involved in visual memory search, and not just attention to the original visual stimulus. Moreover, since the reactivity was strongest over occipital and posterior parietal areas, it suggests that the same areas of cortex involved in the processing of primary sensory visual information, as revealed by evoked responses, also contribute directly to specific cognitive functions, as indexed by changes in rhythmic activity. Indeed these changes may, like their 40 Hz counterparts, indicate a coordination of activities between neocortex and thalamic or limbic areas.

The limitations of the single-dipole-per-time approach loom large in these attempts to characterize rhythmic activity. However, whole head systems and new developments in the modeling of multiple sources (Salmelin and Hari 1994), as well as in the modeling of extended sources, are being brought into play with regard to these problems.

CONCLUSIONS

Magnetic Source Imaging is becoming a valuable addition to the methods of functional imaging employed in the exploration of mechanisms of human cortical function and dysfunction. Its unique combination of spatial and temporal resolution makes it suitable for the direct measurement and localization of neural activity. Innovative studies of cognitive processes and other functions measured by PET and fMRI (Kwong et al.

1992) may well provide guidelines for the next generation of studies using MSI. The advantage of these imaging methods over MSI lies in their capacity to detect activity in central regions of the brain, regardless of the geometry or orientation of the area involved. However, PET, SPECT, and functional MRI measure changes in blood chemistry or metabolism, which are necessarily slower in response than the locally summed post-synaptic potentials measured with MEG or EEG. Possibly these limitations would become even more profound with higher cognitive testing, let alone more subtle cognitive events. The need is evident to add functional methods able to resolve sources separated by milliseconds in time or millimeters in space, which underlie sequences of cognitive processes. Mapping the dynamics of these sequences may well serve to distinguish normal from abnormal cortical cognitive processing.

ACKNOWLEDGEMENTS

This work was supported by the Armstrong McDonald Foundation, the McDonnel-PEW Foundation, the Pasarow Foundation, and by a cooperative agreement with Biomagnetic Technologies, Inc.

REFERENCES

Chapman, R. M., Ilmoniemi, R., Barbanera S., and Romani, G. L. 1984. Selective localization of the alpha frequency activity in human subjects. *Society for Neuroscience Abstracts* 15(1):121.

Eisenberg, H. M., Papanicolaou, A. C. et al. 1991. Magnetoencephalographic localization of inter-ictal spike sources: Case report. *Journal of Neurosurgery* 74:660–64.

Galaburda, A. M., and Kemper, T. M. 1979. Cytoarchitectonic abnormalities in developmental dyslexia: A case study. *Annals of Neurology* 6:94–100.

Gallen, C. C., Schwartz, B. J., Bucholz, R., Malik G., Barkley, G. L., Smith J., Tung, H., Copeland, B., Bruno, L., Assam, S., Hirschkoff, E., and Bloom, F. 1995. Presurgical localization of functional cortex using magnetic source imaging. *Journal of Neurosurgery* 82:988–94.

Gallen, C. C., Schwartz, B. J., Rieke, K., Pantev, C., Sobel, D., Hirschkoff, E., and Bloom, F. E. 1994. Intrasubject reliability and validity of somatosensory source localization using a large array biomagnetometer. *Journal of Electroencephalography and Clinical Neurophysiology* 90(2):145–56.

Gallen, C. C., Sobel, D. F., Waltz, T., Aung, M., Copeland, B., Schwartz, B. J., Hirschkoff, E. C., and Bloom, F. E. 1993. Noninvasive pre-surgical neuromagnetic mapping of somatosensory cortex. *Neurosurgery* 33(2):260–68.

Gallen, C. C., Hampson, S., Young, W., and Bloom, F. E. 1989. Reactivity of neuromagnetic alpha frequency activity in human subjects. *Society for Neuroscience Abstracts* 15(1):121.

Geschwind, N., and Behan, P. O. 1982. Left-handedness: Association with immune disease, migraine and developmental learning disorders. *Proceedings of the National Academy of Sciences USA* 79:5097–5100.

Hari, R., and Kaukoranta, E. 1985. Neuromagnetic studies of somatosensory system: Principles and examples. *Progress in Neurobiology* 24:233–56.

Hari, R., and Makela, J. P. 1987. Evidence for cortical origin of the 40 Hz auditory evoked response in man. *Electroencephalography and Clinical Neurophysiology* 66:539–46.

Hari, R., Reinikainen, K., Kaukoranta, E., Hamalainen, M., Ilmoniemi, R., Penttinen, A., Salminen, J., and Teszner, D. 1984. Somatosensory evoked cerebral magnetic fields from Sl and Sll in man. *Electroencephalography and Clinical Neurophysiology* 57:254–63.

Ioannides, A. A., Fenwick, P. B. C., Lumsden, J., Liu, M. J., Bamidis, P. D., Squires, K. C., Lawson, D., and Fenton, G. W. 1994. Activation sequence of discrete brain areas during cognitive processes: Results from magnetic field tomography (Short communication). *Electroencephalography and Clinical Neurophysiology* 91:399–402.

Kaufman, L., Schwartz, B., Salustri, C., and Williamson, S. J. 1990. Modulation of spontaneous brain activity during mental imagery. *Journal of Cognitive Neuroscience* 2(2):124–32.

Kaufman, L., and Williamson, S. J. 1986. The neuromagnetic field. In *Evoked Potentials: Frontiers of Clinical Science*, eds. R. Q. Cracco and I. Bodis-Wolner. New York: Alan R. Liss.

Kwong, K. K., Belliveau, J. W., Chesler, D. A., Goldberg, I. E., Weisskoff, R. M., Poncelet, B. P., Kennedy, D. N., Hoppel, B. E., Cohen, M. S., Turner, R., et al. 1992. Dynamic magnetic resonance imaging of human brain activity during primary sensory stimulation. *Proceedings of the National Academy of Sciences* 89(12):5675–9.

Niedermeyer, E. 1993. The normal EEG of the waking adult. In *Electroencephalography. Basic Principles. Clinical Applications and Related Fields*, eds. E. Niedermeyer and F. Lopes da Silva. Baltimore: Williams and Wilkins.

Okada, Y. 1986. Physiological basis of magnetoencephalography. *Biomedical Engineering* 14:84.

Paetau, R., Hamalainen, R., Hari, R., Kajola, M., Karhu, J., Larsen, T. A., Lindahl, E., and Salonen, O. 1994. Magnetoencephalographic evaluation of children and adolescents with intractable epilepsy. *Epilepsi* 35(2):275–84.

Pantev, C., Gallen, C., Hampson, S., Buchanan, S., and Sobel, D. 1991. Reproducibility and validity of neuromagnetic source localization using a large array biomagnetometer. *American Journal of EEG Technology* 31:83:101.

Pantev, C., Lehnertz, K., Lutkenhoner, B., Anogianakis, G., and Wittkowski, W. 1988. Tonomotpic organization of the human auditory cortex revealed by transient auditory evoked magnetic fields. *Electroencephalography and Clinical Neurophysiology* 69:160–70.

Pantev, C., Makeig, S., Hoke, M., Galambos, R., Hampson, S., and Gallen, C. 1991. Human auditory evoked gamma-band magnetic fields. *Proceedings of the National Academy of Sciences* 88:8996–9000.

Pratt, H., and Starr, A. 1981. Mechanically and electrically evoked somatosensory potentials in humans: Scalp and neck distributions of short latency components. *Electroencephalography and Clinical Neurophysiology* 51:138–47.

Ramachandran, V. S. 1993. Behavioral and magnetoencephalographic correlates of plasticity in the adult human brain. *Proceedings of the National Academy of Sciences USA* 90:10413–20.

Ribary, U., Ioannides, A. A., Singh, K. D., Hasson, R., Bolton, J. P. R., Lado, F., Mogliner, A., and Llinas, R. 1991. Magnetic field tomography (MFT) of coherent thalamo-cortical 40 Hz oscillations in humans. *Proceedings of the National Academy of Sciences* 88:8996–9000.

Romani, G. L., Williamson, S. J., and Kaufman, L. 1982. Tonotopic organization of the human auditory cortex. *Science* 216:1339–40.

Salmelin, R., and Hari, R. 1994. Characterization of spontaneous MEG rhythms in healthy adults. *Electroencephalography and Clinical Neurophysiology* 91:237–48.

Schwartz, B. J., Gallen, C. C., Hampson, S., Hirschkoff, E. C., Sobel, D. F., and Rieke, K. 1992. Reliability of somatosensory neuromagnetic source localizations using a multisensor biomagnetometer. In *Biomagnetism: Clinical Aspects, Proceedings of the 8th International Conference on Biomagnetism*, eds. M. Hoke, S. N. Erne, Y. Okada, and G. L. Romani. Amsterdam: Elsevier Science Publishers.

Singer, W., Gray, C. M., Engel, A., Konig, P., Artola, A., and Brocher, S. 1990. Formation of cortical cell assemblies. *Cold Spring Harbor Symposia on Quantitative Biology* 55:939–53.

Sobel, D. F., Gallen, C. C., Schwartz, B. J., Waltz, T. A., Copeland, B., Yamada, S., Hirschkoff, E. C., and Bloom, F. E. 1993. Locating the central sulcus: Comparison of MR anatomic and magnetoencephalographic functional methods. *American Journal of Neuroradiology* 14:915–25.

Sutherling, W. W., Crandall, P. H., et al. 1987. The magnetic field of complex partial seizures agrees with intracranial localizations. *Annals of Neurology* 21:548–58.

Sutherling, W. W., Crandall, P. H., Darcey, T. M., Becker, D. P., Levesque, M. F., and Barth, D. S. 1988. The magnetic and electric fields agree with intracranial localizations of somatosensory cortex. *Neurology* 38:1705–14.

Tallal, P. 1991. Hormonal influences in developmental learning disabilities. *Psychoneuroendocrinology* 16:203–11.

Tallal, P., Stark, R. E., and Mellits, E. D. 1985. Identification of language-impaired children on the basis of rapid perception and production skills. *Brain and Language* 25:314–22.

Vieth, J., Grummich, P., Sack, G., Kober, H., Schneider, S., Abraham-Fuchs, K., Kerber, U., Ganslandt, O., and Schmidt, T. 1990. Three-dimensional localization of the pathological area in cerebro-vascular accidents with multichannel magnetoencephalography. *Biomedical Engineering* 35(2):238–9.

Williamson, S. J., and Kaufman, L. 1987. Analysis of neuromagnetic signals. In *Handbook of Electroencephalography and Clinical Neurophysiology (Revised series. Vol. 1)*, eds. A. Gevins and A. Remond. Amsterdam, Elsevier Science Publishers.

Woldorff, M. G., Gallen, C. C., Hampson, S. A., Hillyard, S. A., Pantev, C., Soble, D., and Bloom, F. E. 1993. Modulation of early sensory processing in human auditory cortex during auditory selective attention. *Proceedings of the National Academy of Sciences* 90(18):8722–26.

Yang, T. T., Gallen. C. C., Ramachandran, V., Cobb, S. J., Bloom, F. E., and Schwartz, B. J. 1994a. Sensory maps in the human brain. *Nature* 368:592–3.

Yang, T. T., Gallen, C. C., Ramachandran, V. S., Cobb, S., Schwartz, B. J., and Bloom, F. E. 1994b. Noninvasive detection of cerebral plasticity in adult human somatosensory cortex. *NeuroReports* 5(6):701–704.

Yang, T. T., Gallen, C. C., Schwartz, F. J., and Bloom, F. E. 1993. Noninvasive somatosensory homunculus mapping in humans by using a large-array biomagnetometer. *Proceedings of the National Academy of Sciences USA* 90:3098–3102.

INDEX